Timely discharge from hospital

Other books from M&K include:

Nurses and Their Patients: Informing practice through psychodynamic insights
ISBN: 9781905539314

Developing Advanced Assessment Skills: Patients with Long Term Conditions
ISBN: 9781905539185

The Primary Care Guide to Mental Health
ISBN: 9781905539109

Research Issues in Health and Social Care
ISBN: 9781905539208

Identification and Treatment of Alcohol Dependency
ISBN: 9781905539161

Spiritual Assessment in Healthcare Practice
ISBN: 9781905539277

The Clinician's Guide to Chronic Disease Management for Long-Term Conditions:
A cognitive-behavioural approach
ISBN: 9781905539154

Therapy Skills for Healthcare: An introduction to brief psychological techniques
ISBN: 9781905539581

Timely discharge from hospital

●

Edited by

Liz Lees

RGN; Dip.N; Dip.HSM; BSc (hons) first class; MSc
Consultant Nurse in Acute Medicine

Timely Discharge from Hospital
Liz Lees

ISBN: 978-1-905539-55-0

First published 2012

British Library Cataloguing in Publication Data
A catalogue record for this book is available from the British Library

Notice

Clinical practice and medical knowledge constantly evolve. Standard safety precautions must be followed, but, as knowledge is broadened by research, changes in practice, treatment and drug therapy may become necessary or appropriate. Readers must check the most current product information provided by the manufacturer of each drug to be administered and verify the dosages and correct administration, as well as contraindications. It is the responsibility of the practitioner, utilising the experience and knowledge of the patient, to determine dosages and the best treatment for each individual patient. Any brands mentioned in this book are as examples only and are not endorsed by the publisher. Neither the publisher nor the authors assume any liability for any injury and/or damage to persons or property arising from this publication.

To contact M&K Publishing write to:
M&K Update Ltd · The Old Bakery · St. John's Street
Keswick · Cumbria CA12 5AS
Tel: 01768 773030 · Fax: 01768 781099
publishing@mkupdate.co.uk
www.mkupdate.co.uk

Designed and typeset by Mary Blood
Printed in England by H&H Reeds, Penrith

Contents

Acknowledgements

To Tracy Kelly – thank you for your invaluable administrative support throughout the compilation and many adaptations of this seemingly epic book and for keeping me on track.

To Kelly Davis – having moaned about my authors for not providing adequate referencing, I find myself humbled at having been picked up for my own referencing at times by my 'hawk-eyed' copy editor! Thank you for your perseverance in editing this rather large compilation of chapters.

I would also like to extend a huge thank you to Mr John Deutsch for his contribution to the design of the book cover.

List of contributors

Liz Lees (Introduction and Chapters 1, 3, 10 and 29)
Consultant Nurse and Clinical Dean,
Heart of England NHS Foundation Trust, Birmingham

Sam Foster (Chapter 2)
Deputy Director of Nursing,
Heart of England NHS Foundation Trust, Birmingham

Lorraine Longstaff (Chapter 4)
Matron for Safeguarding,
Heart of England NHS Foundation Trust, Birmingham

Ruth Eley (Chapter 5)
Director, Flynn and Eley Associates Ltd
Formerly: Older Persons Lead, Older People and Dementia,
Social Care Local Government Care Partnerships, London

John O'Brien (Chapter 6)
Senior Partner, Adaptive HVM, Dublin, Chief Executive,
Mount Carmel Private Hospital, Dublin
Formerly: National Director, Health Service Executive, Ireland

Antoinette Doocey (Chapter 6)
Independent Healthcare Management Consultant
Formerly: Programme Director, Integrated Services Development,
National Transformation Programme

NHS Wales (Chapter 7)
Innovation House, National Leadership and Innovation Agency for Health, Bridgend

Ros Moore (Chapter 8)
Chief Nursing Officer for Scotland,
Health and Social Care Directorates of the Scottish Government,
St Andrew's House, Edinburgh

Dr Deirdre McCormick (Chapter 8)
Nursing Officer, Children and Vulnerable Families,
Health and Social Care Directorates of the Scottish Government,
St Andrew's House, Edinburgh

Graham Monteith (Chapter 8)
CAMHS Nurse Adviser,
Health and Social Care Directorates of the Scottish Government,
St Andrew's House, Edinburgh

Sian Wade (Chapter 9)
District Nurse, part time (semi-retired), Stratford-Upon-Avon

Marie Mackenzie (Chapter 10)
Corporate Nursing Team, Heart of England NHS Foundation Trust, Birmingham

Jo Brady (Chapters 11 and 23)
Lead Occupational Therapist, REACT Team,
Heart of England NHS Foundation Trust, Birmingham

Karen Richardson (Chapter 12)
Lead Pharmacist, Pharmacy Department, Warwick Hospital

Dr Mark Temple (Chapter 13)
Consultant Renal Physician,
Heart of England NHS Foundation Trust, Birmingham

Dr Philip Dyer (Chapter 13)
Clinical Physician, Diabetes and Endocrinology
and Lead Consultant, Acute Medical Unit,
Heart of England NHS Foundation Trust, Birmingham

Jamie Emery (Chapter 14)
Patient and Public Involvement Manager,
Heart of England NHS Foundation Trust, Birmingham

Ann Saxon (Chapter 15)
Principal Lecturer for Post-graduate Studies, School of Health,
University of Wolverhampton

Denise Price (Chapter 16)
Director of Nursing and Quality, Trust Headquarters,
South Birmingham Primary Care Trust

Vanessa Lockyer-Stevens (Chapter 17)
Faculty Principal Educator, Faculty of Nursing and Midwifery,
Heart of England NHS Foundation Trust, Birmingham

Sarah Coombes (Chapter 18)
Lead Nurse, Surgery and Nurse-Facilitated Discharge,
Mid Cheshire Hospitals NHS Trust, Crewe

Melanie Webber-Maybank (Chapter 19)
Ward Manager, Cardiff and Vale NHS Trust, Cardiff

Helen Luton (Chapter 19)
Ward Sister, Cardiff and Vale NHS Trust, Cardiff

Mr John Deutsch (Chapter 20)
Consultant Ophthalmologist, Hereford County Hospital, Hereford

Bree Coleman (Chapter 20)
Junior Sister, Hereford County Hospital, Hereford

Viv Hoare (Chapter 20)
Staff Nurse, Hereford County Hospital, Hereford

Julie Young (Chapter 20)
Staff Nurse, Hereford County Hospital, Hereford

Claire Craige (Chapter 20)
Staff Nurse, Hereford County Hospital, Hereford

Claire Whittle (Chapter 21)
Faculty Quality Manager, Portfolio and Curricula,
Marston Green, Solihull

Jill Main (Chapter 21)
Registered Nurse
Formerly: Safeguarding Adults Team, South Birmingham Community Health,
Bromsgrove

Corrina Hulkes (Chapter 22)
Senior Clinical Nurse, Addenbrooke's Hospital, Cambridge

Dr Kiaran Flanagan (Chapter 24)
Clinical Director, Acute Medicine,
University Hospitals Coventry and Warwickshire NHS Trust

Ann-Marie Cannaby (Chapter 24)
Director of Nursing, University Hospitals Coventry and Warwickshire NHS Trust

Dr Ola Erinfolomi (Chapter 25)
Consultant in Emergency Care, Emergency Department,
Heart of England Foundation NHS Trust, Birmingham

Dr Neil Fergusson (Chapter 26)
Consultant Geriatrician,
Heart of England NHS Foundation Trust, Birmingham

Dr Benjamin J. Porter (Chapter 27)
Acute Care, Common Stem Trainee,
Heart of England NHS Foundation Trust, Birmingham

Dr Steven Close (Chapter 28)
Consultant in Acute Medicine,
Acute Medicine Unit, Aberdeen Royal Infirmary

Fiona Dey (Chapter 28)
Advanced Nurse Practitioner,
Acute Medicine Unit, Aberdeen Royal Infirmary

Anne Strafford (Chapter 30)
District Nurse, Washwood Heath District Nurse Team,
Birmingham

Maggie Shepley (Chapter 31)
Complex Discharge Matron,
Calderdale Royal Hospital, Halifax

Sheila Kalanovic (Chapter 31)
Complex Discharge Matron,
Calderdale Royal Hospital, Halifax

Diana Milligan (Chapter 32)
Clinical Lead,
Intermediate Care Birmingham East and North Primary Care Trust,
Sutton Coldfield

Janet Knight (Chapter 32)
Clinical Practice Teacher for District Nursing (IV Therapy)
Washwood Heath District Nurse Team, Birmingham

Introduction

This book represents an ambitious compilation of work on the subject of patient discharge from hospital. The vision for the book was to capture a multidisciplinary and multidimensional view of discharge planning. Throughout the text, the focus is on how to make discharge practice timelier. There are 32 chapters in all, written by a number of authors. This makes it possible for the reader to consider and appreciate different aspects of discharge planning practice in a range of clinical settings, of which they perhaps have no prior experience. Hospitals are rife with systems and processes that tend to counteract integrated working and a whole-system approach where we understand each other's issues. It is hoped that many of the tips in this book will become transferable learning points, creating a mutual respect for the broader implications of patient discharge in clinically interfacing areas. In this way, it should help to promote greater understanding and more integrated discharge practices.

Many aspects of discharge practice have been tried in practice without proper evaluation or review, and this lack of evaluation is often criticised by those in search of robust evidence. For example, the practice of estimating (or predicting) dates for discharge is being adopted across the NHS, in the hope that it will reduce length of stay. It may not reduce length of patient stay but it is the very least that patients should expect – if we are to engage them in timelier discharge. Discharge practice needs to become more sophisticated and responsive to patient needs and organisational complexities. Hence this book showcases practical elements of service provision, discharge roles and care pathways to stimulate new ways of thinking about common problems and to explore possible solutions to familiar problems.

We need to challenge our thinking about discharge practice, and move away from living comfortably with problematic patient discharges to (perhaps uncomfortably) finding a solution through change of practice. There is no such thing as the perfect book on any subject but there are those books that dare to explore what others have not. This is such a book.

The text is aimed at practitioners working in acute, community, intermediate and ambulatory care settings; and all these areas of practice are featured. Each section covers a particular theme; and each chapter is written so that it stands alone, allowing the reader to dip in and out as they wish.

As the editor, I have brought a vision of who to invite to contribute to this book in order to create an appropriate balance of work that represents different areas of practice. To this end, I have compiled and edited other people's work to showcase many different perspectives. The process has required a lot of patience – to get all the chapters together and encourage people to write. I have discovered there are a lot of people in the NHS who are doing fantastic work but don't want to write it up for publication – because they don't think anyone will be interested and they don't think it will be good enough. I have allowed their ideas to unfold, and in some cases I have helped them to describe their work.

This book has only been made possible through the hard work and dedication of all the contributors. The individual chapters are truly representative of each author's field of expertise. It has been an absolute privilege to work with them to help to develop their chapters. Some of the authors have not been previously published; but they have been encouraged to share their experience, thus adding to the body of information regarding discharge practice. In doing so, they have enabled many dimensions of discharge practice to be encompassed, to give a comprehensive perspective on a huge, complex and challenging subject.

I have written four of the chapters. I would like to have written more but a book has to be kept on schedule, and this would have caused delays with the numerous edits to the 28 other chapters. I didn't want to be diverted away from editorial work too much. My chapters include an updated nurse-led discharge perspective, and explorations of best discharge practice, discharge coordination and role comparisons, and discharge from an acute medical unit.

Section 1: The fundamentals of discharge practice

The first four chapters set the scene, giving the current context for discharge of patients from hospital. The principles of best discharge practice are explored, including strategic implementation of practice with senior nurse support, nurse-led discharges and safeguarding adults. Each of these topics is high profile at present, and without consideration of these aspects discharge policy would not be properly embedded and could not evolve in response to changing circumstances.

Section 2: The UK perspective on discharge policy and practice

These four chapters demonstrate policy perspectives, the reality of practice, and progress in discharge planning in England, Ireland, Scotland and Wales. This is perhaps the greatest challenge: to present current thinking, along with the future vision for the direction of discharge services policy. This section gives a unique insight into the strategic thinking that underpins the evolution of discharge practice throughout the UK.

Section 3: Multi-professional discharge practice considerations

These seven chapters explore the contribution made by different professional areas to timely discharge practice, including nursing coordination and complex discharge issues, pharmacy, patient advocacy liaison services, medicine, occupational therapy and bed management.

Section 4: Education for discharge planning

These three chapters combine theory with practice, supporting those practitioners who are engaged in developing discharge education and training. There are more training tools available today than ever before, including multi-professional training, e-learning and competence frameworks. All these mechanisms provide alternatives to 'learning on the job' or 'learning in the classroom', which were previously thought to be the only ways to learn about discharging patients.

Section 5: Discharge practice case studies

This final section includes 15 case studies, which illuminate practice points from a clinical perspective. They illustrate some of the challenges that occur in everyday practice and offer solutions that have been actively implemented and audited. The case studies proved to be very popular with readers of my previous book, *Nurse Facilitated Hospital Discharge*. Readers of this book networked with the authors of the present book in a synergistic way, creating a shared pool of knowledge far greater than the authors alone could have hoped to provide.

So, in these challenging times, with change and the need to make financial savings being constant features within the NHS, I offer you, the reader a thought:

'The faster the speed at which you are travelling, the further ahead you need to look'.

As the pace of work increases in the NHS, we need to anticipate the changes required and be prepared to constantly adapt current practice, while looking into the future to respond to needs effectively.

Liz Lees
Consultant Nurse and Clinical Dean
Heart of England NHS Foundation Trust

Editor's note:
The terms 'Accident and Emergency Department' and 'A&E' are no longer used in most British hospitals. We have therefore replaced them with 'Emergency Department' and 'ED' throughout.

I dedicate this book to Mom and Dad, who have taught me to be organised, to have the tenacity to keep going when the going gets very tough, and most of all to encourage others to succeed. Also to Freda and Alan Parsons. Thank you.

Section I

The fundamentals of discharge practice

Chapter 1

What is best practice for timely discharge?

Liz Lees

This chapter discusses the principles of best practice in discharge planning and transfer, and offers suggestions regarding the application of 'Ready to go?' (DH 2010a) in clinical practice (Lees 2010). For each of the ten steps in the discharge process, the Lean methodology (which improves flow and eliminates waste) has been systematically applied (NHS Institute, www.institute.nhs.uk).

In early January 2010, the Department of Health published a new policy: 'Ready to go? Planning the discharge and transfer of patients from Hospital and Intermediate Care' (DH 2010a). The title of this document leaves readers in no doubt that the scope of discharge practice has undergone permanent change. 'Discharge and transfer' are presented as synonymous, and there are planned discharge pathways, with a series of coordinated steps in the process of planning a patient's discharge or transfer from 'Hospital and Intermediate Care'. As with any health policy, 'Ready to go?' needs to be considered in conjunction with other policies that have preceded its development (DH 2003, DH 2004, NLIAH 2008, HSE 2008).

The 'High Impact Changes for Nursing and Midwifery' policy document (NHS Institute 2009) is also crucial, incorporating a standard for 'ready to go – no delays'. This is where nurse-led discharge and the skill of estimating dates for discharge should come to the fore, supporting an array of existing measures aimed at reducing overall length of patient stay and seven-day working (Lees 2004, Lees 2007, Webber-Maybank and Luton 2009). While the simplicity and clarity of 'Ready to go?' has revitalised the whole discharge debate, readers should not be lulled into a false sense of complacency regarding the ease of implementing its recommendations (DH 2010a).

'Ready to go?' specifically explores ten principles or steps, which – if adopted – would promote timely patient discharge from hospital (see page 7). The ten steps require tenacity and sustained commitment to achieve and embed appropriately, throughout the wide range of services where they will be applied.

The context in which 'Ready to go?' will be applied to discharge practice

Although the principles of discharging patients from hospital have not changed for many years, the process and pace of discharge planning have changed beyond all recognition. These changes have come about as a result of cultural, political and financial pressures on the NHS, which is required to provide for an increasingly ageing population with sometimes complex needs.

The discharge process now encompasses a great many services, which collectively aim to reduce the length of patient stay and expedite their discharge. These new services are predominantly at the front door of the hospital, and some may adopt innovative methods of assessing and referring patients. There are in-reach and outreach services, rapid access clinics interfaced with acute medicine, surgical admission units and Emergency Departments, all aiming to increase the pace of discharge or transfer. At the same time, we have developed a whole new vocabulary in order to talk about the discharge and transfer of patients; we now commonly use terms such as: capacity, flow, pathway, variation, predictability and breaches.

Clinical areas can no longer be introspective, simply looking after their own issues and ignoring others. Discharging a patient from hospital requires each clinical area involved in the patient's discharge – (from pharmacy to transport services) to collaborate with others in order to reduce overlap, waste and the frustrations caused by needless delays. Finally, to create effective and efficient discharge practice, clinical staff (including managers) have to understand all the new terminology, new technology, new services and new process steps, in the context of a whole-system approach (DH 2010b). This is a key theme of future workforce planning and role design – to promote responsiveness to patient needs well into the future, when readers of this book will probably have become consumers of the services they help establish.

Discharge practice and older people

Numerous health and social care policies were introduced in 2009, perhaps demonstrating the complexity and challenges faced by the health and social care services in providing appropriate care for patients with dementia while also accommodating safe discharge and transfer (DH 2009a, 2009b). Importantly, these earlier policies have significant implications for the implementation of 'Ready to go?', which must be carefully considered when planning a patient's discharge from hospital (DH 2010a). For example, discharge and transfer for patients with dementia may require a new breed of healthcare worker and new support services, to encompass the whole pathway of care for a society that is growing older and living longer, with increasing frailty (DH 2009a). General awareness of these issues needs to be increased, and dementia care must become mainstream within acute and intermediate care settings, rather than forever being viewed as the domain of 'specialists' (DoH 2009b).

I labour this point because there is currently a shortage of services needed to adequately accommodate patients with dementia, despite frequent reviews of service provision and self care. Even the most innovative services frequently have criteria that exclude patients with dementia. For example, discharge lounges often have inadequate facilities and lack of appropriate equipment for people with dementia. In such cases, it may be concluded that the problem is the dementia, when it is in fact a lack of the infrastructure that should support a discharge plan for a person with dementia.

Two questions to answer before you start the ten steps

Before embarking on the implementation of the ten steps, two preparatory questions need to be answered, which are not cited in the Department of Health guidance:

1. Can you define your discharge process steps?

2. Can you define your multidisciplinary team membership?

1. I firmly believe that the discharge process should be clearly identified. Firstly, from a corporate perspective, the process should be identified within the Trust Discharge Policy. The question is: What are the core steps in your discharge process? Answering this question will inevitably raise issues relating to Step 2 in the ten steps (see page 7) – differentiating between simple and complex discharges.

Also, from an individual ward perspective: Are there any added stages, or does what you do broadly fit under each process heading?

For simple discharges, which are carried out at ward level, the process used should be standardised throughout an entire hospital. If standardisation is incomplete or not properly embedded, simple things often get missed, making discharge a lot more complex than it really needs to be. And simple things that are missed can have a big impact in practice, especially if they involve duplications or omissions of care.

The key to making a simple discharge process work consistently in your organisation is to adapt it to fit existing systems and clinical processes with which it will interface. The key to making it happen in practice is to ensure that the process is widely disseminated and to establish firm expectations about its implementation. This adaptation process will be easier if there is a willingness to learn on the part of patients, carers and family members, who will help design a system that is fit for purpose. Patients and their carers are, after all, the ones who experience the process in action.

2. Although it is widely accepted that discharge planning needs to be carried out by a multidisciplinary team (MDT), following a recognised process, the composition of the MDT will vary according to the clinical setting. For example, some wards may have access to their own social worker, while others will rely on area social workers or the emergency duty service. Sadly, there is no consistency. The table below illustrates some of the other potential changes in team composition, according to the environment. The clinical scope of each staff member depends on their situation. They may work in an acute hospital ward, or in the community, or they may have both perspectives because they alternate between areas. What is critical is that each MDT member should respect the knowledge of their fellow team members, and the way in which they may work, albeit differently, to help bring about effective discharge.

Potential MDT members

Acute MDT	Intermediate MDT	Community MDT Consultants (Specialists)
Consultants (Specialists)	Geriatrician	General Practitioner (GP)
Junior doctors (FY1 and 2)	GP with special interests	GP with special interests or GP in training
Ward nurses	Mixture of district nurses and ward nurses	District nurses Practice nurses
Hospital pharmacists	Mixture of district nurses and ward nurses	Commercial pharmacists
Occupational therapists	Occupational therapists and enablement assistants	Occupational therapists
Physiotherapists	Physiotherapists and enablement assistants	Physiotherapists and enablement assistants
Flow coordinators (admission and discharges) Discharge coordinators	Liaison nurses	Case managers – possibly employed jointly by health and social care services
Ward social worker		Area social workers

Implementing the ten steps

Having answered these two contextual questions, the ten steps can be perhaps more easily considered in practice (see below).

The ten steps

Adapted from 'Ready to go?' (DH 2010a)

1	Start planning for discharge or transfer before or on admission.
2	Identify whether the patient has simple or complex discharge and transfer planning needs, involving the patient or carer in your decision.
3	Develop a clinical management plan for every patient within 24 hours of admission.
4	Coordinate the discharge or transfer of care process through effective leadership and handover of responsibilities at ward level.
5	Set an expected date of discharge or transfer within 24–48 hours of admission and discuss with the patient or carer.
6	Review the clinical management plan with the patient each day, take any necessary action and update progress towards the discharge or transfer date.
7	Involve patients and carers so that they can make informed decisions and choices that deliver a personalised care pathway and maximise their independence.
8	Plan discharges and transfers to take place over seven days to deliver continuity of care for the patient.
9	Use a discharge checklist 24–48 hours prior to discharge or transfer.
10	Make decisions to discharge and transfer patients each day.

You will notice some overlaps and interfaces between some of the steps, which may be quite subtle. For example, Step 6 and Step 7 suggest patient involvement at two levels, firstly by being adequately informed to be able to make a choice, and secondly (where required) to assess their progress according to the choices made. Patient choices need to be enabled by advocates, who are members of the multidisciplinary team. These advocates must have the skills and knowledge required to navigate through available and appropriate services with the patient (Birmingham 2009). Furthermore, Steps 6 and 7 are dependent on Step 3 (the clinical management plan) being in place. Step 8 and Step 10 are inextricably linked but, by looking at them separately, we can consider two different perspectives: the organisational processes required to make seven-day services available; and the clinical infrastructure needed to include senior clinical decision-makers across a spectrum of care (RCPL 2007).

After each step, I have included some tips for the implementation of that step in practice. These tips include 'no-no's' (major stumbling blocks), 'nice ifs' (helpful changes if you are able to make them), 'niggles' (minor problems that often occur) and 'nuggets' (main lessons or golden rules).

While the ten steps are not prescriptive, they should all be considered. If not, the effect will be like 'a house of cards', where one vital 'card' (part of the process) being absent will result in the inevitable collapse of the whole process. The ten steps form the framework for an audit and review of the discharge process. They can also tell us where improvements in quality need to be made. Clinical areas where steps may be routinely missed, or where implementation has failed, or where there is entrenched opposition to any of the ten steps, should be exposed and explored when consolidating or redesigning processes to expedite patient discharge and transfer.

Step 1: Start planning for discharge or transfer before or on admission

If we first consider elective care, this step can be implemented in the preoperative admission phase, and may take the form of a screening tool, risk assessment or care pathway. The aim is to anticipate potential delays, and to respond by managing those potential delays in a proactive manner. With the advent of the Liverpool Care Pathway and the renewed focus on end-of-life issues, care pathways have been developed to facilitate rapid discharge for patients at the end of life – on admission to acute services (National End of Life Care Programme 2009).

Conversely, in emergency (unscheduled) care, advance planning is not possible. Robust systems to gather patient information have to be in place – and the information must then be shared with all members of the multidisciplinary team to ensure early engagement in the process. Rich sources of information often get missed in the activity surrounding assessment and transfer (Helleso 2006); pivotal sources include the GP and primary care team and carers, who may have been providing most of the support but receive little mention. Further complexity is added by the numerous types of documentation used in hospitals and intermediate care settings to catalogue discharge communications. If each ward uses its own type of documentation, this will slow the process of retrieval and discharge from hospital (Lees 2010).

Practice tips for implementing Step 1

No-no's	Not acting upon information gathered in a timely manner
Nice ifs	Information could be shared at a central point such as an electronic handover system
Niggles	Lack of continuity of documentation between wards and departments
Nuggets	Create a user-friendly screening tool or discharge risk assessment tool

Step 2: Identify whether the patient has simple or complex discharge and transfer planning needs, involving the patient or carer in your decision

The aim of this step is to identify the likely patient pathway from the outset, at admission or earlier. This should make it possible to recognise the point at which a simple discharge becomes complex. A simple discharge is one that can be executed at ward level with the MDT. A complex discharge involves funding issues, change of residence and/or increased care needs negotiated between health and social care (provision of care packages). Taking the time to predict whether a discharge will be simple or complex is infinitely preferable to an insidious deterioration of the patient's condition while in the 'waiting process', with risk issues perhaps not being recognised before the discharge date is set (HSE 2008). It may also prevent some 'failed discharges' and help all those involved to understand what to expect.

Practice tips for implementing Step 2

No-no's	Lack of decision at the outset as to whether the discharge will be simple or complex
Nice ifs	'Simple' or 'complex' could be included on ward patient journey boards
Niggles	If this step is not integrated into a clinical management plan
Nuggets	Develop a clear definition of 'simple' and 'complex' in your discharge policy

Step 3: Develop a clinical management plan for every patient within 24 hours of admission

Most patients admitted by junior medical staff will have an outline (initial) management plan. The extent of the MDT involvement will depend upon the time of day of the patient's admission. For example, admissions after 5 pm will be reviewed by the whole team the next day on the ward round. Ward rounds therefore become inextricably linked to management plans (Lees *et al.* 2006). Ultimately a management plan should engage and focus the whole MDT, *with* the patient, to plan the aspects of care required, leading to discharge. Clinical management plans do not have to be prescriptive – they should serve as a guide and be revisited as the patient moves through the continuum of care (Lees & Delpino 2007, Thompson *et al.* 2004). For those patients on a care pathway, there will be different stages of care that mark progress through the ongoing plan. The care pathway is a vital element in the handover between clinical settings (including nursing homes, intermediate care and GPs), and should prevent delays or lack of clarity regarding which stages of care have or have not been completed.

Practice tips for implementing Step 3

No-no's	Following basic clerking instructions and daily changes of care, in the absence of an overall plan
Nice ifs	The management plan could be created by the MDT and shared at MDT meetings
Niggles	The absence of stages in a plan, and failure to determine whether or not they have been completed
Nuggets	Have a management plan proforma developed and available for download on the Intranet

Step 4: Coordinate the discharge or transfer of care process through effective leadership and handover of responsibilities at ward level

The pace of discharge and transfer is such that most clinical areas have developed systems in which they have a discharge coordinator allocated to this role. There is a lot of disparity between these systems, with some using clerical staff to coordinate simple tasks and others employing up to Band 7 nurses (see Chapter 10 on discharge coordinator roles). Some clinical areas rotate nurses in a daily shift coordinator role, while others hold the full-time role of discharge coordinator. Certainly, a 'one size fits all' approach cannot accommodate all simple and complex discharges. Communication, MDT working and assessment are three key roles for discharge coordinators (Rose *et al.* 2009). In addition, they need to look after the transfer of information, which may otherwise be missed (Helleso 2006). Paradoxically, the setting up of coordinator roles to manage complexity in discharge planning, promoting flow and increased capacity, may sometimes cause a loss of the skills and experience required to carry out discharge planning across the nursing team. Nevertheless, this concern should be balanced against the fact that communication and coordination are the essence of good practice in achieving effective, timely discharges (Macleod 2006, Pethybridge 2004).

Practice tips for implementing Step 4

No-no's	Tackling day-to-day discharges without a strategic approach on the wards
Nice ifs	Assessment of need and process mapping were to be carried out – planning of ward needs to involve MDT
Niggles	Lack of leadership when staff shortages occur and coordinators are 'counted in the numbers', which means that they are not freed up to coordinate
Nuggets	Prepare job descriptions aligned to Knowledge and Skills Framework (KSF) to reinforce the role of coordinator – also consider involvement of allied health professionals

Step 5: Set an expected date of discharge (EDD) or transfer within 24–48 hours of admission and discuss with patient and carer

This area of practice has proved incredibly difficult to implement and embed within organisational philosophy. Essentially, the patient's discharge date is estimated or predicted, and this EDD is intended as a guide for the patient in the discharge planning process. It is not intended to be exact, and it will need to be refined as the patient's progress, set against the clinical management plan, is reassessed towards the anticipated discharge date (Webber-Maybank and Luton 2009).

There is also some confusion of terminology evident in practice areas, with use of similar but subtly different terms such as 'predicted length of stay', 'estimated length of stay' and 'estimated date of discharge' (Lees 2008). Regardless of what we choose to call it, if the EDD is to have any meaningful application in practice its underpinning principles must be understood at three levels:

1. Strategically – to predict overall hospital capacity
2. Operationally – to assess progress and outcomes of clinical plans
3. Individually – for patients to understand expectations, limitations and what engagement is required from them in the process of planning discharge (Lees & Holmes 2005, DH 2004).

The third point, 'patient engagement', is often absent from the process or conducted on a very superficial level (Sargent *et al.* 2007). This is where I believe the greatest improvement could be made in the whole process of estimating a discharge date.

Estimating dates for discharge requires a change of mindset for both health and social care professionals towards a culture where 'time' is of the essence, and lost 'time' (or waiting) in the process of discharge planning should be minimised. Time can, after all, be translated into money. In estimating length of patient stay, the aim is to focus on planning the time carefully and accounting for variance (except for deterioration in the patient's condition).

Practice tips for implementing Step 5

No-no's	Not estimating a date of discharge
Nice ifs	Patient could be involved from the outset in the planning of the date
Niggles	Estimating a date of discharge without clarification from the MDT of what is achievable
Nuggets	Improve staff understanding in order to improve compliance with EDD – and conduct patient surveys to assess extent of patient involvement in the process

Step 6: Review the clinical management plan with the patient each day, take any necessary action and update progress towards the discharge or transfer date

Provided that the clinical management plan was commenced on admission, reviewing it with the patient should be a relatively straightforward process. Review, action, progress (RAP) is the process suggested (NLIAH 2008). The important aspect is to update the plan with input from the MDT *and* the patient (Efraimsson *et al.* 2003). Clinical management plans will reflect progress towards both medical and therapy milestones. In some cases, the management plan may also form part of an MDT meeting or will be utilised in an MDT meeting, depending on the frequency of these. Ideally there should be only one plan, which is central to the discharge process, to avoid confusion and duplication of documentation and to ensure transparency.

Practice tips for implementing Step 6

No-no's	Having more than one management plan
Nice ifs	Clinical management plan could be used in MDT meetings or SMART (specific, measurable, attainable, realistic and timely) ward rounds
Niggles	Management plans tend to exclude nursing actions and nursing plans
Nuggets	Incorporate EDD, simple or complex discharge, and the anticipated destination (home, nursing home, etc.) in the plan

Step 7: Involve patients and carers so that they can make informed decisions and choices that deliver a personalised pathway and maximise their independence

This step is aimed at managing patient/carer expectations and understanding potential issues, involving therapy, nursing, medicine and predominantly (but not exclusively) social care partners, who should be guided by the clinical referrals and actions in the clinical management plan (Sargent *et al.* 2007). There needs to be careful consideration of patient choice to utilise supporting services in intermediate care, care pathways and/or dementia care. Involvement is an ongoing core principle, not a one-off action. Patient involvement may require experience and patience, with a series of meetings being arranged with the patient's carers, the MDT and social care services. It is about genuine and meaningful engagement with patients throughout the entire discharge planning process. It requires nurses not simply to deliver care, as members of the team, but to represent the patient and understand their own barriers to truly shared decision-making (Milton-Wildey

& O'Brien 2010). Patients should be assisted to understand and embrace their responsibilities, with support, and they may need to be helped to ask the appropriate questions (Borthwick *et al.* 2009; see also Chapter 14 on patient involvement). One suggestion is to ask carers if they feel they can cope or if they anticipate problems (Princess Royal Trust 2007).

Practice tips for implementing Step 7

No-no's	Excluding the patient and making decisions based only on input from the MDT
Nice ifs	Integrated care pathways could be established
Niggles	Lack of understanding of patient involvement strategies
Nuggets	With complex discharges, establish a key worker who coordinates the discharge plan

Step 8: Plan discharges and transfer to take place over seven days to deliver continuity of care for the patient

This step relies upon engagement from services that support discharge. Some of these may not be ward based (for instance, therapy services, x-ray services, transport, district nursing, and intermediate care services). Only by means of seven-day working on the part of hospital and community services will continuity over seven days of the week be possible (DH 2004). For example, generally therapists only work Monday to Friday, although this is slowly changing in some areas of practice, such as acute medical units. This means that the discharge plans that have been put in place have to continue at the weekend with nursing staff support – although in some areas with early supported discharge schemes. This step is vital, and seven-day services should be established as new contracts, posts or services are established.

Practice tips for implementing Step 8

No-no's	Drawing up plans that accommodate organisational capability rather than responding to patient needs
Nice ifs	Nursing and support workers (healthcare assistants) could continue the therapy plan over weekends – mobilising the patient, etc.
Niggles	Insistence on five-day working from some essential services
Nuggets	Analyse your high volume groups – what services are required by this group? Work to ensure that weekend provision of those services becomes available, to enable seven-day working and discharges

Step 9: Use a discharge checklist 24–48 hours prior to transfer

The discharge checklist has proved to be a difficult area of practice to sustain. The principle of a checklist is not new (Lees 2006). What is new is the concept of uniformity, of one checklist being used across a whole trust/organisation, and ensuring that it is developed with input from both the primary care trust (PCT) and social care services. Such checklists are more commonly seen in integrated care pathways, often for surgical conditions. Their purpose is not to duplicate information but to ensure that, amid all the heightened activity before discharge, vital planning aspects are not missed or forgotten.

If used appropriately, a discharge checklist can counteract complaints about the discharge process, and assist compliance with the standard for discharges within the Clinical Negligence Scheme for Trusts – 'The organisation has an approved documented process for managing the risks associated with the discharge of patients that is implemented and monitored' (NHSLA, Standard 4, Criterion 10, 2010/2011). There is potential for the checklist to be merged with the discharge letter and carbonated, to enable copies to be given to the patient upon discharge from hospital.

Practice tips for implementing Step 9

No-no's	Not using any form of pre-discharge checking process, which is recorded and shared with the team
Nice ifs	Audit could be carried out, concentrating on completion to embed process. Do discharge checklists reduce complaints? Do they improve the quality of discharge process?
Niggles	Each ward developing its own discharge checklist
Nuggets	Develop the checklist with input from social care services and PCT; keep it to one page; provide copies for patients

Step 10: Make decisions to discharge and transfer patients each day

The key difference between this step and Step 8 is the requirement to make a decision. Many publications have dealt with issues surrounding safety, suggesting that the consultant's decision is critical to safe, effective discharge (RCPL 2007). This raises a whole new debate, concerned with the reduction in junior doctors' working hours, and changes in roles and responsibilities required across a team to support this change (RCPL 2007). Each clinical area needs to decide on a discharge structure for the future, which takes into account decision makers regardless of profession.

The High Impact Changes (NHS Institute for Innovation and Improvement 2009) reiterate earlier publications and have made nurse-led discharge a key deliverable. Nurse-led discharge will never replace the role of the MDT and senior clinical decision-makers such as consultants, but well thought out implementation will support the MDT to deliver services over seven days (Macleod 2006, Lees 2007). The evidence base is gradually increasing – but it is crucial that the nursing profession grasps the opportunity to develop this new way of working as part of the existing discharge process (Lees 2004; see also Chapters 3, 18, 22, 24 and 28).

Practice tips for implementing Step 10

No-no's	Attempting to introduce nurse-led discharge without supporting education or time to embed
Nice ifs	Medical champions could assist the process and work towards delegated decision-making with nurses and MDT
Niggles	There are pockets of excellent practice – but they are not shared
Nuggets	Start work in an area with relatively simple discharges; identify high volume condition groups

Conclusion

It is often quite a challenge to know where to start implementing a new policy. However, the clarity of the ten steps enables specific areas to be audited in order to focus on where work should be undertaken on particular points in the care pathway. Equally, it is very important to look at what the current process consists of, and in doing so understand the obstacles that staff might face on a day-to-day basis, in order to design a sustainable discharge process. For example, if there is no clinical management plan, this alone may cause staff to dismiss the process and 'execute discharge in their own way'.

The process used on each ward must be the same, underpinned by 'specialist' aspects of discharge planning pertaining to the individual area. For example, adding to the process may be acceptable but leaving out parts of the process will delay the eventual discharge – if not in the clinical area where it was started then further on, at a later stage in the care pathway. The discharge process must work out of hours and must not include delays caused by lack of availability of transport, medications, and so on. The discharge policy must also support the process – and a wise step may be to reconsider the elements within your discharge policy. For example, you could ask: does the policy include the ten steps?

If we can consider and start to conquer these problems at a micro level, policies at a macro level (supporting organisational safety, patient satisfaction and a reduction in length of stay) should start to become integrated within practice. The discharge process at all levels is central to the efficiency and effectiveness of any healthcare organisation; and on this basis it is well worth a systematic review, using the ten-step approach outlined in this chapter.

References

Birmingham, J. (2009). Patient choice in the discharge planning process. *Journal of Professional Case Management.* 14 (6), 296–309, Maryland: Lippincott Williams & Wilkins, Inc.

Borthwick, R., Newbronner, L. and Stuttard, L. (2009). 'Out of Hospital': a scoping study of services for carers of people being discharged from hospital. *Health and Social Care in the Community.* 17 (4), 335–349.

Department of Health (2003). 'Discharge from hospital: pathway, process and practice'. London: HMSO.

Department of Health (2004). 'Achieving simple timely discharge from hospital: a multidisciplinary toolkit'. London: HMSO.

Department of Health (2009a). 'Living well with dementia: a national dementia strategy implementation plan'. London: HMSO.

Department of Health (2009b). 'Joint commissioning framework for dementia'. London: HMSO.

Department of Health (2010a). 'Ready to go? Planning the discharge and transfer of patients from hospital and intermediate care'. Department of Health, Quarry House, Leeds.

Department of Health (2010b). 'Liberating the Talents: Developing the healthcare workforce: a consultation on proposals'. Department of Health, Quarry House, Leeds.

Efraimsson, E., Rasmussen, B.H., Gilje, F. & Sandman, P. (2003) Expressions of power and powerlessness in discharge planning: a case study of an older woman on her way home. *Journal of Clinical Nursing.* 12 (5), 707–716.

Health Services Executive (2008). Code of Practice for Integrated Discharge Planning. 31–33 Catherine Street, Limerick, Ireland. www.hse.ie

Helleso, R. (2006). Information handling in the nursing discharge note. *Journal of Clinical Nursing.* 15 (1), 11–21.

Lees, L. (2004). Making nurse-led discharge work to improve patient care. *Nursing Times.* 100 (37), 30.

Lees, L. & Holmes, K. (2005). Estimating a date of discharge at ward level: a pilot study. *Nursing Standard.* 19 (17), 40–43.

Lees, L. (2006). 'Not Just another sheet of paper: discharge checklists'. The Communicator, RCN discharge planning and continuing care forum. Summer 2006, 4–5. www.rcn.org.uk/liaisondischarge

Lees, L., Allen, G. & O'Brien, D. (2006). Using post-take ward rounds to facilitate simple discharge. *Nursing Times.* 102 (18), 28–30.

Lees, L. (2007). *Nurse Facilitated Hospital Discharge.* Keswick: M&K Publishing.

Lees, L. & Delpino, R. (2007). Facilitating timely discharge from hospital: Combining patient name boards and discharge planning information. *Nursing Times.* 103 (29), 30–31.

Lees, L. (2008). Estimating patients' discharge dates: applied leadership, *Nursing Management.* 15 (3), 30–35.

Lees, L. (2010). Exploring the principles of best practice discharge to ensure patient involvement. *Nursing Times.* 106 (25), 10–14.

Macleod, A. (2006). The nursing role in preventing delay in patient discharge. *Nursing Standard*. **21** (1), 43–48.

Milton-Wildey, K. & O'Brien, L. (2010). Care of acutely ill older patients in hospital: clinical decision-making. *Journal of Clinical Nursing*. **19** (9–10): 1252–1260.

NHS Institute for Innovation and Improvement (2009). 'High Impact Changes for Nursing and Midwifery'. Coventry House, University of Warwick Campus CV4 7AL. www.institute.nhs.uk

NHS Litigation Authority (2010/2011). *The risk management handbook supporting the risk management standards*. www.nhsla.com

National Leadership Innovation Agency for Health Care (2008). *Passing the Baton – A Practical Guide to Effective Discharge Planning*. The Welsh Assembly.

National End of Life Care Programme (1 October 2009). *Liverpool Care Pathway: response to media reporting*. http://www.endoflifecareforadults.nhs.uk/case-studies/lcp.

Pethybridge, J. (2004). How team working influences discharge planning from hospital: a study of four multidisciplinary teams in an acute hospital in England. *Journal of Interprofessional Care*. **18** (1), 75–80.

Princess Royal Trust for Carers (2007). Out of Hospital Project, Report from Stage 1. Malton, York: Acton Shapiro Consultancy and Research.

Rose, M., McCarthy, G. & Coffey, A. (2009). Discharge planning: the role of the discharge coordinator. *Nursing Older People*. **21** (1), 26–31.

Royal College of Physicians of London (2007). 'Acute medical care: the right person in the right setting first time – report of the acute medicine task force'. London: Royal College of Physicians of London.

Sargent, P., Pickard, S., Sheaff, R. & Boaden, R. (2007). Patient and carer perceptions of case management for long-term conditions. *Health and Social Care in the Community*. **15** (6), 511–519.

Thompson, A.G., Jacob, K., Fulton, J. & McGavin, C.R. (2004). Do post-take ward round proformas improve communication and influence the quality of patient care? *Postgraduate Medical Journal*. **80**, 675–676.

Webber-Maybank, M. & Luton, H. (2009). Making effective use of predicted discharge dates to reduce the length of stay in hospital. *Nursing Times*. **105**, 15.

Chapter 2

How senior nurses can maintain strategic organisational momentum in safe discharge practice

Sam Foster

The first line of the professional Nursing and Midwifery code states: 'The people in your care must be able to trust you with their health and wellbeing' (NMC 2008). It is therefore the responsibility of the senior nurse, when leading the practice of safe discharge, to develop local policy that is fit for purpose, and to ensure that this policy is successfully implemented. The senior nurse also needs to monitor the policy, to ensure that patients and their families and carers have a safe, high quality experience.

This chapter relates to both the strategic and the clinical practice considerations that guide senior nurses in maintaining strategic momentum in discharge practice. It will review policy development, implementation and monitoring processes.

Local policy development

When developing local discharge policy, it is essential that the senior nurse reviews relevant national policy drivers and related regulatory standards; and that lessons learnt from any complaints or patient safety incidents relating to discharge are integrated as guidance/protocols.

In recent years, safe, high quality patient care has been the guiding principle of all policy drivers and regulatory standards aimed at setting the direction for the NHS. The Department of Health White Paper 'Equity and excellence: Liberating the NHS' (DH 2010) launched the government's plans for a new direction for the NHS. The paper outlined an ambitious programme of reforms, starting with revisions to 'The Operating Framework for the NHS in England' (DH 2011). The Framework recognised the challenges involved in implementation. The first full year of the transition was seen as a critical period that would require all parts of the NHS to respond positively to the principles and purposes set out in the White Paper, whilst ensuring that service quality, productivity, efficiency and financial performance were maintained and improved. Furthermore, a new requirement was included in the Framework, which identified safe discharge as an area for improvement.

The challenge for an Acute Trust now is that hospitals will no longer be reimbursed for emergency readmissions within 30 days of discharge, following an elective admission. All other readmission rates will be subject to locally determined thresholds, with a 25 per cent decrease in activity desired where achievable. Strategically, NHS organisations now need to balance the potential financial penalty against the requirement to deliver patient safety by ensuring that length of stay is appropriate to patient need. Estimating dates for a patient's discharge from hospital plays a crucial part in getting this balance right (see also Chapters 13 and 27).

The Care Quality Commission (CQC) provides a regulatory function for all health services and adult social care services in England. In order to provide health or social care services, organisations are required to register with the CQC, and make a formal declaration of compliance with a set of standards. A number of these standards include the need to ensure safe discharge. Organisations must declare compliance in the following areas:

- Cooperating with other providers to ensure safe transfer of care or discharge
- Ensuring that a patient's length of stay will be as short as possible in order to meet their needs, or as required by legal restrictions
- An organisation's accommodation must not limit patients' freedom any further than is agreed in their plan of care, wherever possible
- Patients should know the names and job titles of the people who provide their care, treatment and support, and how to contact them
- Patients must have adequate plans in place for when they leave the service and be fully involved in this planning, where they have the capacity and the wish to do so.

(CQC 2010, Regulations 24 and 9)

The National Health Service Litigation Authority handles negligence claims and works to improve risk management practices in the NHS (NHSLA 2010/2011). It has a framework of standards by which it assesses the level of risk that organisations pose in their delivery of care, based on the level achieved (0–3). Organisations pay a premium and the NHSLA provides an indemnity. (See NHSLA standard 4 (2010/11), relating to discharge.)

Standard 4 - Criterion 10: Discharge of Patients

Acute Trusts and Independent Sector organisations: The organisation has an approved documented process for managing the risks associated with the discharge of patients that is implemented and monitored.	
Level 1	**Minimum Requirements**
1.4.10	As a minimum, the approved documentation must include a description of the: a. Duties b. Definition of all patient groups c. Discharge requirements which are specific to each patient group d. Documentation to accompany the patient upon discharge e. Information to be given to the patient f. Process for discharge out of hours g. Process for monitoring compliance with all of the above.
Level 2	**Minimum Requirements**
2.4.10	The organisation can demonstrate compliance with the objectives set out within the approved documentation described at Level 1, in relation to the: • Discharge requirements which are specific to each patient group • Documentation to accompany the patient upon discharge. The assessor will select two patient groups at random to assess the organisation's compliance with the above minimum requirements.
Level 3	**Minimum Requirements**
3.4.10	The organisation can demonstrate that it is monitoring compliance with the minimum requirements contained within the approved documentation described at Level 1, in relation to the: • Discharge requirements which are specific to each patient group • Documentation to accompany the patient upon discharge. The assessor will select two patient groups at random to assess the organisation's compliance with the above minimum requirements. Where the monitoring has identified deficiencies, there must be evidence that recommendations and action plans have been developed and changes implemented.

The NHS Confederation is the independent membership body for the full range of organisations that make up the NHS. The Confederation works to influence policy in the interests of patients, the public and NHS staff. It supports leaders to deliver strong and innovative leadership within the NHS. Part of the Confederation's work is ensuring that users of the NHS know their rights. Through a variety of media, such as the NHS Choices website, it clarifies patients' rights to safe discharge, stating:

- In England, you should not be discharged from hospital until your care needs are assessed and arrangements made to ensure that you will receive any necessary services when you are discharged.
- Any assessment should take into account your wishes, the wishes of your family and of any carer. You should be kept fully informed and involved, be given sufficient time to make decisions, and be told how to seek a review of any decisions made. You can ask for a reassessment of your needs if circumstances change in the future.

(NHS Choices website: http://www.nhs.uk/Pages/HomePage.aspx)

If patients, their families or carers are not satisfied with discharge plans, NHS Choices reminds them:

- Before discharge takes place, you, or your family, carer or representative, have the right to ask for a review of the decision, which has been made, about your eligibility for continuing NHS care. In England, you can also ask for a review after discharge.

To summarise, patient safety and the quality of patient experience underpin all current political and regulatory drivers. This in turn must influence all senior nurses involved in local policy development and ratification, to ensure that local policy is fit for purpose (see Chapter 14).

Local policy implementation

The method of implementing local policy is crucial for sustainability. John Overtveit (cited in Maher *et al.* 2007) stated: 'The challenge is not starting, but continuing after the initial enthusiasm is gone' (p. 23).

Evidence shows that change is most successful if it is locally owned. However, a practitioner's enthusiasm, once gained, has to be channelled to ensure action. This can only be achieved by having an organisational strategy, supported by local information and involvement. The strategy must be linked to organisational strategic plans and translated into meaningful objectives for nurses.

Senior nurses need to ensure that there is strong organisational support for improving discharge practice, and this support must be explicit to bring about a change in culture. However, too much central control will lead to less ownership at ward level so it is important to ensure involvement and genuine representation. Devolution of responsibilities should be accompanied by a training strategy so that nurses are equipped to implement changes. The role of the senior nurse is to make sure that the training strategy is realistic, deliverable and linked to the business planning process, in order to accurately identify the need for resources. Meeting educational needs is discussed further in Section 4 (Chapters 15, 16 and 17).

When considering local policy implementation, it is crucial that key stakeholders are identified and that the overarching safety aim is explicit. In 2004, the Department of Health (DH 2004a) said that, in addition to support from the multidisciplinary team (MDT), executive-level sponsorship was central. Board-level nurses are professionally accountable for all nursing staff, and frequently have professional responsibility for allied health professionals within an organisation. Therefore they will also need to focus on non-medical multidisciplinary working.

Responsibility for the delivery of a safe discharge process lies with the entire MDT (DH 2003, 2004a) and thought should be given to the needs of different wards and departments, where it may be more appropriate for leadership to be provided by other members of the MDT (Pethybridge 2004b).

The coordination of safe discharge lies centrally with the ward nurses, led by the ward sister, who have patient contact 24 hours a day, seven days a week (see Chapter 10 for more on discharge coordination). Traditionally, nurses have been anxious about discharging patients too early, in the belief that patients are better off in hospital. However, this fear contradicts research findings, which show that longer stays in hospital can result in deterioration in a patient's condition and an increase in mortality (Steel, Gertman, *et al.* 2004, Clarke 2002). In addition, there is some cynicism regarding national targets, which are often perceived as being driven by financial pressures rather than patient need (Drake, Bore, *et al.* 2004). However, in relation to discharge, a shorter hospital stay will actually benefit most patients. Goodacre (2006, p. 253) goes so far as to say:

'Emergency doctors often decide whether to advise hospital admission or discharge by assessing whether a decision to discharge home is considered safe. This implies that hospital admission may be recommended on the basis of exceeding an arbitrarily defined risk of adverse outcome, rather than weighing the potential benefits, risks and costs of hospital admission. This approach is likely to lead to irrational decision-making, unnecessary hospitalisation and unrealistic expectations regarding risk. Instead of using the concept of a safe discharge, we should take a more rational approach to decision making, weighing the benefits, risks and costs of hospitalisation against a default option of discharge home. Hospital admission should be recommended only if the expected benefits outweigh the risks and can be accrued at an acceptable cost. Guidelines should be developed using this approach and used to promote and support rational decision-making.'

Changing the culture at ward level

In order for safe, effective discharge to form a timely part of everyday practice, the focus on discharge has to be part of the ward culture. This requires synergy between the roles of doctors and nurses at ward level, as well as with allied health professionals, in order to make a difference to discharge in practice.

Effective team working is crucial, as junior doctors often assume a large proportion of responsibility for discharge planning, but have many other commitments. In practice, discharge planning may not be a high priority amongst those competing commitments, especially when they have too many jobs to do – in too little time. In recent years, discharge initiatives that aim to free up hospital beds have become commonplace. However, new systems (such as bed management) have left many nurses feeling disengaged from patient admission and discharge. The increasing focus on bed capacity and patient turnover can make junior doctors and nurses feel pressurised into speeding up patient discharge, and this may also make them feel distanced from their primary role of caring for patients.

Berwick (2003) describes three pre-conditions required for improvement to take place:

- Face reality
- Seek new designs
- Involve everyone.

Facing reality is about identifying what it is that needs to be changed. What is the gap between the current situation and what you want to achieve? Seeking new designs is self-explanatory. What is important is to acknowledge that ideas can come from anyone and enabling that to happen. Involving everyone should take place at each stage of the improvement or change in practice. Although it can be time-consuming, each clinical team needs to identify gaps in their own performance and what needs to change. This can also be problematic as individuals and teams may not accept the problem as being theirs and will often attempt to blame others. For example, 'Pharmacy is responsible for the delays in discharge because we have to wait so long for the tablets to be dispensed' or 'Ambulance is responsible because they don't pick the patient up on time.' Valid, believable data is important in order to persuade individuals to 'face reality'.

A local policy that reflects national policy and regulatory requirements will not change practice on its own. The senior nurse will also need to lead the MDT to behave in a certain way; and the MDT members need to be enthused, and have their hearts and minds won over. Bibby et al. (2009) introduced the social movement leadership theory to the NHS, defining social movement as 'A voluntary collective of individuals committed to promoting or resisting change through coordinated activity' (p. 25). Framing is seen as the most important element in applying social movement thinking to healthcare. Framing is described as 'hooks' for pulling people in or 'springboards' to mobilise support that taps into the energy of individuals. Senior nurses need to consider how previous bad framing (such as 'you must follow this policy as it is a CQC requirement') needs to be replaced with positive framing (for example, 'patient safety comes first; discussing estimated date of discharge on your ward rounds will promote safe planning').

The 2003 Department of Health publication 'Modern matrons – Improving the patient experience' (p. 5) lists the matron's ten key responsibilities (not to be confused with the ten key roles for nurses) as:

1. Leading by example
2. Making sure patients get quality care
3. Ensuring staffing is appropriate to patient needs
4. Empowering nurses to take on a wider range of clinical tasks
5. Improving hospital cleanliness
6. Ensuring patients' nutritional needs are met
7. Improving wards for patients
8. Making sure patients are treated with respect
9. Preventing hospital-acquired infection
10. Resolving problems for patients and their relatives by building closer relationships.

Whilst discharge processes are not directly mentioned, they could actually be incorporated within the quality of care and clinical tasks. For instance, ensuring that patients' nutritional needs are met while in hospital as well as giving due consideration to their needs after discharge home, and resolving problems for patients and their relatives by building closer relationships, would arguably reduce length of stay and expedite discharge.

There is a clear expectation that matrons will provide strong leadership and act as a conduit between board-level nurses and clinical practice. Nurses at board level have a responsibility to make sure that nursing meets Trust objectives; the role of the matron is to incorporate these objectives in practice.

The matron's role

The matron's role is to provide leadership, momentum and motivation for the nursing team. He or she should be involved in the development of an organisational strategy and will thus be able to translate the strategy into directorate plans and help ward sisters translate the plans into team objectives. Matrons need to involve ward-based practitioners to determine where problems lie and identify local solutions, and ensure they receive regular feedback. The matron will also work with ward sisters to facilitate learning through experience. Matrons tend to be kept busy with processes and reports to pacify senior nurses, and this can create a management and practice gap when implementing new discharge procedures. However, if matrons monitor practice at a local level, alongside ward sisters/charge nurses, this gap can be closed.

Implementing policy at ward level

Whilst new roles and initiatives can be valuable, changing the way nurses engage with discharge is key. In November 2009 the NHS Institute for Innovation and Improvement published a list of eight high-impact actions for nursing and midwifery. 'Ready to go – no delays' is the high impact action pertinent to safe discharge. It said that, if implemented across the NHS, these actions could save over £9 billion a year, whilst improving the quality of care (see Chapter 1).

The NHS Institute has now published a selection of case studies from different settings, demonstrating successful initiatives relating to each action, and a range of other supporting material.

Berwick (2003, p. 449) recognised the need to improve the systems within which we work. He recommended that 'The most effective route to improvement is through changing systems, not yelling at them'. A management system may be used across organisations, to provide a structured approach to implementation and to support the monitoring of improvement and sustainability.

Using a management system to manage change in the discharge process

A number of management systems can be used, including the Business Excellence Model provided by the European Foundation for Quality Management (EFQM). The EFQM was formed in 1988, by the presidents of a number of major European companies. It now has over 850 members, including some healthcare organisations. The excellence model comprises eight concepts:

1. Results – the needs of all stakeholders are met

2. Customers – the customers' needs are known and met

3. Leadership – there is a clear direction which is known throughout the organisation

4. Management by process – all activities are managed in a systematic way

5. People development – there is a culture of trust and participation

6. Continuous learning – there is sharing of knowledge, and innovation is encouraged

7. Partnership development

8. Public responsibility – there is a relationship with the community, which is advantageous to both.

(British Quality Foundation 2000)

The EQFM model uses Six Sigma, Lean and Balanced Scorecard methods. These methods have been used in businesses across the world and are being adopted in healthcare organisations in the United Kingdom. A more detailed explanation of Six Sigma and Lean is given in the NHS Institute for Innovation and Improvement publication 'Lean Six Sigma Some Basic Concepts' (2005).

Six Sigma uses statistical tools to reveal variation and implements changes to reduce the variation. Its stages are (D)MAIC (Define, Measure, Analyse, Improve, Control) and it is based on the 'Plan, Do, Study, Act' (PDSA) cycle, originally developed by Dr W. Edwards Deming, and now promulgated by the Institute of Innovation and Improvement (formerly the Modernisation Agency) as a tool for change.

When applied to hospital discharge, the Six Sigma framework would require the collection of data relating to the patient pathway, and reduction of variations, thus reducing length of patient stay.

Lean thinking is focused on reviewing work systems and processes, and looking at opportunities to remove or reduce waste and improve flow. In relation to discharge, this would mean reducing the delays that lengthen the average patient stay. The Theory of Constraints is another popular model, as it helps us understand the way a system functions and identify those elements that constrain the system and prevent it from achieving its goals.

Monitoring

One of the biggest challenges in implementing new practices is maintaining momentum and improvement. Senior nurses (both matrons and board-level nurses) need to know that changes in practice are being implemented, that improvements in performance are being made, and that the changes are sustainable.

The DH 'Next Stage Review' (2008) showed a commitment to quality measurement. Griffiths *et al.* (2008) appraised methods of measuring quality. Griffiths and his co-authors were tasked with finding ways to measure nurse-delivered outcomes and patient experience. Below is a summary of what makes a good indicator.

What makes a good indicator?

- Indicators must be measurable with available data at reasonable cost
- There must be evidence of variability associated with nursing and this variability must be substantial
- For process or structure measures, evidence must support links to important health outcomes
- The indicator must be recognised as important (by the public, managers and nurses) and the contribution of nursing must also be recognised by nurses and by others
- Nurses must have responsibility for actions that lead to the outcome in terms of legitimate authority, self-perception and sphere of practice
- There must be sufficient knowledge to inform remedial action
- Measures should be chosen to minimise the risk of gaming, where improving performance on the indicators detracts from overall performance
- Measures need to be risk adjusted to ensure comparability across settings

Source: State of the art metrics for nursing 2008 Kings College London

Once a measurement is designed, the senior nurse must implement a robust reporting mechanism. The reporting mechanism must allow learning and not be seen as a punitive process, as this can have a negative impact on morale. The diagram below shows the Seven Steps to Measurement, advocated in the High Impact Actions methods.

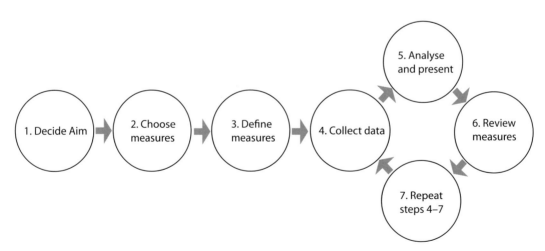

Figure 2.1
Seven Steps to Measurement 2010
adapted from NHS Institute for Innovation and Improvement

The frequency of reporting will depend on the measure but must take into account the need for monitoring and reporting at Trust board level. The Secretary of State for Health put this role firmly in the hands of the matron, but board-level nurses need to recognise that some matrons need help to put these systems in place (DH, 2010a).

Conclusion

At the beginning of this chapter, the need to deliver service quality, productivity and efficiency and financial performance was highlighted. As we have seen, in order to deliver quality care, local policy must be fit for purpose, a strong implementation plan is required and robust monitoring must be designed.

The key to maintaining momentum at organisational level is through MDT working, strong leadership and local involvement. It can be difficult to strike a balance between centralisation and devolution, and getting this wrong can lead to a failure in implementation – either at the beginning or later on, when the change in practice should have become part of everyday working.

When carrying out improvement initiatives, it is vital to assess whether the outcomes achieved are worth the cost of making the improvement. This can be determined through a simple return on investment (ROI) calculation, which is typically a cost benefit analysis that gives the net gains as a percentage of the costs. Using this approach will give safety improvements some currency. Usually, the main costs involved in making a service improvement will be staff time and training, along with any materials and equipment purchased. The benefits to be measured should include, as a minimum, any changes in quality, patient experience and cost, and should be assessed against the aims of the initiative.

Board-level commitment and effective senior nurse leadership are necessary to help overcome the barriers to success. Frequent and accurate feedback about progress (and lack of progress) is vital, in order to maintain the enthusiasm of practitioners and the support of executives. A lack of progress can be used to identify where further changes need to be made and to promote learning. It should not be used in a punitive way. Finally, the senior nurse must ensure that progress is reported both to nurses and the Trust board to give assurance, and to sustain and support best practice.

References

Berwick, D.M. (2003). Improvement, trust and the healthcare workforce. *Quality and Safety in Healthcare*. **12**, 448–452.

Bibby, J., Bevan, H., Carter, H., Bate, P. and Robert, G. (2009). *The Power of One, the Power of Many – Bringing Social Movement Thinking to Healthcare Improvement*. Coventry: NHS Institute for Innovation and Improvement.

British Quality Foundation (2000). *The Model in Practice*. London: British Quality Foundation.

Care Quality Commission (2010). *Essential Standards of Quality and Safety.* Care Quality Commission.

Clarke, A. (2002). Length of in-hospital stay and its relationship to quality of care. *Quality and Safety in Healthcare.* 11, 209–210.

Department of Health (2000). 'The NHS Plan'. London: HMSO.

Department of Health (2002). PL/CNO 2002/5. London: HMSO.

Department of Health (2003). 'The Knowledge and Skills Framework and Related Development Review'. London: HMSO.

Department of Health (2004a) 'Achieving timely "simple" discharge from hospital toolkit'. London: HMSO.

Department of Health (2004b). 'An Evaluation of the Matron Role: The Royal College of Nursing Institute and The University of Sheffield School of Nursing and Midwifery'. London: HMSO.

Department of Health (2008). 'High Quality Care for All: NHS Next Stage Review' final report. London: HMSO.

Department of Health (2010). White Paper. 'Equity and Excellence: Liberating the NHS'. London: HMSO.

Department of Health (2011). 'The Operating Framework for the NHS in England'. London: HMSO.

Drake, L., Bore, J., Humm, C. and McMahon, B. (2004). Down with targets. *Nursing Standard.* 19 (9), 22.

Fenton, K., Maher, I. and Ward, I. (5 July 2010). How nurses can implement the high impact actions to improve quality and cost effectiveness. *Nursing Times.net.*

Goodacre, S. (2006). Safe discharge: an irrational, unhelpful and unachievable concept. *Emergency Medicine Journal.* 23, 753–755. (doi: 10.1136/emj.2006.037903)

Griffiths, P., Jones, S., Maben, J. and Murrells, T. (2008). *State of the art metrics for nursing: a rapid appraisal.* National Nursing Research Unit. Kings College London.

Maher, I., Gustafson, D. and Evans, A. (2007). 'Sustainability Model and Guide'. Coventry: NHS Institute for Innovation and Improvement.

NHS Institute for Innovation and Improvement (2005). 'Lean Six Sigma: Some Basic Concepts'. Coventry: NHS Institute for Innovation and Improvement.

NHS Institute for Innovation and improvement (2010). 'High Impact Actions for Nursing and Midwifery: The Essential Collection'. Coventry: NHS Institute for Innovation and Improvement.

NHSLA 'Risk Management Standards for Acute Trusts, Primary Care Trusts and Independent Sector Providers of NHS Care (2010/11)'. London: NHS Litigation Authority.

Nursing and Midwifery Council (2008). 'Nursing and Midwifery Council – The code: Standards of conduct, performance and ethics for nurses and midwives'. London: Nursing and Midwifery Council.

Pethybridge J. (2004). How team working influences discharge planning from hospital: a study of four multi-disciplinary teams in an acute hospital in England. *Journal of Interprofessional Care.* 18, 29–40.

Steel, K., Gertman, P.M, Crescenzi, C. and Anderson, J. (2004). Iatrogenic illness on a general medical service at a university hospital. *Quality and Safety in Healthcare.* 13, 76–80.

Thompson, C., McCaughan, D., Cullum, N., Sheldon, T., Mulhall, A. and Thompson, D. (2001). The accessibility of research-based knowledge for nurses in United Kingdom acute care settings. *Journal of Advanced Nursing.* 36 (1), 11–22.

Ward, L., Fenton, K. and Maher, L. (2010). The high impact actions 8. Ready to go – no delays. *Nursing Times.* 106, 34 (early online publication).

Chapter 3

Implementation of nurse-facilitated discharge from hospital

Liz Lees

This chapter discusses nurse-facilitated discharge in the context of NHS acute hospitals. Of course, nurses facilitate the process of patient discharge from many other settings, and the principles outlined throughout this chapter are clearly transferable to different situations. Since nurse-facilitated discharge was first mooted in 2000, many different approaches to it have been tried, yet it would seem that nurse-led discharge has failed to make a major impact in practice, in hospitals (DH 2000). When considering the reasons for this, we need to look at both the medical model of patient care and the methods used to introduce nurse-facilitated discharge.

Firstly, hospitals and other organisations interested in promoting nurse-facilitated discharge need to work with the professionals involved in discharge planning, at ward level, to promote different approaches. Each ward will have evolved aspects of care that are unique to its own area. While these may broadly fit with organisational policy, there will be differences and perhaps overlaps that need to be considered to ensure the success of new approaches. These approaches should engage and integrate other professionals and agencies as closely as possible at the start of the discharge planning process. This will enable us to move away from a purely medical model of patient care, based on diagnosis, treatment and cure. Consultants must be engaged in the discharge process if they are to understand the broader implications and benefits of smoothing the patient pathway and expediting discharge from hospital. Chapters 18, 20, 23 and 28 expand upon this aspect, showing nurses taking the lead in discharge, with involvement from consultants and other professionals.

Secondly, while researching this book it has become apparent that nurse-facilitated discharge may not have been supported in practice to the extent that was required to embed this approach. For example, in some hospitals, nurse-facilitated discharge coordinators were introduced, to project-manage the scheme of work identified. However, once the scheme of work was introduced, it was assumed that it required no support or maintenance (Lees 2010a). Hence, some excellent nurse-led initiatives (Lees 2007) were left to languish when staff vacated their project posts. This left projects vulnerable to 'breakdown', as they could not be sustained without the support of staff.

This approach has only served to reinforce a pre-existing NHS culture of short-termism, whereby projects are rapidly established in order to meet policy changes but don't continue in the long term. Moreover, nurse-facilitated discharge was viewed as a totally separate activity from mainstream discharge coordination or planning. Some Trusts, anxious to reduce delays in the discharge process, explicitly embraced nurse-facilitated discharge as a 'quick fix'. In some cases, there was little integration or flexibility of organisational practices (both old and new) to accommodate such change.

Conversely, some nurses have been facilitating patient discharge for many years. In such cases, this has become normal practice to the extent that they have not even recognised it or measured its impact as part of service delivery. In the example described in Chapter 20, the nurse's role in the discharge of patients was conducted in accordance with the outcome required as part of the ophthalmology care pathway, rather than being seen as new practice. Although much new evidence has become available in the last few years (Lees 2007), it cannot possibly represent the enormous amount of work that has actually been undertaken, as many isolated pockets of excellent practice are not mentioned in the literature.

Overview

This chapter begins by reviewing policy initiatives that have created renewed impetus for the implementation of nurse-facilitated discharge – in particular, the 'High Impact Actions for Nursing and Midwifery' (Institute for Innovation and Improvement 2009). It then explores what is required for nurse-facilitated discharge from hospital to be embedded in practice. For example, leadership, responsibility and accountability will be discussed, in relation to other factors that should be taken into account when planning to introduce nurse-facilitated discharge. Distinctions will be drawn between nurse-led, nurse-facilitated, bespoke and criteria-led discharge, with examples. Key questions will be offered, to identify some of the systems and processes that need to be in place, in order to implement nurse-facilitated discharge planning. (Some of these points will be further illustrated in Chapters 18, 22 and 23, which offer case studies of nurse-facilitated discharge in practice.) Inevitably, some of the issues discussed will be inter-related and may, at times, overlap, but they all play an important part in discharge planning.

Policy developments

The principles underpinning discharge planning remain largely unchanged, despite the evolution of the NHS and all its governing policies. 'Discharge planning should start on admission' is understood as the key principle; but discharge planning is a hugely complex topic, affecting almost every aspect of inpatient care and all new service developments. In the face of such scope and complexity, the key principle may not always be remembered or achieved. The way that services are delivered is changing rapidly, often involving multiple stakeholders and service commissioners, who are keen to influence service provision (DH 2010a).

Hence, if nurse-facilitated discharge is to have any impact on innovation and improving healthcare services, it cannot be instigated in isolation from the current NHS changes. Perhaps the biggest challenges arise from shorter lengths of patient stay, the need to increase patient throughput, and the acuteness of the medical condition of patients admitted to hospital (Institute for Innovation and Improvement 2010). Often forgotten are the gradual and sustained advances in medical science that impact upon development of services, particularly home and outpatient-based services. Where most patient services were once inpatient based, art and science have played a part in adapting the way the NHS plans and delivers patient discharge from hospital.

Nurses are a large staff group, who are also responding to changes in the way care is delivered. Quality and safety are leading priorities, in discharge practice as in all other areas, and workforce development is required (DH 2004b, 2010b). Of all NHS staff, nurses have the greatest level of interaction with patients, and it is a logical progression that they should facilitate patient involvement, leading to nurse-led discharge.

Moreover, patient/carer expectations are being made more explicit, guiding the commissioning of services and stimulating further changes in discharge planning practice (Lees 2010b, DH 2010a, CarersUK 2008, Brown *et al.* 2006). Policy documents are reflecting these changes by becoming more specific in their emphasis on individual areas of discharge practice and, in particular, the partnership elements within those areas (DH 2008, DH 2010c). Patients and carers alike are no longer content to be passive recipients of care; they expect to be kept informed and involved in the discharge planning process (ADASS 2010, DH 2005a, 2005b; see also Chapter 14). To this end, anyone introducing nurse-facilitated discharge needs to ensure that patient satisfaction and feedback mechanisms are integral from the outset (Lees & Chadha, 2011).

Finally, the talk of timely discharge to stimulate simple discharges from hospital saw the introduction of a Toolkit. This reasserted and embraced the nurse's leading role, as the staff member who has the most patient contact time and as a member of the multidisciplinary team that facilitates timely discharge from hospital (DH 2004a, DH 2010c). The Toolkit was also cited in a review of literature, by the Office of Public

Management, among the top ten pieces of work fitting its search criteria (OPM 2010). The Toolkit offered competencies (a core set to build on) and a guide to implementation in practice. It differed from most documents published at the time, in that it presented the whole picture of hospital discharge, both simple and complex, augmented by estimated dates for discharge – at the time merely a debating point!

Are we making progress with nurse-facilitated discharge?

In most cases, NHS policies aim to stimulate innovative ways of working. In others, they may endorse mechanisms for additional support. The additional 'support' for nurse-facilitated discharge arrived in the form of a timely reminder and deadline for implementation of key actions – 'Ready to go?' (DH 2010c). The publication of this policy document meant that the nurse's role in discharge planning was in the spotlight yet again, shortly after the launch of the 'High Impact Actions for Nursing and Midwifery' (Institute for Innovation and Improvement 2009).

These 'high impact actions' built on the ten key roles (or functions) of nurses set out in 2000, one of which was 'admitting and discharging patients' (DH 2000). Many believed that it would only be possible for nurses to fulfil this admission and discharge function if care pathways, protocols and services in general were originally established with it in mind. Existing services and pathways had to be adapted and this created inertia in practice. Often there is an abundance of NHS policy, which is not necessarily followed through with the level of organisational scale changes required; and, in this case, making some of these adaptations in actual healthcare settings continues to be a challenge.

So, are we really any further forward with implementing nurse-facilitated discharge? Published evidence reveals that disparate practice is rife, ranging from well-developed work to small-scale projects with little strategic support to sustain good practice (Lees 2004, Lees & Field 2011). Hence, to reiterate an earlier point, the published research does not reflect the true level of activity that has taken place.

A review of evidence regarding nurse-led discharge was conducted in 2010 by the Office of Public Management and submitted in a report for the NHS Institute (OPM 2010). Although 57 potentially relevant sources referring to nurse-facilitated discharge were found through the literature review, only ten met the review criteria and were included for analysis of work published between 2001 and 2009. These included local case studies, a toolkit, a non-systematic literature review, cost-effective studies, a systematic review and a service improvement paper. The areas where practice had developed and been cited were breast surgery, gynaecology and emergency with integrated early discharge services. Apart from this, nurse-led services within inpatient units, which are a rare breed, accounted for the remainder of the literature reviewed.

The use of predictive discharge dates is inextricably linked with nurses facilitating patient discharge and was cited in the literature review (OPM 2010). Estimating or predicting discharge dates is one aspect of good discharge practice (Webber-Maybank & Luton 2009, Lees 2008, Lees & Holmes 2005). Moving the time of a patient's discharge forward, ahead of forthcoming admissions, was one measurable benefit of nurse-facilitated discharge. This time shift, even if it is only an hour earlier, may provide essential bed capacity at a critical time of the day – for example, when emergency referrals into non-elective capacity exceed the volume of discharged patients. So, nurse-facilitated discharge works well with other components of a good discharge process, such as estimating dates for discharge (see Chapters 13 and 27).

Likely cost savings achieved as a direct result of introducing nurse-facilitated discharge can only be accurately estimated if appropriate benchmarks are put in place prior to commencing the work (Lees & Field, 2011). The evidence in the 2010 case review was relatively poor. Costs must be considered for every element of holistic service provision (OPM 2010). For example, there were additional costs for provision of a service to support the patients following early discharge. However, the early discharge did reduce length of stay, thus releasing beds. In addition, the costs of any investments need to be balanced against the patient quality of care agenda. In doing so, we need to consider the longer-term savings that are likely to be made through investing in work, which will in turn stimulate sustainable changes in practice. Moreover, sustainable changes can be refined and will evolve over time, expanding the evidence base for this area of work.

Moving forward with this knowledge means that we have ample opportunity for new research to be carried out in this area. This is where Trusts must support evidence-based processes and demonstrate their impact in practice (Lees & Field 2011). The route to the sustainable introduction of innovative ways of delivering discharge practice rests firmly with the nursing profession, even though they may perceive it as being dominated by new paperwork and systems of collecting data. To realise the magnitude of change required, NHS directors, consultants and service/operational managers, responsible for patient services, must be prepared to move away from rhetoric, examine their working practices for the benefit of patients, and join in with the process of change equally. Organisational readiness is imperative in order to support nurses, who cannot on their own achieve the scale of change required to implement the concept of nurse-facilitated discharge (see Chapter 2).

Policy implementation and changes in practice

The publication of 'High Impact Actions for Nursing and Midwifery' (Institute for Innovation and Improvement 2009) has created new opportunities and increased responsibilities, depending on the extent to which nurses and midwives are proactively involved in discharge planning and the implementation of nurse-led discharge. This change process is stimulating the development of new organisational policy, protocols and training, which will serve to protect the employing organisation and also the individual practitioner in expanding their role and taking on new practices (NMC 2008, DH 2004a, Lees & Emmerson 2006). It will also instigate innovative ways of working to benefit the patient.

Finally, the scale of change will demand integrated working practices in teams outside hospitals, encompassing a range of different organisations and agencies that deliver health and social care services supporting patient discharge. Agreements regarding service provision will need to include at least two core groups of staff, namely district nurses and GPs, who will feel the impact of earlier discharges from hospital or discharges over seven days of the week (see Chapter 1). Their involvement will primarily be required to ensure that there is no duplication of services or added layers of administration for patients to negotiate and service commissioners to fund (Lees 2010a).

Despite this positive perspective, 'change' can be quite a frightening prospect for some professionals; and changes may not be readily adopted in the area of discharge practice (Lees & Field, 2011). For example, it is evident that protective mechanisms are sometimes adopted by individual professionals to secure the status quo, regarding their particular professional role (Lees 2010a). This tendency is often reinforced by oppressive strategies used to deliberately slow down the pace of change, especially if the proposed change is seen to adversely affect role development (Lees 2008, Leason 2003). If a method of facilitating the change is not used, it is often easy to misinterpret the implications, giving rise to tension.

To counteract possible misapprehension and fragmented practices (moving from reactive to proactive discharge planning), organisations should develop a culture of sustaining new practices, rather than adopting a 'must do by the end of' mentality, which may constrain development or shorten the 'shelf life' of the change. Therefore, change must be managed effectively, and preparation, planning and discussion are crucial to ensure successful implementation. This is particularly important when change is occurring because of wider agendas and priorities, which may not seem apparent at practice level.

Developing the culture: perspectives on leadership

Passion, drive and commitment are three essential requirements when developing a culture of nurse leadership, irrespective of the particular subject being explored (Martin 2009).

Passion about discharge planning may arise from knowledge of the subject and the desire to carry out the role. Drive may be increased by understanding the organisational goals; this will help to give nurses a sense of ownership and a desire to be proactively involved in patient discharge. Drive and commitment go hand in hand, particularly regarding discharge planning, where it is crucial to track the progress of the problem or issue until it is resolved. For example, rather than leaving an issue 'to chance', handing it over to others, or disowning the issue altogether, successful implementation requires follow-through, regardless of shift pattern or which professional it may have been handed to.

Early discharge, promoted through a nurse-facilitated approach, will mean that another acutely ill patient can be admitted to the ward, instead of waiting at home or in another care setting. The increasing acuteness of patients' medical conditions when they are admitted, and the complexity of care they require, make it notoriously difficult to keep track of who did what, what the result was, and its implications for the patient's care. Ultimately, all these issues impact on the discharge plan and possibly the length of stay. Nurse-facilitated discharge must be promoted alongside the quality and safety agenda in nursing, and not simply viewed as a means of creating capacity or to assist other target-driven initiatives. Hence, it requires a significant commitment from the nurse to take responsibility and focus upon creating discharge plans, as a priority, amongst the many other aspects of nursing care that require prioritisation and delivery. Leading the plan requires a sustained commitment to review the patient's progress regularly and to assert control over timing and inputs.

Case study: What plan?

Junior doctors on an acute medical ward had made a physiotherapy request for an oxygen saturation assessment and mobility assessment. They had written the request in the medical records on a ward round early in the week. On chasing up the referral later in the week, they discovered that the physiotherapist had already reviewed and discharged the patient (earlier in the week) from her care.

The physiotherapist conducted a board round of new patients every day and did not wait for referrals from the junior doctors. This meant that the physiotherapist did not refer to the medical notes for referrals. The processes of referral and action were not linked. The physiotherapist had not documented the outcome of the assessments in the medical records. Each outcome had been noted on the whiteboard instead – only to be removed by a nurse once the action had been completed. The nurses were aware of the board rounds but they had not checked the patient notes for referrals or outcomes either.

In this case the central elements in the discharge plan were not stated at the outset of the patient care pathway; and there was no actual overall 'plan'. There was a list of actions to be completed but the anticipated outcome and length of stay were not stated or clear; nor were the responsibilities of the members of the multidisciplinary team.

Staff members had been waiting for a series of unconnected events to take place, leaving the outcome, or desired outcome, uncertain/open-ended. Thus, a 'time lag' was created between each action carried out and patient review.

If the time lag after the saturation assessment and mobility assessment (caused by poor communication and different systems of planning being in place) had been removed, the length of stay could have been reduced by three days.

The change in leadership expectations requires nurses to review the way they organise themselves alongside other professionals to deliver care. Nurses assert that they feel overwhelmed by competing patient activities and tasks; but good organisation and leadership at ward level help to create valuable time. For example, in the case of discharge planning and the busy acute hospital environment, perhaps we get too tied up in individual tasks, rather than understanding where we are in the overall discharge process and therefore which tasks will achieve the biggest impact in the time we have? There is an overwhelming need to be able to clarify, with all professionals involved, the patient's care, over an approximate timescale, in a discharge plan (Lees *et al.* 2006a, Lees & Holmes 2005, Kuockkanen & Leino-Kilpi 2000, Ward *et al.* 2008). This must be supported by fundamental planning principles (see below), which also constitute stages in the process, leading to the desired outcome.

Fundamental principles of discharge planning

1. Having knowledge of the specific disease process or condition
2. Estimating how long recovery might take, or if recovery is a realistic outcome
3. Communicating with, and involving the patient, family and carers in the planning process
4. Proactively dealing with issues and difficulties that may arise
5. Engaging in a process that involves the roles of the MDT (meetings)
6. Communicating and contemporaneous documentation of the plan with the MDT (avoiding duplication and confusion)
7. Making appropriate referrals and following through outcomes
8. Coordinating and owning the discharge information in a plan, identifying names responsible for each action, and in complex cases identifying one case leader

9. Being decisive and carrying out discharge activities

10. Reviewing and updating the progress of the plan

11. Disseminating accurate information to all involved

Evidence reviewed from the case notes for patients who have had reasonably short lengths of stay (perhaps less than three days) indicates that stages 2, 3 and 11 of the process are quite commonly overlooked. If these three aspects were addressed routinely, nurses planning discharge from hospital could assert a greater degree of control and ownership of the discharge process, which would benefit patients. With finite resources available (notably professional time), critical aspects of discharge planning should be addressed in a timely manner with relatives and carers. Visiting times can be a good time for staff to engage with family members and avoid important issues being left to languish. If this is not possible, appointments with key members of the planning team should be made. Collectively, such actions will promote the principles of working in partnership with the patient, family and multidisciplinary team towards effective nurse-facilitated discharge (DH 2004).

Best practice in discharge planning

Since the publication of *Nurse Facilitated Discharge from Hospital* in 2007, it has become increasingly clear that, unless the core elements of good discharge planning are in place, it will not be possible to introduce nurse-facilitated discharge. Discharge planning transcends many areas of practice, which each have unique clinical characteristics. However, the core elements of discharge planning (see below) are consistent across an organisation.

The core elements of discharge planning

- A comprehensive hospital discharge policy (referenced for ease of use and communicated widely to staff)
- Clarity regarding out-of-hours provision (e.g. transport and medications)
- Clarity regarding the roles of individual members of the MDT in planning discharge
- A discharge process, with all stages of the process clearly understood by staff
- A summary of the discharge standard(s) expected
- Ward coordination, with identified roles or individual functions
- Discharge training – including specifics at ward level
- Communication of discharge information to patient and relatives/carers
- Evidence that discharge planning has taken place – the patient should have a copy of their discharge plan

This list is certainly not exhaustive, but it will help Trusts to meet NHSLA criteria for discharge planning (NHSLA 2011/12). When these aspects can be assured, nurse-facilitated discharge can be considered. If the discharge process is unclear or variable or not engaged with, nurse-facilitated discharge will not improve the situation. Resolution of issues should be sought before embarking on any new work. For example, if tablets to take home are delayed through the process used (such as long ward rounds and junior doctors completing them afterwards), nurse-facilitated discharge cannot resolve this issue, unless changes are made to the original discharge planning process.

Debating the name: nurse-led or nurse-facilitated?

Nursing literature has focused a great deal on terminology when it comes to the subject of nurses leading the discharge process (Rudd & Smith 2002, Lees 2004). Evidence from structured workshops suggests that the name adopted is incredibly important to some medical colleagues. For example, 'nurse-led' implies a uni-disciplinary activity, entirely controlled by nurses. The use of this term can generate bad feeling and fear that patients will be discharged without appropriate management from medical colleagues and allied health professionals. Even within nursing, this term can cause ramifications, including discharge being seen as an exclusive role and the domain of a privileged, adequately prepared/trained minority. While the process of defining the concept can be time-consuming, opening up this debate does serve a useful function by unifying agreement and making explicit the intended goal(s). Moreover, in the process of determining organisational discharge policy, it paves the way for the implementation of new and innovative practices.

Nurse-facilitated

The term 'nurse-facilitated' is derived from the actions required to complete the process. For example, it refers to 'a process where nurses adopt specific responsibilities (within a predetermined scope of practice) for the proactive management of activities aligned with a patient's discharge plan'. (The plan will be multidisciplinary, with nurses engaged to ensure it takes place in a timely manner.)

Nurse-led

The term 'nurse-led' has been further defined as 'nurses leading the whole process of discharge planning following decisions made by nurses, using criteria, protocols or given set of principles'. (The plan may be multidisciplinary, with the nurse's role in the care pathway clearly defined to expedite the plan in a timely manner.)

(Adapted from Lees 2006, cited in Lees 2007)

Regardless of which name is adopted, this discharge role should not be seen as unique to senior nurses (such as matrons, nurse specialists, discharge coordinators or nurse consultants). Nor should it be assumed that it can be conducted in isolation, without the support of all appropriate members of the multidisciplinary team.

Perhaps some of the fear amongst other healthcare practitioners can be managed appropriately if the concept is explored in terms of explicit factors, such as what nurses should and should not do when they are involved in the discharge process.

Nurses facilitating discharge should not:

- Follow a series of instructions as indicated by the medical team (this is arguably what the nurse and the MDT would ordinarily do)
- Decide a patient is fit for discharge without consulting the relevant professionals involved with the patient's care
- Defer discharge decisions to the doctor and wait for him/her to make a decision, for which the nurse has had the relevant training/knowledge
- Discharge a patient according to different rules depending who is in charge of the ward and on duty
- Discharge patients without adequate preparation to accommodate bed capacity issues.

Nurses facilitating discharge should:

- Initiate and lead the discharge process with the involvement of all relevant professionals to expedite discharges, and assist bed and capacity management across the whole hospital
- Carry out regular and ongoing patient assessments/evaluation to assist timely and appropriate discharges
- Progress-chase the results of investigations that require the nurse's decisions to expedite discharge
- Review results and make decisions based upon the results within given bespoke parameters applicable to the individual patient
- Proactively engage the MDT at appropriate points in the patient's care
- Proactively promote and discuss discharge decisions, in collaboration with the family and MDT to promote discharges
- Follow up the patient (in and out of hospital) and review progress, according to the discharge plan
- Act as the patient's advocate
- Endorse the system or process being used to carry out discharge practice
- Take ownership of education and training needs at a local level

(Adapted from Lees 2004, Lees & Field, 2011)

The fundamentals of discharge practice

It is suggested that nurses should learn new ways of behaving, and reframe their professional image, role and values. In reality, nurses facilitating patient discharge from hospital are trying to achieve clearly defined roles and responsibilities along the multiple stages of the discharge process. This clarity will benefit patients firstly and the organisation, a very close second.

Inevitably, a minority of NHS organisations have changed their nurse-facilitated discharge processes in an extreme way, transferring the vast majority of patient discharge decision-making, previously undertaken by junior doctors, to nurses. Some nurses see the expansion and gradual adjustment of their roles as the natural evolution of the caring process, while others argue that they are effectively carrying out doctors' duties for a nurse's pay.

Nonetheless, nurse-facilitated discharge provides a positive step forward. The diagram below places 'nurse-facilitated' and 'nurse-led' discharge on a continuum of development. With this in mind, nurses need to have a good understanding of their parameters of practice and be aware of their individual responsibility and accountability (NMC 2008).

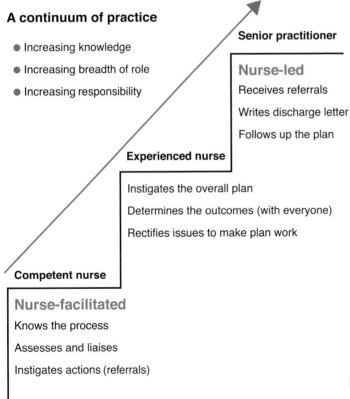

A continuum of practice

- Increasing knowledge
- Increasing breadth of role
- Increasing responsibility

Senior practitioner

Nurse-led
Receives referrals
Writes discharge letter
Follows up the plan

Experienced nurse

Instigates the overall plan
Determines the outcomes (with everyone)
Rectifies issues to make plan work

Competent nurse

Nurse-facilitated
Knows the process
Assesses and liaises
Instigates actions (referrals)

Figure 3.1
A continuum of practice

This diagram attempts to visualise the nurse's progress through a trajectory of learning in practice, and begins to distinguish 'nurse-facilitated' from 'nurse-led' behaviours. Nevertheless, it is not necessarily easy to measure at exactly which point the nurse's progress through a series of increasing responsibilities puts her on the level of a senior practitioner. Clinical exposure is crucial, in order to experience the different facets of practice required. Encouraging nurses to take on greater responsibility requires a governed framework that promotes safe practice.

Exploring responsibility and accountability

There is sometimes a reluctance to embrace nurse-facilitated discharge. For instance, practice and attitudes may differ from ward to ward, even within a single organisation. Part of the reason, until recently, was the absence of organisational policies and protocols to support nursing actions in practice. However, there are no longer any legal or professional reasons to prevent nurses taking increasing responsibility for the discharge process, including the decision to discharge a patient, provided that they are competent and can demonstrate the experience needed to do so (DH 2004).

Responsibility

It may be the individual interpretation of 'nurse-facilitated discharge' that adds an extra layer of caution, which becomes self-limiting. Evidence suggests that nurses may fear the 'responsibility' of being left alone to contemplate a discharge decision, where perhaps not all the issues have been resolved or further clarity is required. Moreover, guarded behaviour is evident when nurses believe the responsibility is not 'theirs' to take. This issue is compounded when junior and senior members of the medical teams fear their patients will be discharged without their prior knowledge or consent!

Conversely, in some areas it is considered an insult to nurses to suggest that they have ever practised any other way. In these cases, they do indeed lead and coordinate all discharges from hospital in their area of practice, with the absolute support of their medical colleagues. The degree of decision-making responsibility required will vary tremendously, depending on the expertise of the particular nurse facilitating the discharge. The same can be said of junior doctors, who may sometimes 'admit' patients as a safeguard or even delay a discharge decision, until their senior colleagues are present. Furthermore, with the inception of new protocols and policies, the opposite of nurse-facilitated discharge may occur. For example, nurses may need to elicit safer discharges, which are well informed and appropriate. In some cases, this may mean that patients are not discharged and the plan has to be revisited. The most important aspects to understand are outlined below:

- Knowledge of the patient is prerequisite
- Training is required (identified within own clinical area)
- Experience of discharge process and discharge planning is essential
- Discharge is not a uni-disciplinary activity
- The patient must be reviewed and be medically fit for discharge

Accountability

The Nursing and Midwifery Council (NMC 2008) has set out the professional standards that underpin the foundation of practice. Central to these standards are nurses' decisions to act or not act, and to act in the best interests of the patient. These are guiding principles that can be applied to nurse-facilitated discharge from hospital. Understanding what nurse facilitation involves is a prerequisite in order to understand whether sufficient preparation has been undertaken.

Equally, interpretation of the accountability framework is a good place for nurses to start, rather than fearing consequences, litigation or possible removal from the register. Nurse-facilitated discharge involves assessing the patient, liaising with the multidisciplinary team, and planning timely discharge based on the agreed plan of care (DH & RCN 2003, DH 2004a, Lees 2004). Writing or contributing to discharge letters, making follow-up calls and advising patients, carers and other professionals are all within the scope of the nurse's role in discharge planning (NMC 2008, DH 2004, DH & RCN 2003).

Nevertheless, making decisions within agreed parameters requires experience and professional judgement. However, this degree of experience and judgement is not necessarily indicated by a nurse's pay banding or job title. This is why it is not possible to include nurses within Band 5 (or exclude them from Band 5), as they may have a great deal of experience to offer, depending on how long they have been in that role. Experience in the role through proven activities is desirable, though some discharge issues are multifaceted and require supreme confidence to deal with effectively.

Implementation of nurse-facilitated discharge

Before nurse-facilitated discharge can be successfully implemented, it is absolutely essential that the existing discharge process is mapped and fully understood by all participating. Existing issues must be resolved first.

Critical questions (before, during and after implementation)

1. Is your existing discharge process an efficient one?
2. Why do you want to introduce nurse-facilitated discharge?
3. Where do you need to make changes in the process for it to be nurse-facilitated?

4. Where do you need to add in support or training or competencies?
5. What are the desired outcomes (measures of success)?
6. Who is responsible for auditing the discharge process?

Methods applicable in elective and non-elective care

Any of the methods outlined below can be used to introduce a nurse-facilitated discharge process, but it is essential to be clear about which method has been chosen to drive practice forward.

Bespoke discharge management plans (useful in non-elective services)

A bespoke discharge plan is written specifically for a particular patient, who may have multiple investigations taking place and multiple problems to resolve. In such cases, it may not be possible to set out a specific care pathway. Such a plan has the following characteristics:

- It may be agreed on a ward round, with set parameters for discharge.
- It works best when there is an agreed estimated or predicted date of discharge.
- A discharge checklist should always be used, to demonstrate who discharged the patient and what actions were carried out.
- It does not necessarily require additional documentation, but the documentation must demonstrate that the parameters were met prior to discharge.

Discharge checklists with variance measured against the norm (useful in elective care)

Having explored the existing discharge process (see 'critical questions', p. 44), and made changes to accommodate nurse-facilitated discharge, a simple additional checklist is very useful in elective care. This list would include aspects that need to be checked before the patient is discharged, such as: oozing from wound sites, pain score, vomiting, and so on. The following points need to be remembered:

- A discharge letter will still be required.
- A process must be put in place to enable tablets to take out to be supplied in a timely manner.
- Documented evidence will be required that the patient was fit to be discharged.

Protocol- or criteria-led discharges (useful for patients with specific conditions, both elective and non-elective)

This type of discharge is useful when the patient has a specific condition or has had a particular procedure or operation performed. It will provide a framework for what needs to be done prior to discharge and to ensure fitness for discharge. For example, a patient with asthma that is responding well to treatment may be following a treatment plan, which has clearly defined stages of care such as:

- Wean from oxygen by 2 litres until discontinued
- Make pre- and post-peak flow checks
- Ensure temperature is below 37.5°C
- After evening dose of nebuliser, transfer on to inhalers (teach inhaler technique)

It should not be necessary to write this plan separately for each patient. Instead, if the parameters align with the usual care protocols/guidance for that particular condition or group of conditions, the same criteria can be applied and followed to execute the discharge plan. Of course, as with any plan, it can be adjusted by adding to the stated criteria.

Apart from criteria-led plans, some settings have established protocols to guide the discharge of their patients. Protocols tend to have their origins in national guidance and will be referenced as such. While researching this book, protocols have been located for gynaecological conditions and frequently for termination of pregnancy and vomiting during pregnancy. The common features are that the specifics of each condition are clearly stated, as are the parameters to be achieved before discharge home.

Patient care pathways

Finally, there are care pathways, in which discharge planning is automatically part of the pathway and will have been agreed by those involved. Care pathways are usually developed for specific operations or procedures, as well as end of life and the management of chronic conditions. In such cases, there are partnership agreements that may span different organisations and a range of professionals delivering the care. Discharge planning is implicit throughout the pathway – especially when the pathway may be ambulatory or an outpatient-based service (see Chapters 18–21). In such cases, the process leading to discharge planning usually (but not exclusively) begins in the preoperative assessment phase. At this stage, elements that need to be present post-discharge are put in place.

There are always exceptions to criteria and pathways, and complex, acute medical and older patients may have many potential variables, which make it difficult to employ a protocol-managed approach. In this situation, a bespoke management plan and estimated date of discharge will provide the central structure.

On the other hand, using a management plan alone can encourage a reductionist approach, whereby the nurse may be tempted to rely entirely on the plan (especially in a fast-moving acute hospital environment) and not use other tools that are available, such as the single assessment process or other assessments that have been carried out since admission.

Regardless of the specific speciality or the approach taken, it is worth remembering that a patient enters the discharge process when they are admitted to hospital. This approach should not be undermined, and the discharge should not be viewed as a single task or checklist.

Conclusion

At present, discharge planning is very high profile across the NHS, with systems and practices constantly playing catch-up in their attempts to integrate policy into practice settings. Nurse-facilitated discharge from hospital is multifaceted. The time is right to bring about the developments needed, along with new systems of working to support far-reaching NHS changes. At the very least, we should be able to look back (over time) and realise, irrespective of the exact terminology used to frame the policy, that our actions have improved care for our patients. This will require knowledge that goes way beyond discharge planning, transcending different expert knowledge bases and different organisational agendas. Healthcare professionals working in hospitals must draw on their experience and share it openly in order to provide the best care in the patient's acute phase. This requires a truly integrated approach, both professionally and organisationally.

References

Association of Directors of Adult Social Services (February 2010). 'Carers as partners in hospital discharge: A review paper'. Warwickshire: ADASS.

Brown, D., McWilliam, C. & Ward-Griffin, C. (2006). Client-centred empowering partnership in nursing. *Journal of Advanced Nursing*. **53** (2), 160–168.

CarersUK (February 2008). 'Coming out of Hospital: a guide for carers'. Fact sheet.

Department of Health (2000). 'The NHS Plan: a plan for improvement, a plan for reform'. London: HMSO.

Department of Health & Royal College of Nursing (2003a). 'Freedom to Practice: dispelling the myths'. London: HMSO.

Department of Health (2003b). 'Discharge from Hospital: pathway process and practice'. London: HMSO.

Department of Health (2004a). 'Achieving timely "simple" discharge from hospital toolkit'. London: HMSO.

Department of Health (2004b). 'The NHS Knowledge and Skills Framework (NHS KSF) and the Development Review Process'. London: HMSO.

Department of Health (2005a). 'Creating a patient led NHS: delivering the improvement plan'. London: HMSO.

Department of Health (2005b). 'Commissioning a patient led NHS'. London: HMSO.

Department of Health (2008). 'High quality care for all: NHS Next Stage Review'. Command paper, final report. London: HMSO.

Department of Health (2010a). 'Equity and excellence: Liberating the NHS'. London: HMSO.

Department of Health (2010b). 'Liberating the NHS: Developing the workforce: a consultation on proposals'. London: HMSO.

Department of Health (2010c). 'Ready to go? Planning the discharge and the transfer of patients from hospital and intermediate care'. London: HMSO.

Efraimsson, E., Rasmussen, B., Gilje, F. & Sandman, P. (2003). Expressions of power and powerlessness in discharge planning: a case study of an older woman on her way home. *Journal of Clinical Nursing*. **12** (5), 707–716.

Institute for Innovation and Improvement (2009). 'High Impact Actions for Nursing and Midwifery'. University of Warwick.

Institute for Innovation and Improvement (2010). 'Quality and Improvement tools: return on investment calculator'. www.institute.nhs.uk/quality_and_service_improvement

Kuockkanen, L. & Leino-Kilpi (2000). Power and empowerment in nursing: three theoretical approaches. *Journal of Advanced Nursing*. **31**(1), 235–241.

Leason, K. (2003). Delay tactics. *Nursing Standard*. **17** (24), 16–17.

Lees, L. (2006). Emergency Care Briefing Paper: Modernising discharge from Hospital, updated version January 2006. National Electronic Library for Health.

Lees, L. (2007). *Nurse Facilitated Hospital Discharge*. Keswick: M&K Publishing.

Lees, L. (2008). Estimating Patients' Discharge Dates: applied leadership. *Nursing Management*. **15** (3), 30–35.

Lees, L. (2010a). A practitioner's guide to service development. *Nursing Management*. November 2010, **17** (7), 30–36.

Lees, L. (2010b). Good postoperative care means setting personal goals for patients: comment on practice. *Nursing Times*. 16 February 2010.

Lees, L. & Chadha S. (2011). Factors to consider in designing a patient satisfaction survey. *Nursing Management*. **18** (7) In press.

Lees, L. & Field A. (2011). Board to Ward – lessons learned implementing nurse facilitated discharge. *Nursing Times*. In press.

Lees, L. (2004). Making nurse led discharge work to improve patient care. *Nursing Times*. **100** (37), 30–32.

Lees, L. & Holmes, C. (2005). Estimating date of discharge at ward level: a pilot study. *Nursing Standard*. **19** (17), 40–43.

Lees, L., Allen, G. & O'Brien, D. (2006). Using post-take ward rounds to facilitate simple discharge. *Nursing Times*. **102** (18), 28–30.

Lees, L. & Emmerson, K. (2006). Identifying discharge practice training needs. *Nursing Standard*. **20** (29), 47–51.

Martin, R. (2009). *The Design of Business: Why Design Thinking is the Next Competitive Advantage*. Boston, MA: Harvard Business Press.

NHSLA (2010/11). Risk Management Handbook 2010/11. Standard 4, Criterion 4.10 – discharge and transfer of patients. London: NHS Litigation Authority.

Nursing and Midwifery Council (2008). 'The NMC Code of Professional Conduct: standards for conduct, performance and ethics'. London: Nursing and Midwifery Council.

Office for Public Management (2010). 'Nurse-led discharge: extracts from literature review – High Impact Actions for Nurse and Midwives, Report to the NHS Institute'. London. http://www.opm.co.uk

Rudd, C. & Smith. J. (2002). Discharge Planning. *Nursing Standard*. **17** (5), 33–37.

Ward, L., Fenton, K. & Maher, L. (2008). Nurse led discharge improves care: the high impact actions for nursing and midwifery, ready to go – no delays. *Nursing Times*. **106**, 34.

Webber-Maybank, M. & Luton, H. (2009). Making effective use of predicted discharge dates to reduce the length of stay in hospital. *Nursing Times*. **105**, 15.

Chapter 4

Safeguarding issues for the transfer of patients

Lorraine Longstaff

This chapter will specifically address safeguarding adults in relation to discharge planning from hospital. Mental capacity will be taken into consideration but will not be addressed in depth. The author's expertise lies in safeguarding and in dealing with cases that arise in a large NHS Foundation Trust. The chapter begins with a discussion of what we mean by the term 'safeguarding adults', which adults are vulnerable, and what constitutes 'abuse'. Examples will be used to demonstrate salient points.

'Safeguarding' isn't new, but over the last decade professionals have taken on safeguarding as a new role when caring for inpatients. They now have to take responsibility for recognising patient issues and taking action when necessary, especially in the light of increasing complexity of care and recent high-profile inquiries. Three reports spanning the last ten years have emphasised the importance of safeguarding adults and children and the fact that lessons have to be learnt (Mencap 2007, DH 2000, Parliamentary and Health Service Ombudsman 2011).

What do we mean by the term 'safeguarding adults'?

Safeguarding adults is defined by the Department of Health (2010) as: 'Safety from harm and exploitation', which is one of our most basic needs. Being or feeling unsafe can undermine our relationships and our self-belief. 'Safeguarding' refers to actions aimed at upholding an adult's fundamental right to be/feel safe. It is of particular importance for people who, because of their situation or circumstances, are unable to assure their own safety. Hence, 'safeguarding vulnerable adults from abuse and harm is everyone's business and is now becoming an important part of everyday healthcare practice' (DH 2010).

Which adults are 'vulnerable'?

There is no formal definition of vulnerability within healthcare, although some people receiving healthcare may be at greater risk of harm than others, sometimes as a complication of their presenting condition and their individual circumstances. The risks that increase a person's vulnerability should be appropriately assessed and identified by the healthcare professional at the first contact and continue throughout the care pathway.

The Safeguarding Vulnerable Groups Act (2006) recognises that any adult receiving any form of healthcare is potentially vulnerable. 'No Secrets' (DH 2000) defines a vulnerable adult as a person aged 18 years or over, 'who is or may be in need of community care services by reason of mental or other disability, age or illness; and who is or may be unable to take care of him or herself, or unable to protect him or herself against significant harm or exploitation'.

However, a person's disability or age does not in itself make the person vulnerable. An adult's ability to protect themselves and safeguard their well-being will be influenced by many factors:

- Personal circumstances such as physical disability; learning disability; mental health; illness; frailty AND
- Risks arising from the person's environment – social contacts; quality of care; physical environment COUNTERED BY
- Resilience factors – personal strengths; social supports; environmental supports

(DH 2011)

Eligibility for social care (community care services) focuses upon the immediate or longer-term risk to a person's independence and well-being. A patient's need for social care will vary by degree and across time but many may fall within the scope of adult protection. Levels of independence and well-being may be temporarily or permanently affected by health-related conditions. A patient's health condition may reduce the choice and control they have, as well as their ability to make decisions or to protect themselves from harm and exploitation. Consequently, the definition of 'vulnerable adult' may apply broadly within healthcare (DH 2011).

What is 'abuse'?

The term 'abuse' can be subject to wide interpretation. However, 'No Secrets' suggests the starting point for a definition is the following statement:

'Abuse is a violation of an individual's human and civil rights by any other person or persons' (DH 2000).

Furthermore, abuse may consist of a single act or repeated acts. It may be an act of neglect or an omission to act. Examples of when abuse may occur are (1) when a vulnerable person is persuaded to enter into a financial or (2) sexual transaction to which he or she has not consented, or cannot consent. Nonetheless, abuse can occur in any relationship and may result in significant harm, or exploitation of, the vulnerable person (DH 2000).

What are 'safeguarding adults concerns'?

Safeguarding adults concerns vary according to the nature of the harm, the circumstances in which it arose, and the people concerned. Three points to consider are:

1. The degree of harm
2. The type of harm
3. The source of harm

Degree of harm

Some concerns may be minor in nature at the point they are highlighted or recognised. At this stage, they may pose no particular danger but provide an opportunity for early intervention, such as the chance to give early advice and thus prevent a minor problem escalating.

Other safeguarding concerns may be more serious and will require a response through multi-agency procedures and possible statutory intervention through regulators, the criminal justice system or civil courts.

Type of harm or abuse

Examples of the types of harm that may occur are listed below.

The main forms of abuse are:

- Physical abuse, including hitting, slapping, pushing, kicking, misuse of medication, restraint, or inappropriate sanctions
- Sexual abuse, including rape and sexual assault or sexual acts to which the vulnerable adult has not consented, or could not consent or was pressured into consenting
- Psychological abuse, including emotional abuse, threats of harm or abandonment, deprivation of contact, humiliation, blaming, controlling, intimidation, coercion, harassment, verbal abuse, isolation or withdrawal from services or supportive networks
- Financial or material abuse, including theft, fraud, exploitation, pressure in connection with wills, property or inheritance or financial transactions, or the misuse or misappropriation of property, possessions or benefits

- Neglect and acts of omission, including ignoring medical or physical care needs, failure to provide access to appropriate health, social care or educational services, the withholding of the necessities of life, such as medication, adequate nutrition and heating
- Discriminatory abuse, including racist or sexist abuse, or that based on a person's disability, and other forms of harassment, slurs or similar treatment

Neglect and poor professional practice also need to be taken into account. This may take the form of isolated incidents of poor or unsatisfactory professional practice at one end of the spectrum, through to pervasive ill-treatment or gross misconduct at the other. Repeated instances of poor care may be an indication of more serious problems and this is sometimes referred to as 'institutional abuse'.

Source of harm and abuse

Harm or abuse can take place in a wide range of settings, ranging from regulated services to people's own homes. The cause of harm and abuse may be similarly wide-ranging. For instance, harm may be caused unintentionally by an unsupported carer; or neglect could be caused by staff or a service; or abuse may be caused through recklessness or may be intentional. One example of harm that has a huge interface with safeguarding and abuse is the development of pressure ulcers (see below). The prevalence of such problems is under close scrutiny.

Pressure ulcers

Pressure ulcers may be seen to have developed as a result of neglect or institutional abuse. However, some pressure ulcers are unavoidable, even with the highest-quality care; therefore it is inappropriate to report all pressure ulcers as safeguarding cases. The principle should be to determine whether the pressure ulcer was avoidable and if the care was neglectful. Robust reporting and an investigation process must be instigated according to the organisation's policy. In addition, local Safeguarding Adults Boards have thresholds/triggers that can assist the multidisciplinary teams in deciding whether or not the incident should be referred to the multi-agency safeguarding process.

In order to prevent a charge of neglect or institutional abuse regarding pressure ulcers, staff must ensure that they accurately assess and grade the pressure ulcer: what is the cause – is it really pressure? For example, a leg ulcer is not caused by pressure and cannot be graded. Detailed knowledge is required in order to discriminate and refer appropriately.

When the ulcer has been assessed and graded, the staff must implement and adhere to the care plan, evaluate any deterioration, document clearly within the notes, inform and involve other members of the multidisciplinary team. It is important to understand the broader ramifications – pressure ulcers are not a uni-disciplinary or solely a nursing issue. In this way, a culture can be developed where there is a zero tolerance approach to hospital-acquired pressure ulcers, or there is strict reporting of these during the admission process if a patient is brought to hospital with an ulcer.

Finally, and of particular importance to discharge planning, the patient's condition must be communicated clearly to social workers, district nurses and (where relevant) nursing staff/carers from nursing homes or rest homes. They should all be kept updated to ensure transparency of issues upon discharge; assessment and reassessment are critical aspects of this process.

Assessment considerations

The seriousness or extent of abuse is often not clear when anxiety is first expressed. It is important, therefore, when considering the appropriateness of intervention, to approach reports of incidents or allegations with an open mind. The following factors need to be considered:

- The vulnerability of the individual
- The mental capacity of the vulnerable adult
- The frequency, duration and effect of the alleged abuse
- The nature and extent of abuse
- The degree of immediate risk
- Whether others may be at risk
- Whether safeguarding is the most appropriate and proportionate response to the situation

The investigation process

Each organisation will have developed guidelines for reporting and investigating incidents, and these guidelines will be based on the national safeguarding adult policies. All staff must be familiar with their organisation's internal policy and procedure. In particular, nurses should understand how to deal with any safeguarding concerns, when to take action and where to get help. Three R's may help to focus attention on three vital stages in the process:

- Recognise (know the indicators of abuse)
- Respond (ensure the person is safe/risk assess)
- Report (inform your senior and follow Trust procedure)

Two important points to consider throughout the process are 'consent' and 'involvement'. An adult's legal right to consent marks the fundamental difference between approaches to safeguarding adults and approaches to safeguarding children ('No decision about me without me' DH 2011). The vulnerable adult must be central to this investigation process.

Safeguarding investigation meetings

If you are asked to attend an investigation/strategy meeting or case conference it is imperative that you attend. Such meetings can often be arranged at very short notice, with the responsibility for co-ordinating the safeguarding process belonging to the local authority via the Social Work Team Manager, who will call together all the relevant agencies.

The meeting attendees will differ with each individual case. Within an acute hospital setting, the list may be as follows: team manager from social services as the chair; representative from police (depends on the case); Care Quality Commission (CQC); social worker; carers from the nursing home/rest home; member of the family; tissue viability nurse; ward manager or deputy from the ward; matron; discharge liaison nurse; other members of multi-disciplinary team such as OT; physiotherapist. In addition, a speech and language therapist and a dietician may be asked, depending on the stage of the investigation or the concerns being addressed.

The expectation is that all the relevant information will be shared and will contribute to any action plan developed. These meetings can be challenging, and other agencies may well perceive the situation in very different ways. This is a learning opportunity for all involved. Most importantly, such instances serve to protect patients and ensure the right outcome. We therefore need to work effectively together and learn to keep an open mind.

How can nurses reduce the risk of harm or abuse?

Prevention, prevention, prevention – this should be our primary goal. Safeguarding is not an isolated topic; it overlaps with 'dignity in care' issues, whistle-blowing and safe recruitment processes. Staff will need to keep up to date with a broad range of issues and be ready to access different sources of knowledge.

It is vital that we maintain standards, adhere to policies and procedures, and challenge poor and outdated practice. Safeguarding adults is not hard to do but good teamwork, culture and leadership are crucial to maintain the impetus.

We need to work with patients and their carers to help them reduce risks to their safety. We should also listen and learn from patients and their relatives. In one ward area, staff put up posters saying 'Your Opinion Matters' to encourage relatives, patients and carers to communicate their concerns. Some of the relatives said: 'We have difficulty finding someone to talk to during visiting times'. The organisation responded by saying: 'We will change staff break times so that the nurses are on the ward during visiting hours.'

Discharge planning and safeguarding

It is important to assess and identify the risks that increase a person's vulnerability. This should be done from the first contact (on admission or preadmission) and assessments should continue throughout the patient care pathway. Safeguarding assessment must also be an integral part of the discharge process, regardless of whether the individual is a day patient or an inpatient. It must not be seen as an afterthought, separate from the discharge process itself.

If there is a safeguarding investigation in progress then the discharge cannot go ahead, unless there is an agreement, or an alternative plan from the relevant social worker involved in the case. If a safeguarding alert has been raised, it may be thought that this will increase the length of stay and cause delays. However, such delays can be avoided by using a proactive approach, attending the relevant strategy/investigation meetings, and working with the social work teams.

Considering individual circumstances

When discharging a patient with possible safeguarding issues:

- Consider the risks and how they can be managed
- Consider the mental capacity and decision-making ability of the individual involved

Communication, communication, communication (both written and verbal) is always vital for effective discharge planning.

If there are wound care issues and pressure ulcers, you will need to complete body maps. Give a clear summary of the patient's care needs and how they are now. If they have a bruise caused by a cannula or clexane injection, let the staff at the nursing home/rest home know. This may seem 'petty' but if they are discharged with unexplained bruising/marks on their body that weren't there before admission, a safeguarding alert may well be completed by them against your ward. It is important to remember that we would be expected to do the same for patients if they came into hospital with unexplained bruising or marks.

We also have to recognise that there may well be times when we disagree with a particular decision that is being made. But we have to remember that this is about the patient and we should be working towards outcomes the person wants, and respecting their choices. Not everyone's lifestyle and belief system are going to be the same as our own.

Four examples are given in the following case studies to illustrate the dynamics of safeguarding and abuse in relation to discharge planning.

Case study 1: A patient discharged to a residential home

Staff at a residential home raised concerns that a patient of theirs had been discharged back to them from the hospital with no walking frame, not enough medication, extensive bruising over her body and no skin integrity paperwork and that the discharge letter had very little information on it.

A review was undertaken by the matron and ward manager and it was noted that the patient had been confused throughout the admission. She was at high risk of falls and had several falls, which accounted for the bruising. Incident forms had been completed and actions to try and prevent/manage the falls had been implemented. On one occasion, she sustained a laceration to the right elbow, which again was clearly documented in the medical notes. However, there was no documentation from the physio regarding a frame for discharge. As the patient had been wandering around the ward and not compliant with using the frame, this may be why one wasn't sent with her. During her admission, her medication had been reviewed and changes were made but were not included in the tablets for home.

Recommendations made

- Completion of body map and skin integrity documentation
- Communication (both verbal and written) to the staff at residential home
- Communication from the physio to the ward staff regarding equipment for discharge
- Improve completion of discharge transfer sheets and ensure staff give a clear and concise picture of the care and treatment given during admission. For example, if medication is changed then this must be included.

Case study 2: Inpatient standards of care

Situation

A safeguarding alert was raised regarding the care and treatment received by a patient whilst in an acute hospital setting.

Background

An elderly gentleman was admitted with increased confusion secondary to a urinary tract infection. He had a history of dementia. A relative expressed concerns about the attitude of nurses, lack of dignity, basic standards of nursing care not being met, delays in responses to buzzers, and continence and hydration issues.

Assessment

The case was investigated by the ward manager and the Matron for Safeguarding Adults. A strategy meeting was held and an action plan was devised.

Recommendations made and lessons learned

- This safeguarding incident could have been prevented if staff had done what they were supposed to have done and communicated clearly with the family.

- The action plan identified several key themes to be addressed – staff attitudes, documentation, accountability and responsibility, pain management, tissue viability, and response to patient buzzers. Leadership was vital to the successful implementation of this plan, and the ward has since improved significantly. This was monitored on a regular basis by the head nurse and matron.

- Human resources support was enlisted to help challenge poor performance and attitudes.

Case study 3: A daycare patient

An elderly female patient attends the day hospital for a follow-up appointment and discloses to the consultant that she hasn't been sleeping very well, as she is scared of a relative who has recently moved in with her. The relative has been verbally abusive towards her and continually asking for money. The consultant listens to her concerns and, as this lady does have capacity* to make decisions, asks her what she wants to happen and for permission to discuss these issues with other colleagues. The lady agrees and the consultant contacts the Matron for Safeguarding Adults and asks for advice and support. There is then a discussion about the risks/safety of the patient and the process of referral to social services. The main question to be considered: Is the lady safe to go home?

Plan

- Discuss the patient's wishes with the patient. What does she want to happen? And what can we do as a team to support her?

- Contact social services
- Speak to her GP

Outcome

She is happy to return home and it is arranged that a social worker, Vulnerable Persons Officer and GP will do a follow-up visit. It is also arranged that the patient will come back to the day hospital the following week.

*Mental capacity simply means our ability to make decisions. These may be everyday decisions about the food we choose to eat or the clothes we wear. They may be bigger decisions, for example where we live, who we live with, what healthcare treatment we need, or what we spend our money on. Some people have the capacity to make some decisions, such as what to have for breakfast, but cannot make more complex decisions, such as how much of different foods to eat to stay healthy. Some people have 'fluctuating capacity'. This means that they can make decisions some of the time or at certain times of the day but not at other times.

Case study 4: Transfer to a nursing home

Situation

A multi-agency safeguarding alert was raised by staff at a nursing home following the transfer of a patient from hospital. In particular, concerns were expressed regarding nutritional status and skin integrity.

Background

An elderly female patient was admitted with a fractured left neck of femur to a trauma and orthopaedic ward. She had been found on the floor by staff at the nursing home. She went to theatre within 24 hours and had a left dynamic hip screw fixation.

Assessment

It was clear from the review of the nursing and medical notes that this lady had complex needs and required maximum assistance with personal hygiene, elimination, eating and drinking, mobility and management of pressure areas. There were also communication issues: she had dementia and would often scream and cry out. (This had been discussed with the nursing home staff and they said that this was normal behaviour for her.) Physiotherapists were actively involved with her care but it was felt that she was unable to follow their instructions. After regular reviews and assessment, she was deemed high risk and therefore they advised that only hoist transfers would be the safest option for her.

Tissue viability

A hospital-acquired G4 pressure ulcer to the left heel developed and a sore to the right hip. She was assessed as high risk and had been placed on a pressure-relieving mattress, with skin inspections being undertaken daily. However, it was shown that there were discrepancies in the grading and severity of the ulcer. It was also noted that she was often very agitated and staff had difficulty positioning her.

Nutrition

A risk assessment was completed on admission and she scored low risk. However, she began to refuse meals and drinks so a food chart was started. She was also reviewed by the dietician and supplements were recommended. During her stay she had regular episodes of dehydration, which required intravenous fluid management, and continued to refuse meals and the supplements. There were regular reviews by the dietician. However, it was felt to be unlikely that she would tolerate naso-gastric feeding and it was acknowledged that her nutritional needs were not currently being met and were unlikely to be met.

What happened on transfer?

It was clear from the investigation undertaken by the matron and ward manager that there was a lack of communication from hospital staff. Nursing home staff were not made aware of issues that had arisen whilst the patient had been on the ward, notably lack of diet and fluids, or the recommendations made by the dietician. In the documentation of the discharge process, there were no entries relating to conversations between the ward staff and the nursing home. The transfer letter that was sent on discharge was inadequate, with no mention of poor dietary input or the sore to the right hip or the management of the necrotic left heel. It was also not known that this lady resided in the residential part of the nursing home and this would therefore have an impact on her mobility status.

Could a safeguarding referral have been prevented?

In my opinion, a safeguarding referral could have been prevented. Staff in the hospital could have prevented this situation escalating, and the following recommendations were made.

Recommendations made and lessons learned

After the review, it was concluded that poor communication had resulted in poor discharge. The importance of documentation and communication was enforced. Staff were reminded about the need to complete transfer documents and what was required on these documents for a safe and effective discharge. Study days were arranged for registered nurses and healthcare assistants regarding tissue viability and its link with safeguarding. A separate root cause analysis and action plan has also been developed in relation to the pressure ulcers – main lesson is the grading of sores and consistency with the documentation.

Conclusion

This chapter has focused on safeguarding adults in relation to discharge planning from hospital. It has identified some key definitions, including what is meant by 'safeguarding adults', which adults are 'vulnerable', is the meaning of 'abuse' and the different types of abuse that occur.

Safeguarding adults from abuse and harm is everyone's business and an important part of everyday healthcare practice. All staff must therefore familiarise themselves with their organisation's internal safeguarding policy and procedure. In particular, nurses should understand how to deal with any safeguarding concerns, when to take action and where to get help.

Our primary goal should be prevention, and we have to ensure that we maintain standards, challenge poor and outdated practice and work effectively within our teams. Documentation and communication is a challenge for us all. However, with regard to safeguarding, we have to get it right, not just some of the time but all of the time. Above all, we must remember to keep the patient central in the decision-making process. It is every adult's legal right to give or withhold consent, and this marks the fundamental difference between approaches to safeguarding adults and approaches to safeguarding children.

References

Department of Health (2000). 'No Secrets: Guidance on developing and implementing multi-agency policies and procedures to protect vulnerable adults from abuse'. London: HMSO.

Department of Health (2010). 'Clinical Governance and Adult Safeguarding: an integrated process'. London: HMSO.

Department of Health (2011). 'Safeguarding Adults: The Role of Health Service Practitioners'. London: HMSO.

Heart of England NHS Foundation Trust (2010). 'Policy for Safeguarding Adults'. Birmingham: Heart of England NHS Foundation Trust.

Mencap (2007). *Death by Indifference*. London: Mencap.

Mid Staffordshire NHS Foundation Trust Public Inquiry (2010).

Nursing and Midwifery Council (February 2011). 'NMC Update – safeguarding adults – if you don't do something, who will?' London: Nursing and Midwifery Council.

Parliamentary and Health Service Ombudsman (2011). 'Care and Compassion? Report of the Health Service Ombudsman: an investigation into NHS care of older people'. London: HMSO.

Safeguarding Vulnerable Groups Act (2006).

Section 2

The UK perspective on discharge policy and practice

Chapter 5

Discharge policy and practice in England

Ruth Eley

This chapter will consider why hospital discharge In England has had so much political attention over the last 20 years or so, and what this means at a local level for the NHS and for social care. It will then look at why discharge planning is important, and what health and social care practitioners can do to improve the hospital experience of patients and carers.

A brief history of discharge policy

Delayed discharges and discharge planning have been of political interest since the early 1990s. The previous decade had witnessed the growth of private residential care provision funded by the public purse, as increasing numbers of older people were able to access social security funding. The growth in capacity in this sector meant that few people were delayed in hospital. The subsequent report by Sir Roy Griffiths (1988) and the community care reforms that followed in 1993 were largely responses to the fact that many older people were entering community care without an assessment of need other than a financial one. The impact on the social security budget was also significant.

The impact of community care reforms

The community care reforms introduced local authorities to the model of assessment and care management. Individuals would only be deemed eligible for a service after the completion of a community care assessment. Local authorities took on an explicit commissioning role, and most split their purchaser and provider functions. To meet their new demands, bureaucratic procedures were developed, including the establishment of panels in many social services departments to approve funding for packages of care. If the panel only met once a week, a delay was automatically built into the process.

At the same time, hospital social work came under scrutiny, as NHS provision became increasingly specialised. Regional, supra-regional and even national units developed for cardiac, renal and various cancer services, for example, serving patients beyond their immediate local populations, with the expectation that the host local authority would provide the necessary social work support services. The situation was further complicated by the development of NHS Trusts, whose constituent acute hospitals often admitted patients from wide catchment areas that did not coincide with local authority boundaries. Cross-boundary agreements began to break down, and some local authorities withdrew hospital-based social workers completely, opting instead for community-based assessment teams, accessed via generic customer call centres. The House of Commons Select Committee on Health's report *Community Care: the Way Forward* (1993) concluded that one of the key requirements to prevent delays was to establish effective joint arrangements between health authorities and local authorities in order to integrate assessments with hospital discharge planning. The following year, the Department of Health published the *Hospital Discharge Workbook*, a guide to discharge planning (DH 1994).

Data and definitions

The Department of Health began collecting data on delayed discharges in 1997, when the rate of delayed discharges for people over 75 was 15.7%. However, the Department did not issue a standard definition of what constitutes a delay until April 2001:

'A delayed transfer occurs when a patient is ready for transfer from a general and acute hospital bed but is still occupying such a bed. A patient is ready for transfer when:

- A clinical decision has been made that the patient is ready for transfer;
- A multi-disciplinary team decision has been made that the patient is ready for transfer;
  and
- The patient is safe to discharge/transfer'

The 'National Beds Inquiry' (DH 2000a) found that the significant reduction in hospital beds was adversely affecting older people and identified the need for more rehabilitation and recovery beds. The 'NHS Plan' (DH 2000b), which followed, identified the fact that delayed discharges from hospital were a significant problem and set an ambitious target to 'end widespread bed blocking by 2004'. It included an additional investment of £900 million annually for three years for intermediate care and to improve services for older people. The detail was later set out in the 'National

Service Framework for Older People', published the following year (DH 2001). Delayed discharges reached 7,065 in the second quarter of 2001–2, representing 6% of all acute beds.

In 2002, the House of Commons Select Committee on Health reported on delayed discharges (HCSCH 2001–2). They declared that the term 'bed blocking' was offensive to people whose discharge from hospital was delayed, as it suggested that these individuals were to blame, and they urged the Department of Health to reject its use. The committee questioned the reliability of the data on delayed discharges, and noted the wide interpretation of the Department of Health's definition of 'delayed discharge' by individual hospitals and health authorities. They also noted that, although the language of whole systems working was widely used, there was 'a long way to go before the phrase provides an accurate description of what is taking place on the ground, other than in pockets of good practice'.

The report concluded that developing whole systems approaches was 'a highly demanding task' that required 'a redistribution of services at both strategic and operational levels', and that local health and social services organisations needed more help to assess the balance of services in their patch and work out where to make additional investment. The committee also concluded that 'arrangements for the management of discharge need radical overhaul in many hospitals. In our view, best practice involves a multi-agency team actively managing all aspects of the discharge process'. The Select Committee welcomed the establishment by the Department of Health of the Health and Social Care Change Agent Team to tackle delayed transfers of care.

The Change Agent Team, whole systems solutions and reimbursement

The Change Agent Team (CAT) became operational in March 2002 and offered targeted support to local health and social care systems struggling with delayed transfers. When it started its work, 5,700 people were delayed in acute hospital care. The team adopted an overtly whole systems approach, only working with localities where all the relevant NHS and local authority bodies had agreed to the CAT's involvement. The team was funded through the 'Cash for Change' programme, which also allocated money to councils to develop effective local solutions, including investment in new services to maintain the independence of people leaving hospital. These services included, for example, intermediate care and intensive home support, and rapid response services (to prevent unnecessary hospital admission).

In 2002, the CAT commissioned a revision of the *Hospital Discharge Workbook*, to reflect the new policy framework and the impending introduction of reimbursement. This was published by the Department of Health in 2003 as 'Discharge from hospital: Pathway, process and practice' (DH 2003). It focused on the 20% of hospital discharges that are complex and require additional expertise beyond the capacity of the ward-based team. The following year, the Modernisation Agency commissioned a guide on timely discharge for the 80% of discharges that are more straightforward and can be managed at ward level (DH 2004).

In 2002, the government announced the introduction of a system of reimbursement for acute Trusts, where delays were solely the responsibility of social services. This initiative was based on the Swedish model, although the health and care system in that country was significantly different from that of the UK. The proposal was widely seen as controversial. There were fears that it would lead to unnecessary bureaucracy and create a 'blame culture' (to the detriment of social services and social work professionals), undoing much of the good work that had been done to achieve strong partnerships and joint working. The Community Care (Delayed Discharges) Act (2003) introduced the arrangements in shadow form in October 2003, with full implementation in January 2004. The legislation applied to delays in the acute sector only, with an agreement that proposals to introduce reimbursement into mental health and learning disability provision would require further debate by Parliament.

The Department of Health, recognising that the legislation was being met with hostility and confusion in services, used the Change Agent Team's expertise to support implementation and a reimbursement group was quickly established. They liaised closely with Department of Health policy leads and key stakeholders to develop a range of practical support products to explain the notification process, and clarify the new duties for local authorities and the NHS, and highlight best practice. The evaluation of the CAT published in 2004 concluded that 'the reimbursement work was highly successful, not least in contributing to a shift in perception on the ground and an improved understanding of the objectives of the legislation to improve the quality of hospital discharges and ensure that people do not remain in hospital beds needlessly' (Henwood 2004).

Delays had already begun to reduce by the time reimbursement was introduced, partly as a result of the Building Capacity Grant to local authorities. This had the explicit objective of 'developing sustainable long term solutions aimed at eliminating delayed transfers of care'. The sites in which the CAT provided intensive support reported a reduction of 24% in delays in the 12 months since May 2002. This was significantly higher than the reductions across England as a whole. In many localities, acute Trusts, Primary Care Trusts and local authorities drew up joint agreements to re-invest any money raised through reimbursement, rather than see the money disappearing into general NHS coffers. It is therefore difficult to measure the impact of reimbursement, given other initiatives that had also been introduced at about the same time. However, not all localities had effective partnership arrangements, and there is no doubt that reimbursement was effective in getting reluctant partners around the table to discuss and agree implementation and use of the grant. A study commissioned by the Department of Health, to evaluate the effect of reimbursement, found 'quite different styles of implementation at strategic and operational levels, ranging from close adherence to nationally outlined reimbursement processes, to adoption of a partnership agreement with joint investment plan, which obviated the necessity for financial reimbursement' (Godfrey *et al.* 2008).

In 2004, the Commission for Social Care Inspection (CSCI) undertook a review of hospital discharge, following the introduction of reimbursement. Behind the positive news of falling delays, they found a mixed picture in terms of the patient experience. In localities where services to support recovery were under-developed 'efforts to speed up discharge are … disempowering individuals and undermining their potential for improvement and rehabilitation. In these councils … reimbursement has become more a paper chase than a means to an end' (CSCI 2004). They concluded that, although delays were better monitored than many other parts of the health and social care system, few councils had reliable systems in place to monitor the outcomes achieved for individual patients.

No decision has been taken to extend reimbursement to non-acute and mental health settings, although the Department of Health began collecting data through SitRep reporting in 2005. Some would argue that this failure to extend reimbursement has skewed the system, in that, in order to avoid reimbursable delays, patients are transferred to non-acute settings (such as community hospitals) where discharge planning may not be as structured or effective and where the pace of work is less frenetic. In response to similar concerns about the absence of reimbursement incentives in mental health facilities, the Department of Health sponsored Care Services Improvement Partnership published a guide to effective discharge practice from mental health settings (CSIP 2007).

Recent policy initiatives

From a policy perspective, hospital discharge has remained a core element of recent initiatives. 'Putting People First' (Her Majesty's Government 2008) – a concordat between six government departments, the NHS and key partner agencies across healthcare and social care – cited hospital discharge arrangements and the provision of adequate intermediate care amongst key areas that were necessary for 'an integrated approach with local NHS commissioners and providers to achieve specific outcomes'. In 2009, the Department of Health published its prevention package for older people, which included the updated intermediate care guidance 'Halfway Home' (DH 2009). Since the original 2001 guidance, services had developed in a piecemeal fashion and some aspects of the guidance had been misinterpreted. For instance, the expectation that episodes would 'normally' be for no longer than six weeks had become an absolute requirement in some localities, so that people requiring a longer period of rehabilitation (such as frail older people with complex needs or those with dementia) found themselves automatically denied the opportunity. In many cases, they were admitted direct to long-term residential care from hospital without being given the chance to return home again.

In 2009, the National Dementia Strategy was published (DH 2009a). Amongst its 17 objectives is one specifically addressing the need to improve acute care for people with dementia. Their experience is often poor, as few nursing and medical staff receive adequate training in dementia and therefore are often at a loss to know how to respond. The strategy commends the development of multidisciplinary liaison teams for older people's mental health, to provide speedy advice and support to ward teams and to facilitate the timely discharge of patients to more appropriate settings, where their needs can be properly assessed and appropriate support packages put in place. It also recommends the appointment of a senior clinician within the hospital to ensure the development of care pathways for people with dementia and a competent workforce.

A further political initiative relevant to discharge planning is the national Dignity Campaign, launched in 2007. Its aim was to promote dignity and respect for older people and the Dignity Challenge set out ten standards for services to meet, including:

- Listen and support people to express their needs and wants
- Enable people to maintain the maximum possible level of independence, choice and control
- Engage with family members and carers as key partners

All these are highly pertinent to discharge planning and are reflected in the revised Department of Health guide 'Ready to go?' (DH 2010). The Campaign also set out to recruit 'Dignity Champions' to speak up for the dignity of older people and challenge disrespectful behaviour. In September 2010, there were over 20,000 Champions in all sectors, including acute hospitals, and many organisations have appointed individual senior managers or non-executives to take the lead on promoting dignity as part of their core responsibility.

The numbers of delayed transfers of care have continued to fall, reaching about 2,200 in acute care nationally in 2009. However, these figures mask huge regional and local variation, and some localities report no delays at all. Whilst there are undoubtedly examples of excellent practice arising from strong multidisciplinary working and inter-agency co-operation, a degree of scepticism is nonetheless necessary. Certainly, judging from enquiries that come into the Department of Health, much effort seems to have been put into reducing the numbers on paper rather than tackling the issues for patients. Regrettably, some NHS organisations appear to have lost sight of the fact that each of the 5,400 delays recorded in the statistics represents a real individual who is in the wrong place, receiving the wrong type of care.

A new government but discharge planning remains important

The coalition government formed after the 2010 general election confirmed the importance of re-ablement, good discharge planning, post-discharge support and the implementation of the national dementia strategy. However, they have also announced that they will be focusing on outcomes rather than process-driven targets. Government will no longer direct what the NHS and social care should deliver. Instead, it will publish outcome frameworks, against which local health and social care services will publish their plans, and these services will then be accountable to their local population.

The coalition government has also stated its intention to make acute Trusts responsible for post-discharge support for patients for up to 30 days and to apply penalties through the tariff system for people readmitted during this period. Final details have yet to emerge for proposed implementation in April 2012, but there is concern amongst some professionals that such an approach may encourage hospitals to be risk-averse. This may mean that they end up keeping frail patients and those with more complex needs in hospital for longer, rather than discharging them home with support.

Delayed transfers are monitored by the Department of Health through a joint national indicator. It is important to note that the NHS is now responsible for the majority of delayed transfers; the belief that delays are all the fault of social care is mistaken. By January 2011, the number of delays had crept up again slightly, and there is concern that severe cuts in the public sector, especially for local authorities, will result in fewer preventive services that help avoid unnecessary hospital admissions or help enable timely discharge. Local authorities may revert to using long-term residential care for older people, rather than creating imaginative packages of care to support people in their own homes. In times of financial constraint, organisations tend to retreat behind their organisational boundaries and focus on managing their own budgetary challenges, rather than working collaboratively to find whole systems solutions. The proposed organisational changes and the transfer of commissioning responsibility to GP consortia may also have significant effects, as existing strategic relationships disintegrate.

Delayed transfers of care – an important indicator

Delayed transfers of care are a symptom of whole system failure. Effective discharge planning relies on sound professional judgement and decision-making at the individual clinician or practitioner level, ideally through multidisciplinary working. Such co-operation requires a high level of inter-professional trust, effective communication and timely information sharing. However, when a patient's discharge is delayed, they are in the wrong part of the system and receiving inappropriate care. Whilst this may be the result of a practitioner's failure to make or communicate appropriate plans, it may also be that organisational planning and investment through the commissioning process have failed to deliver the right range of services to enable people to be discharged from hospital to the most appropriate place in a timely fashion. These two aspects of effective discharge planning are therefore mutually dependent.

In tackling delayed discharges from hospital, no single agency is usually responsible for the problem; nor does the solution lie in their hands alone. Rather, resolution lies in multi-agency co-operation and decision-making to ensure the most effective use of resources. Healthcare and social care organisations – especially commissioners – need to know the needs of their local population and how well those needs are met by current service provision. There must be high-level, strategic commitment to working together to solve problems and improve outcomes for people. Commissioners need political support in order to be able to disinvest in services that are not delivering good outcomes in a cost-effective way, recognising that deficiencies or changing service configuration in one part of the system will almost certainly have an impact on the rest.

For example, many older people are admitted to Emergency Departments and subsequently become inpatients either because there are no available alternatives or because the professional responding to the crisis at home is unaware that alternatives exist or how to access them, and therefore resorts to a 999 call. Preventing such hospital admissions requires a flexible range of services to be in place that can respond quickly. The introduction of intermediate care services has led to the development of rapid response services that can either maintain people at home or provide a less intense level of care in a residential setting. However, these services remain patchy and, like many types of intermediate care, may not be available to people with dementia – one of the groups most likely to be admitted to hospital in a crisis.

Similarly, there is evidence that many older people are admitted directly to long-term residential care from hospital, without the benefit of rehabilitation through intermediate care or re-ablement. This practice is often based on a mistaken belief amongst acute sector staff that frail older people, especially those with dementia or other mental health needs, require more complex care than can be provided in their own homes by community health and social care services and that residential care is therefore the only possible option. The updated intermediate care guidance 'Halfway Home' (DH 2009) stated explicitly that: 'all older people at risk of entering care homes, either residential or nursing, should be given the opportunity to benefit from rehabilitation and recuperation and for their needs to be assessed in a setting other than an acute hospital ward'.

Moving into long-term residential care is a life-changing decision; yet we expect older people and their families to make such decisions in a matter of days. An acute hospital ward is an inappropriate setting in which to assess whether an older person, who may be recovering from a serious acute illness, surgery or injury, is able to manage in their own home or with less intensive care. We have to remember that older people do get better, but that they may need a bit of help and more time to do so. Some local authorities, in partnership with their PCTs, have adopted policies in accordance with the intermediate care guidance (DH 2009). For example, no one in Croydon is discharged from hospital to a different residence from the place from which they were admitted without an Intermediate Care assessment based on a model of recovery/re-ablement. This has resulted in a reduced number of admissions to residential care. Coventry has adopted a similar approach. Such high-level strategic commitments have to be followed up with clear operational procedures, sufficient resources to meet the demand and rigorous monitoring of performance, to ensure that services are delivering the desired outcomes.

Systems factors affecting effective discharge and what can go wrong

One of the building blocks for a whole systems approach to effective discharge is reliable data. This must be much more than just the high-level data collected as part of the weekly SitRep reporting process. Organisations need to be able to monitor and evaluate the causes, length and type of delays that follow the patient through the system, and how the rest of the system is performing to support the discharge process. The following are suggested data fields:

- Detailed reasons for delays
- Length of time people are delayed
- Numbers of emergency admissions
- Numbers of readmissions within 7 days and 30 days
- Use of rapid response and intermediate care services
- Number of admissions from hospital to long-term residential care
- Numbers of people admitted to intermediate care to prevent hospital admission
- Numbers of admissions to intermediate care from hospital
- Number of people still at home 3 months, 6 months and 12 months after completion of a period of intermediate care
- Comparative use of bed-based and home-based intermediate care

- Detailed reasons for people being delayed in non-acute settings such as community hospitals or mental health units

The collection, analysis and monitoring of such data will enable the health and social care system to identify trends and problem areas, and to make investment decisions about where best to target resources. At ward level, managers and clinicians should review patients' length of stay regularly, using the 'estimated day of discharge approach' to highlight extended stays, and ensure regular discussion by the multidisciplinary team of all patients who have been in hospital over an agreed period, such as 10 days.

Referral processes are another essential feature of discharge planning. All too often, referrals are made for assessments by key professionals – particularly therapists and social workers – too late in the patient's hospital stay, often at the point at which they have been declared 'medically fit' by the consultant team. Planning a hospital discharge is akin to planning a dinner party; no cook in their right mind would think of cooking the key elements of the meal in separate, sequential steps. The key is to have various dishes cooking simultaneously so that the finished product comes together at the right time, and diners are not left waiting for a particular vegetable or the sauce that will provide the finishing touch to the meal.

The NHS has a statutory duty under the 2003 Community Care (Delayed Discharges) Act to inform social services of any patient who is likely to need community care services on discharge. Such notifications should take place as soon after hospital admission as possible, and the same principle applies to referrals for other professional assessments. Social services departments that only accept referrals once patients are declared 'medically fit' are doing them a disservice, as this practice almost certainly leads to delays in discharging them from hospital. Part of the skill in making a social care assessment is to gather information about the individual's circumstances, ascertain their wishes and those of key people in their lives and help them make decisions about their future support needs. Details overlooked at this stage can cause distress and delay in the discharge process. Early referral means that assessment and planning can take place over a more manageable time period, and avoids the possibility that the patient will be perceived as ready to leave hospital by the rest of the multidisciplinary team and that it is only social care that is holding things up. These principles apply equally to people directing their own care through personal budgets or Direct Payments.

Sharing information and involving patients and carers in decisions

Patients regularly complain that one of the most tiresome experiences for them is having to tell their story several times, repeating information that has already been given to other professionals involved in their care. This can include preadmission questionnaires, which can take a considerable time to complete but that are then ignored or not even collected from the patient when they are admitted to the ward. Patients expect that professionals involved in their care will talk to each other and share information to make sure their care is co-ordinated and efficiently delivered. Ward teams should therefore ensure that they have effective systems in place for sharing key information and for minimising duplication of effort, particularly assessments. Effective multidisciplinary working involves a high level of trust between the various professionals involved.

Patients and carers also want to be involved in decisions that affect them. All too often, practitioners merely inform patients and carers of decisions that have already made about their care or treatment. This can make them feel disempowered and isolated – hardly a recipe for speedy recovery and a sense of well-being! Carers may find that they have to be strong advocates for their loved ones – because they are unable to take good planning and communication for granted: 'For family carers, the discharge process was often very stressful and at points they felt a sense of both powerlessness and of having to fight to achieve what they considered would be best for their relatives' (Godfrey *et al.*2008).

The Department of Health good practice guide, 'Ready to go? – Planning the discharge and the transfer of patients from hospital and intermediate care', includes a detailed section on how to involve patients and carers throughout the discharge process (DH 2010). Carers have invaluable information about the people they care for. Staff should not take their input for granted but work with them as key partners in the patient's care and not make assumptions about how services on discharge should be organised. For example, discussion with working carers may reveal that they prefer a weekend discharge from hospital, as this means they can be available to settle the patient back home, ready for care services to start up on Monday morning. It is also important to remember that some carers will have their own support needs and that they are entitled to an assessment in their own right.

Lack of trust does not only occur between different professionals in acute settings. It can also be a feature of relationships between staff in acute and primary or community care settings. Poor communication, inaccurate or late information and lack of knowledge of the skills and capacity of community-based services to support people with complex needs may all contribute to a mutual wariness. Although most qualified doctors and nurses working in community settings will have done a stint in acute hospitals, the reverse does not apply to clinicians in acute care. These clinicians may therefore assume that illness and frailty are inevitable consequences of old age, and that such needs can only be met by full-time residential care.

References

Care Services Improvement Partnership (2007). *A Positive Outlook: a good practice guide to improve discharge from inpatient mental health care.* London: HMSO.

Commission for Social Care Inspection (2004). *Leaving Hospital – the price of delays.* London: CSCI Publishing.

Department of Health (1994). *Hospital Discharge Workbook.* London: HMSO.

Department of Health (2000a). 'National Beds Inquiry (NBI) – Shaping the future NHS: long-term planning for hospitals and related services'. London: HMSO.

Department of Health (2000b). 'The NHS Plan – a Plan for Investment, a Plan for Reform'. London: HMSO.

Department of Health (2001). 'National Service Framework for Older People'. London: HMSO.

Department of Health (2003). 'Discharge from hospital: Pathway, process and practice'. London: HMSO.

Department of Health/Modernisation Agency (2004). 'Achieving timely "simple" discharge from hospital'. London: HMSO.

Department of Health (2009a). 'Living well with dementia'. London. HMSO.

Department of Health (2009b). 'Halfway Home'. London: HMSO.

Department of Health (2010). 'Ready to go? – Planning the discharge and the transfer of patients from hospital and intermediate care'. London: HMSO.

Godfrey, M., Townsend, J., Cornes, M., Donaghy, E., Hubbard, G. and Manthorpe, J. (2008). *Reimbursement in practice: the last piece of the jigsaw?* University of Stirling, University of Leeds, King's College, London.

Griffiths, Sir Roy (1988). *Community Care: Agenda for Action.* A Report to the Secretary of State for Social Services. London: HMSO.

Henwood, M. (2004). *All Change Please – an independent evaluation of the Change Agent Team.* Towcester, Northamptonshire: Melanie Henwood Associates.

Her Majesty's Government (2008). *Putting People First: A shared vision and commitment to the transformation of adult social care.* London: HMSO.

House of Commons Select Committee on Health (1992–3). *Community Care: The Way Forward.* 6th Report. London: HMSO.

House of Commons Select Committee on Health (2001–2). *Delayed Discharges*, 3rd Report. London: HMSO.

National Audit Office (2003). *Ensuring the effective discharge of older patients from NHS acute hospitals.* London: HMSO.

Social Care Change Agent Team/Reimbursement Implementation Team/Department of Health (2003). *Definitions – Medical Stability and Safe to Transfer.* London: HMSO.

Chapter 6

Reforming discharge services in western Ireland

John O'Brien and Antoinette Doocey

The 2003 Health Service Reform Programme (HSRP) in Ireland introduced the greatest change programme in the public sector in over thirty years. The objectives for such a major change programme were clearly outlined in the national health strategy Quality and Fairness (DOHC 2001), with the overall aim of improving healthcare delivery and management and providing better value for taxpayers' money. The HSRP outlined a raft of major structural changes aimed at reducing fragmentation and variance in delivery processes and patient experience, the most significant of which was the abolition of the eight regional autonomous Health Boards and the recommended establishment of a single national delivery system – the Health Service Executive (HSE).

The eight Health Boards had been established under the Health Act 1970 and came into being in 1971. Prior to 1971, the city and county councils (local authorities) doubled as the healthcare authorities. The 1970 Health Act also provided that each of the eight authorities had its own Board, which comprised three groups: (a) elected representatives, i.e. local councillors; (b) representatives of professional groups working in healthcare, such as nurses, doctors and pharmacists; and (c) members appointed directly by the Minister for Health.

The establishment of one overall authority, the Health Service Executive (HSE), somewhat similar to the NHS in the United Kingdom, was informed by a number of key reports commissioned by the Irish government, each recommending major change in a number of areas, including:

- Healthcare structures (Prospectus Report, DOHC 2003a)
- Financial management (Brennan Report, DOHC 2003b)

- Reconfiguration of hospital services (Medical Manpower Report, otherwise known as the Hanley Report, which looked in depth at two former Health Board regions – one being the Mid-West area)

The 2005 Health Act actually provided for the establishment of the Health Service Executive. There is now one governing Board of the HSE, and the members are appointed by the Minister of Health. None of its members are elected public representatives.

Acute hospital services in Ireland

There are 53 acute hospitals in Ireland, serving a population of approximately four million people, with 33 containing Emergency Departments. (The term 'A&E' is no longer used in Ireland. All former A&E departments have been renamed 'Emergency Departments' and are now referred to as 'ED'.) This arrangement of hospitals resulted in 'over-provision' of some services. For example, there were four Emergency Departments in the Mid-West) and duplication of certain services (such as mammography), which led to inefficiencies.

A single system

Professor Brendan Drumm was appointed as the first chief executive officer (CEO) of the HSE in late 2005. One of his early initiatives was the establishment of a major transformation programme 2007–2010, which aimed to improve patient access and increase public confidence in health services.

Six key transformation initiatives were identified as improvement programmes, with the following aims:

1. Integrate services across all stages of the care journey
2. Configure primary, community and continuing care services to deliver optimal and cost-effective results
3. Configure hospital services to do likewise
4. Implement a model for the prevention and management of chronic illness
5. Implement standards-based performance measurement and management throughout the HSE
6. Engage all staff in transforming health and social care in Ireland

Each programme contained a number of specific supporting projects, with a nationally appointed programme manager to coordinate the overall programme. In addition, the CEO established a 'Winter Initiative' in 2006, to begin to address the national ED issue and particularly to respond to the increase in demand during wintertime. A national director was appointed to this role.

A national approach to discharge planning through the Winter Initiative

The initial focus of the Winter Initiative was three fold:

1. Health promotion and prevention
2. Hospital avoidance (e.g. Hospital in the Home in the greater Dublin area; Home Care Packages and Community Intervention Teams)
3. System capacity (e.g. improved access to continuing care, rehabilitation services and intermediate care to effectively manage demand)

In 2007, a fourth dimension was added – work processes and practices. This followed a detailed national report on bed capacity (HSE 2007a), which identified a number of factors in the Irish system that were significantly out of line with international norms and practices. One of the main findings of this report was that there was 'no discharge planning in place for 60% of patients and no estimated date of discharge for 83% of patients'.

Other key findings in that report were:

- The rate of discharge at weekends was significantly below the rate during weekdays
- Over 40% of medical and surgical beds were occupied by patients who would remain in hospital at least 18 days
- 28% of medical and surgical beds were occupied by patients who would remain in hospital for at least 30 days
- day case rates were 12% below the OECD (Organisation for Economic Co-operation and Development) average and the report suggested that changes in certain practices (such as admitting surgical patients on the day of surgery and increasing access to diagnostics) could save a significant number of bed days

A separate study on 'bed utilisation' (HSE 2007b) was undertaken, using the Appropriateness Evaluation Protocol (AEP) tool, which determines whether a particular patient should have been admitted to an acute bed, and whether they should have been occupying that bed on the day of the survey. The findings showed that 39% of inpatients were outside the AEP criteria and could potentially have been treated in a non-acute setting on the day the survey took place, if appropriate facilities had been available.

These reports were the basis for the new national approach to discharge planning commenced by the HSA as the best way to reduce average length of patient stay and to address the process and practice issues that had been highlighted. A national policy document on discharge planning was formally approved by the HSE Management Team in November 2008.

Following this, a service self-assessment process against the national policy document was conducted across the country jointly between all hospitals and their respective community care areas through Joint Implementation Group structures (JIGs). The JIGs used agreed criteria, which included site-specific, explicit time-framed improvement plans that were reported on by each JIG respectively. The improvement plans formed a critical element of the overall National Winter Initiative programme.

A national A&E Forum was also re-activated and renamed the ED Forum. The purpose of this forum was to engage all key stakeholders in the approach to tackling the ED issue. These stakeholders included representatives from HSE Management, the Irish Association of Emergency Medicine, staff representative associations in medicine and nursing, allied health professionals and non-nursing staff.

The ED Forum gave its formal support and approval to the national discharge planning policy, and subsequently supported and endorsed a set of national nursing guidelines to support the implementation of the discharge planning policy from a nursing perspective. These guidelines were also approved by the HSE Management Team. They included:

• The central role of the nurse/midwife in discharge planning
(Criterion-based discharge by a nurse or midwife must be supported by local guidelines agreed with the medical team and specific to the specialist area of practice (Lees 2011).)

• Using estimated length of stay (ELOS)

• The importance of using the discharge plan, against the ELOS, at each handover and in the completion of relevant documentation

• Using 'criterion-based discharge', whereby patients can be discharged by nurses when specific clinical criteria have been achieved (e.g. no raised temperature for 24 hours, wound healed, mobilising safely or/and no evidence of respiratory distress)

A multidisciplinary and inter-disciplinary education and training programme (Lees *et al.* 2010) to support the successful implementation of nurse/midwife-facilitated discharge guidelines was put in place throughout the Republic of Ireland, with the support of the Nurse/Midwife Planning and Development Units of which there are eight in the country. A key focus of this programme was to ensure a significant increase in patient discharges for those who have completed their care and treatment, using the 'home by 11' initiative. This referred to getting patients out of hospital by 11 am each day, where appropriate.

The ED Forum then started to work on drafting a national policy (for agreement with HSE Management) on admission, discharge and escalation, to deal with throughput in EDs across the country. This draft policy contained a number of escalation measures, including Full Capacity Protocol (FCP), similar to that used at Stonybrook Hospital in the USA. FCP and its application/implementation proved very contentious within the ED

Forum. Significant disagreement emerged between emergency medical consultants, who wanted FCP, and nurses and their representatives, who were fearful that medics would use FCP as a 'first response' to overcrowding rather than a 'last resort' when all other escalation measures had been exhausted.

The roll-out of the national policy on discharge planning took place simultaneously across the country, with varying degrees of emphasis and success. In view of the differences between emergency medical consultants and nurses in regard to FCP, the ED Forum supported a focused pilot initiative at five locations to test the implementation of critical aspects of the discharge planning policy. For example, they looked at the time delay in transferring patients to ward areas from EDs, and the efficiency of the discharge process each day.

Reconfiguration in the Mid-West

A major programme to reconfigure acute hospital services commenced in the Mid-West region in early 2009. The HSE Mid-West geographical area encompasses the counties of Limerick, Clare and North Tipperary, serving a population of approximately 350,000, and contains three 'small' acute hospitals (meaning those with no more than 100 beds):

- Ennis Hospital, with 94 beds
- Nenagh Hospital, with 68 beds

(Both these acute hospitals are located about 25 miles from the Regional Centre in Limerick, i.e. the Mid-West Regional Hospital Limerick (MWRHL), which has 375 beds. These two small acute hospitals serve respectively more clearly defined geographical catchment areas in Counties Clare and Tipperary (North) than the third of the smaller hospitals.)

- St John's Hospital (a voluntary hospital funded by the HSE), located in Limerick city, adjacent to the Regional Centre, which has 105 beds

The implementation of the recommendations in the Hanley Report referred to on p. 78 proved particularly problematic, due to public and political opposition. To overcome this opposition, Teamwork Management Services and Horwath Consulting Ireland (Teamwork/Horwath 2009), who had undertaken a review of acute hospital services in HSE North-East area with the emphasis on clinical practice and patient safety, were appointed to carry out a similar review in the Mid-West.

The regional centre in the Mid-West (Mid-Western Regional Hospital, Limerick) was chosen as one of the five pilot sites for this initiative. This was particularly appropriate, as the Mid-West was already proceeding with the reconfiguration of its hospital service as set out below.

The Teamwork/Horwath Report was formally published in January 2009. The main recommendations concerned patient safety (Teamwork/Horwath 2009, p. 22): 'The core specialties of general medicine, general surgery, emergency and critical care are too fragmented, carry increased risks for patients and staff and are not sustainable in their present form'.

The immediate changes proposed by the Teamwork/Horwath report were to:

- Provide a regional tertiary acute centre based in the Regional Hospital in Dooradoyle (MWRHL)
- Move all acute surgery to the tertiary centre
- Centralise all critical care and trauma in the regional centre in Limerick
- Provide an enhanced ambulance service for the region

In addition to the key recommendations in the Teamwork/Horwath Report, a decision was taken in consultation with the HSE Management Team to address the risk issues associated with the Emergency Departments at Ennis and Nenagh (Emergency Departments, PA Consulting and Balance of Care, 4 May 2007), which were open 24 hours a day, seven days a week. (St John's Hospital had already restricted access to its Emergency Department to daytime hours on Monday to Friday.)

This decision was taken on the basis that a separate but concurrent review into two deaths at Ennis General Hospital by the independent Health Information and Quality Authority (HIQA) reported in April 2009, and also raised very serious concerns regarding aspects of patient safety, specifically at Ennis General Hospital. This report also contained a number of recommendations that applied to all hospitals across the country, particularly smaller acute hospitals.

The above recommendation, together with the decision to 'centralise' emergency services, was likely to lead to an increase in patient numbers requiring treatment at the Mid-Western Regional Hospital in Limerick (the regional centre). While some additional bed capacity was made available with the additional funding, the Project Board (which had been set up to implement the changes in the Mid-West) felt the need to examine in further detail the efficiency of the use of existing capacity in the context of the 'reconfiguration programme'.

Making change happen

A number of key steps were taken in the Mid-West in advance of the publication of the Teamwork/Horwath Report, to facilitate an implementation strategy. These included:

- The establishment of a Project Board referred to above
- The assignment of Clinical and Executive 'leads' with a direct line to the CEO of the HSE

- The preparation of a Project Plan
- The assignment of a small number of personnel from both the Mid-West and the national Transformation Programme who possessed both clinical and project management skills, to work on a full-time basis on the project

The Project Board identified a number of key issues likely to impact on the successful implementation of changes one of which was: the need to frame the changes as part of an overall national approach to change and transformation, as in the national policy on discharge planning, the 'Winter Initiative', the Report on Bed Capacity, and a national Bed Utilisation study.

Emergency Departments

The closure of the Emergency Departments at Ennis and Nenagh Hospitals from 8 pm until 8 am, seven days a week, went ahead on 6 April 2009 as planned. The new 8 am to 8 pm service departments were renamed Local Emergency Centres (LECs). The initial impact on ED services in Limerick reflected predictions, indicating an overall increase in monthly attendances of 1.08%, represented by 50.5 additional attendances per month up to mid-January 2010. The largest increase in ED attendances for this period occurred during the out-of-hours times of 8 pm to 8 am, when Ennis and Nenagh LECs are closed. Overall, there was an average monthly increase of around 214 patients (from 1,335.5 to 1,549.6 or 13.2%) going to Limerick ED between the hours of 8 pm and 8 am.

Despite increased Emergency Department activity, there does not appear to have been an associated increase in admissions via ED in Limerick for this period. The average monthly number of patients for admission through Emergency Department (ED) prior to 6 April 2009 was 1,281. This average was reduced to 1,203.7 (a decrease of 77.3). At this stage, it is difficult to ascertain the specific reason for this reduction but there may be a number of contributory factors, given the improved GP referral direct access portals to both acute medical and surgical services that were developed as part of the overall reconfiguration plan.

Acute surgery

On 1 July 2009, the centralisation of acute and complex surgery in the regional centre in Limerick began. Although the ED issue was always likely to attract far more public outcry, the Project Board believed that changes in surgery were likely to present a far greater challenge to the regional centre in Limerick, in terms of its ability to provide sufficient bed capacity and cope with patient numbers.

By October 2009, centralisation of all acute surgery at the Mid-Western Regional Hospital (MWRH) Limerick was completed, and a single Department of Surgery was set up for the region. All major, cancer and complex surgery is now performed in the regional centre. The MWRH Limerick is now on call 24 hours a day, 365 days a year, for all emergencies in the region, which has a population of 365,000. This makes MWRH, Limerick, the busiest acute general surgical hospital in the Republic of Ireland.

A Surgical Assessment Unit (SAU) has been established in the MWRH, Limerick, to provide rapid access to a senior decision-maker for acute surgical patients. GPs can refer directly to the SAU, using agreed criteria and clinical guidelines. Changes in practice by consultant surgeons on call have also been introduced, whereby elective work is curtailed when on emergency call. A 'surgeon of the week' system has been introduced, to enable more rapid processing of emergency patients in both the SAU and ED.

Five-day elective surgery and day surgery are now performed in St John's Hospital, while day surgery is also carried out in Ennis and Nenagh. Day surgery and outpatient clinics in Ennis and Nenagh are currently being expanded and include new specialties such as orthopaedics, maxillo-facial, plastic surgery, ENT and vascular surgery. General surgery is also being expanded in the peripheral hospitals. Further expansion of day services, such as endoscopy, has commenced in Nenagh, where a new facility has become operational and Ennis will follow shortly.

Acute medical assessment

Following the regionalisation of ED services, the Acute Medical Assessment Unit (AMAU) in MWRHL extended its operational time to 12.5 hours daily (on weekdays) and now provides protocol-based direct access for GP referrals. At present, it is seeing up to 30 patients daily, and has an admission rate of less than 15% per day. A retrospective study (Watts 2010) of the first six months of 2010, using the Manchester Triage System (Mackway-Jones 1997), showed that an average of 12.1 patients were treated daily and an additional 14 patients were seen in the AMAU follow-up outpatient clinic. Overall, 12.5% of AMAU patients were hospitalised after initial assessment, 73% entered outpatient pathways and the remainder were either referred to specialist outpatient clinics or discharged directly back to the referring GP.

There are also Acute Medical Units in Ennis, Nenagh and St John's Hospitals, and these are being managed by the medical teams on call. In Ennis and Nenagh, the GPs are still able to admit directly to the hospital over the 24-hour period, using appropriate protocols.

Discharge planning pilot project

Work on the discharge planning 'pilot' project, as part of the national approach to discharge planning referred to previously, commenced in Limerick in August 2009 and was scheduled to continue to the end of December 2009.

The following actions were taken at local level:

- The Hospital Executive (General Manager, Director of Nursing) at the regional centre was designated as the group responsible for implementing changes. These included putting in place a discharge lounge to facilitate more timely discharges from beds; inviting trade union representatives into the Joint Implementation Group (JIG), chaired by the Director of Nursing, whose purpose was to implement national policy on discharge planning; creating awareness among all staff involved in the patient journey; ensuring that the Clinical Director engaged with all medical staff; and arranging staff education and training as appropriate.

- A detailed communication programme on discharge planning and the pilot project was provided for all relevant staff.

- All consultants at the regional centre received a written communication from senior management, outlining the details of the pilot initiative and seeking cooperation.

- A number of measures were put in place, including daily monitoring of potential/ predicted discharges and actual discharges and consultant ward rounds.

The monitoring of consultant ward rounds showed varying patterns and gaps in arrangements. When presented to consultants, this became a very contentious issue, as they took the view that it was unacceptable that nurses were now 'auditing their practice'.

Despite repeated written requests from senior management, it also became clear that consultant practice and process changes required for more effective discharge planning would not be achieved easily or quickly without significant changes. For example, the arrangements regarding ward rounds centred around each individual medical team and required a more coherent system.

The ED in Limerick began to experience significant delays in early December 2009. This occurred against a backdrop of no overall national agreement on the 'escalation' measures and limited support, locally, particularly among medical staff, for the pilot initiative on discharge planning.

Local management took a decision, in consultation with key personnel in the ED, to implement a version of FCP as an early response to ED overcrowding. This was done by placing a limit on the number of 'admitted' patients (eight) in the ED at any given time. 'Admitted' patients over and above eight were distributed to the ward areas. This action led to an immediate reduction of 54 % in patient numbers waiting for admission into the ED.

However, allegations of 'overcrowding' at ward level from the nursing unions (extra patient numbers at ward level amounted to one or two patients per ward) led to a 'work to rule' by nurses, which continued for several weeks on the basis that ward nurses were now having to deal with additional workload. Paradoxically, prior to this, nursing unions locally had contended that there was 'overcrowding' in the ED in Limerick. The 'work to rule' was lifted in February 2010, following a meeting between local management, local union representatives and the joint chairs of the national ED Forum.

The ED in Limerick managed to function during the winter of 2009–2010, despite all the changes and the additional workload for the hospital. The view of emergency consultants was that the implementation of the Full Capacity Protocol (FCP) was critical to enable this. The ED regional medical team gained an additional three ED consultants during this period, and this helped them to cope with the increased workload. Meanwhile, there was also centralisation of major emergencies in Limerick, while strengthening EDs in the peripheral hospitals with more robust clinical governance and management structures.

The actions taken in the Mid-West on FCP proved problematic for the nursing representatives on the ED Forum. However, this tension also proved to be a catalyst for more focused discussion at the ED Forum on the requirement to include FCP as part of the national escalation policy.

Alignment of purpose

As the implementation of changes progressed in the Mid-West, some with difficulty (such as the discharge planning pilot initiative), there was a growing perception that reconfiguration was the cause of the overall problems. For instance, there were issues such as trolley waits in ED and capacity issues at ward level. There was a reluctance to accept that work practices and processes needed to change in a major way, and it was sometimes a challenge to explain the need for these developments. However, over a relatively short time, a closer alignment of common goals and objectives gradually emerged, as described below.

Improving hospital services and processes

There was broad agreement on:

- Improving access to Acute Medical and Surgical Assessment Units (direct GP referrals)
- Improving access to specialist consultants by using a text messaging system (ED)
- Using whiteboards on inpatient beds, displaying expected day of discharge
- The need to develop regional bed management capacity, including long-stay and assessment beds
- The need to appoint a regional Patient Flow Coordinator
- Using assessment beds in all long-stay facilities

- Using Quality (Lean) tools and practices:

  – A Kaizan event was undertaken to reduce the waiting time from 'decision to admit' in ED to 'bed occupancy' on a medical ward. 'Home by 11 am' improved by 100% on this ward.

  – HSE/University of Limerick (UL) Hospital Optimisation Programme Experience (HOPE), a collaborative improvement project: (a) pharmacy rationalisation and automation; (b) Hospital Hand Hygiene improvement programme by 100%; (c) ICU Order Book management and cash flow increase; (d) Patient Flow in ED – develop chest pain pathway; Fractured neck of femur pathway; Pulmonary Embolism and other joint protocols with AMAU working as a collaborative acute medical team; (e) Data management. The HOPE project is supported by seven multidisciplinary teams, agreeing and improving process and practices as the project progresses.

- Piloting the draft national Escalation Framework, including measured use of Full Capacity Protocol
- Piloting nurse-facilitated discharge in a number of wards and specialties

Nursing/midwifery developments

A regional Directors of Nursing and Midwifery Development Group was established and provided a forum for senior nurse managers from all disciplines and services to work collaboratively, in an integrated way, for the first time. Nurse-led service development requirements, including enhanced/specialist (CNS & ANP) nursing roles, were identified and prioritised. More importantly, a significant outcome of this initiative has been the sharing of resources and nurses being enabled to work across traditional boundaries, thereby maximising the potential of scarce specialist resources. Education and training programmes were prioritised, and new service development protocols and governance arrangements were agreed and approved by this group.

Advanced nurse practitioners

Advanced Nurse Practitioner (ANP) site preparation has been completed across the region. Existing nursing positions have again been converted, to appoint two ANPs to the ED at the MWRH Limerick. Four more posts have recently been approved and submitted for advertising.

A regional Care Pathways Group has been established and is progressing the development of care pathways within each acute hospital, between local hospitals and the tertiary centre and also between primary care and acute hospitals.

A regional Infection Control Group has also been established to work collaboratively in improving infection control standards across the region, through integrated working and utilisation of scarce resources.

Community services and responses

A Community Intervention Teams (CITs) service is now in place, covering the entire region. This provides an enhanced nursing service from 8 am to 12 midnight, seven days a week, which supports admission avoidance and early discharge by:

- Providing IV therapies in alternative settings to acute hospital
- Treating exacerbations of chronic disease in the home/community setting
- Medication management

A Discharge to Home Unit has been developed in one of the bigger elderly care hospitals in Limerick. This unit now admits patients who have been treated in the acute hospital and require a short period of non-acute medical care and continued 24-hour nursing before final discharge back home. Strict admission criteria and review processes are in place to avoid inappropriate placement and/or excessive length of stay.

In addition, a number of beds (previously long-stay) in each of the Older Persons Community Nursing Units across the region are now 'ring-fenced' as Community Response Beds. These are provided in order to respond to the needs of patients who require 24-hour nursing care and medical supervision for a short period (no more than five days) and who would otherwise be admitted to an acute hospital bed. One small unit of around 30 beds currently providing this service saved 85 acute hospital bed days in the first three months of operation.

Finally, home care packages are made available as part of both hospital avoidance and early discharge service measures.

Dedicated patient transport

The Emergency and Patient Transport systems in Ireland often become interchangeable and this can result in the neglect, to some extent, of patient transport. For example, patients awaiting transport following discharge often have to spend a number of hours in the acute hospital waiting for an ambulance to become available. In the Mid-West, arrangements were made to separate the two services by providing dedicated staff and vehicles for both emergency and non-emergency patient transport. This has led to more efficient patient discharge. One of the key priorities in the overall reconfiguration project was the enhancement of the ambulance service. A total of 24 additional personnel were employed and now provide a 24-hour advanced paramedic service in both Clare and North Tipperary, where the ED services have been reduced to 12-hour 8 am to 8 pm LEC services. This enabled patients to be rapidly transferred to the regional centre in Limerick where appropriate.

Visible managerial support for discharge planning

The Hospital Executive Team (the Director of Nursing, the Clinical Director and the

General Manager) at the regional centre in Limerick arrange daily meetings each afternoon with senior medical and nursing staff in the Emergency Department and the teams 'on take', to review activity and to ensure that arrangements are in place to absorb the likely workload over the following 24 hours. The measures include reviewing discharge arrangements and the cancellation of electives where appropriate.

The Director of Nursing put an arrangement in place to meet all senior nursing personnel (Clinical Nurse Managers) each morning to review activity at inpatient level and take any appropriate action. For instance, it may be necessary to involve senior medical staff in key decisions and to consult with general management.

The four General Managers in the region (three community and one hospital) set up a weekly meeting to provide additional system-wide support for the nursing managers and medical staff. This assists the patient flow process, for instance by removing obstacles and barriers to patient transfers, by providing immediate access to funding for home care packages.

Evaluation

Two significant independent reviews of the changes in the Mid-West have taken place since the implementation phase commenced in April 2009. One review took place during February 2010, following the discharge planning pilot initiative, while the second looked at emergency care pathways in December 2010 in advance of the national roll-out of the medical programme. The results of these two reviews will inform the next set of changes and improvements and they are summarised below.

Evaluation 1: Pilot project on discharge planning

The evaluation of the five pilot sites in 2010 identified a number of issues, including:

- limited adherence to establishing expected length of stay (ELOS) on admission
- scope to improve the management of the patient journey
- communication deficits between clinical personnel in regard to planned discharges
- limited delegated discharge authority (to nurses) using agreed care protocols
- significant variation in time and frequency of lead clinical consultant ward rounds

The findings from each pilot site were similar in terms of cultural and professional behaviours, and highlighted limitations in effective multidisciplinary team (MDT) discharge decision-making.

A number of key recommendations were made, including:

- ELOS to be identified by the admitting consultant in collaboration with the MDT within 24 hours of admission and revised and updated throughout a patient's journey as required (HSE 2008); the ELOS to be a core component of all handovers

- 'Home by 11 am' to be a standard policy implemented in every hospital and communicated to the public and all external providers and stakeholders
- Internal processes to be improved in line with national HSE policy so that 'waiting time to a bed' is greatly reduced; access to diagnostics is a key issue
- Distinct multidisciplinary groups to be established in each hospital to support effective improvements in patient flow
- Daily ward rounds to be conducted by the MDT, preferably during early morning with delegation to experienced senior qualified staff members where appropriate
- Ongoing development and review of integrated discharge planning processes through audit and reporting on overall patient flow
- Improved communication strategies to include both patients and staff
- Variations in transport and local ambulance practices to be standardised
- Timely organisation and management of discharge and transfer arrangements to continuing care by the discharge/patient flow coordinators
- Ongoing education involving all staff responsible for patient care journeys through the healthcare delivery system

Evaluation 2:
Emergency care pathways at Mid-West Regional Hospital, Limerick

An independent review of hospital practices and processes was commissioned in December 2010 as part of the national roll-out of a new 'Acute Medical Programme' (AMP), designed to treat more medical patients away from hospital settings. (This was a national policy initiative led by the Directorate of Quality and Clinical Care, HSE.) The programme recognises the essential role of large and small hospitals, general practitioners (GPs) and community services. It provides a framework for the delivery of acute medical services that seeks to substantially improve patient care. The Mid-West was the first of three chosen sites to undergo evaluation, which was based on a 'gap analysis' regarding 'state of readiness' to implement the national Acute Medical Programme recommendations.

The Mid-West plan is to centralise acute medical care in MWRH, Limerick, later this year on completion of the construction of a new Critical Care Block and finalisation of a Department of Medicine Clinical Rota covering all four acute hospital sites. In advance of this, one of the Mid-West consultant physicians (based at Nenagh but now retired) led the development and implementation of a standardised systematic evidence-based predictive score for the initial assessment of acutely ill medical patients. The Simple Clinical Score (SCS) was introduced in the ED and the medical floor of Nenagh Hospital in June 2007. This tool has subsequently been adapted in the development of a national standardised assessment tool as part of the AMP.

This evaluation concluded that many components of an effective acute care system are now in place, which bodes well for the future, and recommended strengthening the arrangements for whole system management and service integration. Such a management and clinical leadership structure would become increasingly effective and respected if supported with more timely and relevant performance data and information. The evaluation encouraged the continued development of clear clinical pathways, with models of care focused on patients and consistently delivered, and greater use of the local cadre of senior and experienced nurses who have done so much to make the surgical restructuring and the community integration teams such a success.

Evaluation outcomes

There was acknowledgement of some excellent examples of formal and informal pathways and the systematic whole system transformation of surgery. However, there was also a need for development of systematic pathways of care from ED to Acute Medicine. To support a medical care model, discharge planning was clearly important in achieving standardised, safe, quality patient care. The key findings from the gap analysis are summarised below.

It was acknowledged that the Mid-West Region has a clear and cogent plan for transformation of healthcare, which is understood by all clinical staff. There is evidence of effective implementation of some major changes. The substantial level of clinical engagement was recognised. Plans for a regional medicine programme were considered to be 'sound' and plans to organise medical personnel and service structures were considered fit for purpose. The current capital investment in buildings was viewed as an opportunity to provide improved environments, and local team building shows encouraging progress.

Modelling of demand and capacity across the medical system needs to be improved. Access to diagnostics also needs to improve, to avoid the risk that the behaviours and constraints currently evident may impede implementation of the planned changes. There was also recognition that the local medical assessment unit (MAU) in Limerick needs to develop its role and this has been clearly articulated. Further work with the physicians is required because, although they are engaged with the changes in principle, there are substantial practical concerns about the details of implementation to be addressed.

The AMP programme recommends the implementation of a national early warning score (EWS) and associated protocols to enable early identification of deterioration in patients and how they should best be managed. A similar tool has been in operation since 2007 in Nenagh, as previously stated. However, all four hospitals need to implement the national EWS as soon as possible.

There have also been substantial and effective developments in the whole system bed and capacity management function, and the capacity to manage across the Mid-West region is clearly evident. Arrangements for complex discharge from acute care, optimising the use of all available health and social care agencies in the Integrated Service Area is particularly effective. The access to highly skilled nursing services in both the Community Intervention Teams and Community Response Beds is an added advantage. The Mid-West already has a navigation hub/bed bureau footprint for new build work in place.

However, there is a need for greater clinical governance and team management arrangements, and IT infrastructure to support this. Greater clarity in working practices is also required, and this will involve continued discussions with, and support for, clinicians who are not yet fully engaged in considering all potential local solutions.

The AMP programme recommends the development of acute medicine as a specialty and the establishment of a cadre of acute medicine physicians (meaning physicians with acute medicine as their primary specialty and physicians with a 50/50 acute medicine/specialty interest). To facilitate this, the Royal College of Physicians of Ireland (RCPI) will be establishing a new acute medicine training curriculum. The programme recommends the development of acute medicine as a specialty for nursing.

Key recommendations to address the gap analysis findings

Emergency Department

1. Whole system analysis to be undertaken to develop a more sophisticated demand and capacity model so as to smooth patient flow

2. All acute admitting teams to work together to develop a more responsive and consistent relationship with the ED

3. There needs to be an urgent review of the paediatric pathway into and through the ED, with a clear focus on the needs of the child and family

4. The IT team to work with the ED to enhance the use of the ED patient management system

5. NEWS risk assessment to be trialled, perhaps on patients at time of decision to admit, with re-assessment one hour later, then at appropriate intervals during the wait for a bed

The Medical Assessment Unit and the pathways to medical care

1. The internal proposals for re-organisation of medical resources to support a comprehensive MAU and short-stay facility to be taken forward as a key early component of service

2. Urgent steps to be taken by physicians and senior managers to restore clarity and accountability to clinical and service governance arrangements

Bed management

1. A more robust escalation plan to be developed, with a combination of early triggers to ensure that actions can be taken that will have the maximum impact

2. Review availability and promote provision of pre-assessment clinics for elective surgical patients

3. Develop some tools to enable more accurate prediction of demand to assist with more proactive allocation of patients to beds

Discharge arrangements and links to care in the community

1. Improved internal processes are to be developed using Lean methodologies

2. Access criteria for radiology to be reviewed as a matter of urgency

Measurement of activity and average length of stay 2008–2010

The MWRH Limerick showed a 2.8% increase in emergency medicine activity in 2009 (compared to 2008), and a 1.05% increase in 2010 (compared to 2008). However, there was a 1% decrease in 2010 (compared to 2009), which was in line with overall national trends for this period.

Meanwhile, there was an increase of 2.6% in day case elective surgery in 2009 (compared to 2008), and an increase of 3.9% in 2010 (compared to 2008). Inpatient elective activity decreased at all sites, with the exception of St John's Hospital. This suggests that St John's appears to be developing into the main elective hospital for the Limerick area. Emergency inpatients increased at the regional centre, from 5,547 patients in 2008 to 8,184 in 2010. Meanwhile, there was no emergency inpatient activity at Ennis and Nenagh in 2010. The increase at the regional centre, of 2,637 in the two-year period, almost matches the combined numbers treated at Ennis and Nenagh in 2008, of 2,496.

Average length of stay

For elective admissions, the average length of stay at the MWRH increased at the regional centre from 3.45 days in 2008 to 4.17 days in 2010. Ennis, Nenagh and St John's showed decreases of 0.64 days, 0.84 days and 2.29 days respectively. This suggests that the sickest patients are now being treated at the regional centre, which was the original intention.

For emergency admissions, the average length of stay at the regional centre reduced from 5.23 days in 2008 to 4.93 days in 2010.

Conclusion

Major changes are taking place in the Mid-West region in the delivery of healthcare services, particularly for those who require hospitalisation. This is happening in the context of a programme of transformation at national level.

The overall aim is to include key stakeholders from the outset in the planning, development and implementation of new services and also in the revision of existing services. The introduction of Lean tools and methodologies and closer collaboration with local third-level institutes continues to support a broad range of multidisciplinary service areas in working differently, and smarter, in the interests of improved patient experience.

External analysis and review has been used to reinforce the need for change and to steer the implementation process, in tandem with the national transformation programme and other major changes, particularly in areas of clinical practice, including discharge planning and the acute medical programme.

The removal of barriers between hospital and community, through more joined-up working arrangements and shared approaches to problem-solving, has supported the care continuum and more seamless transfer of patient care across those 'boundaries'.

This approach has enabled the successful establishment of a regional Emergency Department, encompassing four EDs, and also in establishing a regional surgical department and centralising all acute surgery in the regional centre in Limerick. The regional nursing and midwifery forum supports continued flexibility and progress in this regard, particularly as more nurse-led services are developed, which support safe and appropriate patient transfers across the service delivery spectrum.

The next major service changes are the roll-out of the acute medical programme, the centralisation of critical care and coronary care, and the establishment of a regional anaesthetic service, which are all scheduled to take place before the end of 2011.

The on-going challenge will be to implement the changes in work processes and practices highlighted in the most recent 'external' review. This implementation will be informed by the recommendations listed above, and will require a significant shift in culture and mindset at many levels, including political, policy-making, and service delivery, if Ireland is to achieve a world-class health service, as envisioned in the national transformation programme.

There is also a significant challenge for those in the Mid-West who have moved rapidly ahead of other areas in making changes, alongside the inherent risk of policy changes and associated economic circumstances, which may alter the course of the transformation programme.

References

Department of Health and Children (2001). 'Quality and Fairness: A Health System for You'. Dublin: Stationery Office.

Department of Health and Children (2003a). 'Audit of Structures and Functions in the Health System'. Prospectus Report. Dublin: Stationery Office.

Department of Health and Children (2003b). 'Commission on Financial Management and Control Systems in the Health Service'. Brennan Report. Dublin: Stationery Office.

Department of Health and Children (2003c). 'Report of the National Task Force on Medical Staffing'. Hanley Report. Dublin: Stationery Office.

Emergency Departments, PA Consulting and Balance of Care (4 May 2007). A review of acute hospital bed use in hospitals in the Republic of Ireland.

http://www.hse.ie/eng/

Health Service Executive (2007a). 'Acute Hospital Bed Capacity Review: A Preferred Health System in Ireland to 2020'. Dublin: PA Consulting.

Health Service Executive (2007b). 'Acute Hospital Bed Review – a bed utilisation study'. Dublin: PA Consulting.

Health Service Executive (2008). 'National Integrated Discharge Planning Policy'. Dublin.

Lees, L., Price, D. & Andrews, A. (July 2010). Developing discharge practice through education: module development, delivery and outcomes. *Nurse Education Practice*. **10** (4), 210–15. Epub 27 October 2009

Lees, L. (2011). Board to ward: implementation of nurse led discharge. *Nursing Times*. (in press).

Mackway-Jones, K. (ed). (1997). *Emergency Triage – Manchester Triage Group*. 2nd Ed. BMJ Publishing Group.

Teamwork Management Services and Horwath Consulting Ireland (2009). 'Acute Hospital Bed Review'.

Watts, M., Powys, L., Hora, C.O., Kinsella, S., Saunders, J., Reid, L. & Finucane, P. (February 2011). Acute Medical Assessment Units: an efficient alternative to in-hospital acute medical care. *Irish Medical Journal*. **104** (2): 47–49.

Chapter 7

Reforming discharge services in Wales
NHS Wales

This chapter will describe some of the innovative and empowering approaches that have been used to improve discharge and transfer of care processes in Wales. These include:

- Mobilising and tasking over 100 frontline staff to write a guide to good practice on discharge
- Placing emphasis upon the role of discharge liaison nurses, who support the planning of the most complex discharges
- Holding national learning events to help staff gain the knowledge they need in order to understand and navigate their way through the most legally complex situations
- Providing staff with tools and techniques to give them more time to devote to direct patient care and discharge planning

The National Leadership and Innovation Agency for Healthcare (NLIAH) and the Delivery Support Unit (DSU) provide support for NHS Wales to improve the effective use of bed capacity, and improve patients' experience and flow through hospitals. These organisations also support the development of community-based service models that help to prevent avoidable admissions. NLIAH offers support from a service improvement perspective and the DSU provides performance management support. By working closely together and sharing intelligence and resources, these organisations complement each other. In 2010, the Welsh Assembly Government established a National Programme Board to focus on complex care, with particular emphasis on NHS Continuing Healthcare. This chapter reflects some of the innovative work carried out by these bodies to support NHS Wales.

The work described in this chapter has been designed, developed and implemented with the help of colleagues from other support organisations in Wales, such as the Social Services Improvement Agency (SSIA), local authorities, and third and independent sector organisations. Against this background of innovation and support, it is important to note that any direct changes and improvements at ward level are made through the hard work and commitment of all staff.

Background

Over the coming decade, demographic changes will bring significant challenges for public services in Wales. Life expectancy has increased, leading to projections that the proportion of older people in the general population will grow by 11 % over the next decade. This overall trend conceals even higher growth in the very elderly population, with the numbers of those aged 85 and older projected to increase by over one-third by 2020.

Welsh health policies reflect the challenges that an increasingly older population may bring, and collectively describe how statutory agencies will need to work in close partnership to deliver services that support and maximise all opportunities for independent living, and seek to meet people's needs within the most appropriate location. There is growing recognition of the requirement to further develop integrated community-based responses wherever appropriate, maintaining and supporting people as far as possible within their usual residence/care setting.

The effective discharge and transfer of care of patients is an ongoing challenge for NHS Wales. To illustrate the progress and scale of improvement made since 2003, the number of delayed transfers of care (DToCs) has reduced sharply. In 2003, there were in excess of 1,000 patients delayed in hospital in Wales, and by December 2010 this figure had fallen to just 432. DToCs now comprise less than 2 % of all discharges from inpatient care. Whilst low in number, delays tend to demand a disproportionate amount of time to manage and resolve, and can have lifelong implications for those patients who are delayed.

In Wales there is no 'purchaser provider split' in healthcare. There are seven Health Board organisations, responsible to their local catchment areas for primary and community care, secondary care (including some tertiary or specialised services), mental health and learning disability services.

Passing the Baton

In 2008, *Passing the Baton – a practical guide for discharge planning* was published (NLIAH 2008). This guide was developed in response to an absence in Wales of any published good practice guidance for improving discharge or transfers of care processes.

The guide takes the view that effective discharge planning is achieved by many people doing simple things consistently. This guide was conceived, developed and written by over 100 practitioners, representing health and social care organisations across Wales, who participated in a national Community of Practice on discharge planning.

'Passing the baton' is a metaphor, in which 'the baton' stands for the responsibility of ensuring that individuals receive the right care, at the right time, in the right place, supported by the right people. The journey through care, between professions, disciplines and organisations, should be as seamless and smooth as passing a baton in a relay race.

Written for the healthcare service by health service professionals, the guide contains information and advice gathered by practitioners, patients and carers, highlighting what needs to be done in order to improve discharge practice. The view of these frontline staff is that discharge practice will be more effective if all the things that are accepted as good practice are done by every member of staff, all the time. Rather than repeatedly developing new initiatives to improve discharge, these staff feel that good discharge practice should be every patient's experience, all the time.

Passing the Baton provides guidance on a broad range of subjects, from the basic processes of discharge through to the complexities of current legal obligations. In essence, the guide gives the information needed to ensure that individuals experience a safe and timely transfer of care or discharge from hospital. The guide includes a number of simple tools that are recommended for staff to use. As a result of its publication, some Health Boards have redrafted their discharge policies to reflect some of the content and tools within the guide. Others have used the guide as part of their in-house training courses to improve staff knowledge of discharge. The advantage of this guide is that it has been produced by a large number of highly motivated and committed 'doers'. They are able to act as 'Change Agents' in their own right, by promoting their guide to their local colleagues and more widely throughout the organisations within their health and social care community.

Three years on from the publication of the guide, the feedback from staff is that its content is still relevant and important. As of 2011, discussions are progressing with universities in Wales to formally establish the guide as a core element of undergraduate training for health and social care students.

Most importantly, the guide acts as a signpost to staff to show where they can get further knowledge to support their practice. Its overriding value is that it contains information to help staff feel more comfortable and confident when dealing with the complexities of managing discharges. The content of the guide is such that it complements the tools contained in other ward-based improvement programmes, such as Transforming Care.

The three tools described below provide a flavour of the guide's practical content.

The simple/complex matrix

The following diagram contains six generic statements about the person's individual circumstances and the practitioner will need to determine if those statements are 'True' or 'False'. The statements are phrased in positive language towards identifying a simple journey. Therefore more 'True' answers would suggest that the discharge process is more likely to be simple; more 'False' answers and the discharge is probably going to be more complex.

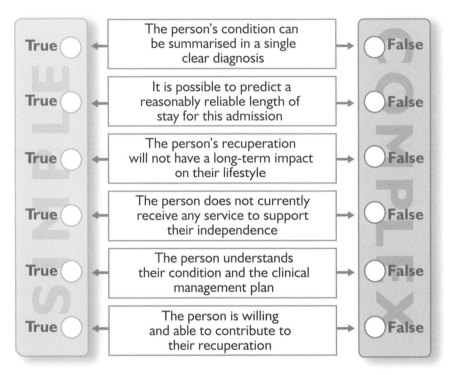

Figure 7.1 The simple/complex matrix

This matrix can be used by the multidisciplinary team throughout the patient journey, to establish whether or not the level of complexity of discharge has changed.

The '4 Ps'

Creating an individualised assessment is the best way to fully understand the patient. This means more than answering a set of predetermined questions and is therefore, difficult to complete in one go. Whereas a great deal of information can be gathered at the first assessment, building a picture of the whole person will require ongoing effort. Over time, the picture will gain additional detail and should reflect changes in the patient's circumstances.

Continuity of assessment

In undertaking individualised assessment it is recommended that professionals consider the '4Ps' principle:

1. Previous   The patient's general circumstances, lifestyle and events leading up to the admission

2. Present   The patient's current condition and how they are dealing with the changes

3. Predict   The factors likely to impact on completing a successful discharge for the patient

4. Prevent   The actions required to overcome problems and prepare the patient for discharge

Using the '4Ps' is like developing the race tactics. It requires an in-depth understanding of physical and emotional strengths and weaknesses, deciding in advance how to run the race on the day and taking responsibility to maximise the chances of success by putting the plan into practice. Think of it as all the things you need to know, to produce your best performance.

Figure 7.2 The '4Ps'

Daily RAP

The 'Daily RAP' (see figure 7.3 on page 102) is a simple and specific face-to-face interaction with the patient for a few minutes every day. It will ensure that the individualised assessment is up to date and that new information can be added. It is also an opportunity to check that the discharge process is progressing as planned. It requires basic observational clinical skills, an effective dialogue with patient and carer, and a personal drive to achieve the best experience for the patient.

To further support the implementation of *Passing the Baton*, a DVD was also commissioned to introduce staff to the content of the guide. Contributors to the guide were interviewed on camera to illustrate the importance of effective discharge planning.

Passing the Baton is still relevant and important in 2011. NHS Wales is fully committed to ensuring that *Passing the Baton* is fully implemented and embedded in practice.

REVIEW	• Ask the patient, 'how do they feel?' • Is the patient responding to treatment? • How is the patient's general condition? • Has there been any change in mental capacity? • Is patient meeting their outcomes and goals? • Is the expected date of discharge accurate?
ACTION	• Talk to patient and carer about progress • Monitor and evaluate care plan • Identify actions required to make progress • Assessment of mental capacity if required • Liaise with multidisciplinary team • Review expected discharge date
PROGRESS	• Advocate on behalf of patient and carer • Check pathway milestones are being achieved • Chase up outstanding actions • Check obligations under Mental Capacity Act • Escalate problems and expedite solutions • Update discharge checklist

Figure 7.3 The Daily RAP

Legal issues

In developing the *Passing the Baton* guide, Morgan Cole Solicitors provided expert help and advice for a specific chapter on the legal issues affecting discharge. This chapter covered topics that included Continuing NHS Healthcare, NHS Choice, and Mental Capacity. The health and social care practitioners involved in writing the guide felt that it was these elements of discharge planning that staff found the most challenging, and which they were least comfortable in dealing with.

To further support staff in dealing with the legal framework relating to assessment and eligibility for complex and/or longer-term care, three national learning events were held in conjunction with Morgan Cole Solicitors. A total of 300 people attended these sessions, with delegates ranging from operational social workers and discharge liaison nurses, to executive nurses and senior managers responsible for commissioning long-term care, including Continuing NHS Health Care.

The main focus was on the legal issues relevant to assessment of complex care needs, decision-making processes and the determination of eligibility for Continuing NHS Health Care, including:

- Patients' rights
- Implications of human rights legislation
- The interface between the law and guidance relevant to complex care
- Continuing NHS Health Care – the primary health need approach, assessment and care planning, decision-making
- Joint funding and pooled budgets – opportunities for innovation
- Mental Capacity Act and Deprivation of Liberty
- The anticipated impacts of the new equality legislation

A key outcome and lesson from these events has been to identify that multidisciplinary team (MDT) working needs to be strengthened. Staff and organisations need to have a clear understanding of the role, responsibilities and accountabilities of the MDT. Work is now underway, through the National Complex Care Forum, to enhance the effectiveness of MDT working to support staff in improving the assessment process.

These events demonstrated that there was variation in terms of how policy was interpreted by organisations and staff. It was also clear that frontline staff only have limited opportunities to keep themselves up to date on the latest versions of an extensive range of policies. Using the 'Knowledge Barometer' tool from *Passing the Baton* (p. 36) to evaluate the experience of the participants, it was possible to see a significant increase in knowledge of the material that was covered.

National Programme Board for NHS Continuing Healthcare (CHC) and the National Complex Care Forum

The NHS Continuing Healthcare National Programme, established in 2010, seeks not only to ensure high-quality, effective service models for those requiring continuing NHS healthcare, but also to develop and support actions that promote independence and manage those people with longer-term and complex needs. This proactive approach helps to prevent an inappropriate slide into dependency and the need for higher-level support services on a long-term basis.

The programme is overseen by a Programme Board, with representation from across the NHS, local government, Welsh Assembly Government policy-makers, and inspection and regulatory bodies. This broad representation ensures that the programme continues to provide a whole systems overview and promotes an integrated approach across the public sector.

High Impact Change	Primary Measure	Source	Recommendation
1. Avoid disruption to the usual care setting	Percentage of people at the same place of residence at the end of an episode of care — reported by team and location of patient	New analysis of existing national data	Improved definition and reporting for type of usual place of residence (UPR) and type of support at UPR
2. Identify complex needs as early as possible	Number of people designated as complex within 48hrs of referral/admission — reported by team and location of patient	Operational process to be developed	Complex Care Bundle: Subject to the development of a complex care definition and screening tool
3. Agreed triggers and timely assessment	Number of complex care assessments initiated within 72hrs of referral/admission — reported by team and location of patient	Operational process to be developed	Complex Care Bundle: Incorporate into local UAP and national review of UAP development of UAP outcomes
4. Effective multidisciplinary working	Percentage of complex patients with an MDT care plan within 10 days of referral/admission — reported by team and location of patient	Operational process to be developed	Complex Care Bundle: Development to identify MDTs aligned with guidance on Effective Multidisciplinary Working
5. Proactive discharge planning	Distribution of length of stay by destination and type of care package on discharge	New analysis of existing national data	Improved standard dataset for reporting subject to updated definitions for HIC1
6. Rapid systems of escalation	Number and type of cases escalated to senior management by category of escalation	Operational process to be developed	Develop standard criteria for clinical escalation of care planning
7. Responsive long-term care	Number of amended community care packages as a result of scheduled and unscheduled reviews — reported by type of care package and UPR	New analysis of existing local data	Align measurement tools for level of need and extent/type of care package
8. Focus on the data for complex care	Number of individually identified MDTs with their own 10 HICs performance report	New analysis of existing and new local data	Development of MDT dashboard to demonstrate outcomes of the 10 HICs
9. Integrated services and effective partnerships	Number of joint packages of care — reported by type, cost and location of patient	New analysis of existing local data	Identify current information on active joint packages of care
10. A workforce designed to serve complex needs	Number and type of staff delivering/qualified in complex care	New analysis of existing local data	Develop a subset of workforce indicators for complex care

Figure 7.4 The 10 High Impact Changes for Complex Care

The *10 High Impact Changes for Complex Care* guide was issued by the Continuing Healthcare National Programme in September 2010 (Welsh Assembly Government and National Leadership and Innovation Agency for Healthcare). This guide sets out the key actions that will support the management of those with complex care needs, helping to maintain people within their usual care setting and avoid crisis admissions to hospital or other residential settings, which can compromise independent lifestyles. There is clear evidence of the damaging effects of an unnecessarily prolonged admission to hospital, with a loss of confidence and rapid functional decline occurring within a matter of days, leading to a potential reliance on higher-level care services in the long term. The best approach is clearly to avoid admission if at all possible, and to encourage timely discharge planning that prevents delays.

For the 10 changes proposed in the guide, the authors have adapted the format used in *10 High Impact Changes for Service Improvement and Delivery: a guide for NHS leaders* (NHS Modernisation Agency 2004). An outcome-based set of metrics is now being developed by the Continuing NHS Healthcare National Programme. This work does not require additional data collection. It is utilising information that has already been collected and reported for a variety of reasons, and collating it into a data set that looks at organisational outcomes through the lens of complex care. The metrics that are being developed will inform service responses that can be focused on supporting independence. The metrics have been designed to capture information and measure improvement across the whole system, and are therefore diverse in nature. Some, for example, will identify information related to discharge from hospital, whilst others capture information on the workforce available to manage those with more complex and longer-term needs.

High Impact Change One is the primary indicator. This High Impact Change is to ensure that services are provided within the usual residence wherever possible, and that in those circumstances where admission to hospital is required, seeks to ensure the person is able to return to their usual setting as soon as possible. An indicator has now been developed, and included within the national performance process – the Annual Quality Framework – for 2011 onwards. Health Boards will be asked to identify the residence prior to admission, and compare this to the location on discharge. This provides MDTs with intelligent management information that will focus on outcomes for individuals, as opposed to outputs – i.e. counting the number of discharges.

Other work being taken forward in the short term seeks to identify and share good practice from across the UK and wider European Economic Community (EEC) countries, related to the management of complex care, including, but not confined to, continuing healthcare. The work is nearing completion and, as anticipated, has concluded that there are no universal solutions to the management of those with complex care needs. However, the service models that have proved most effective are responsive, integrated, community-based models that can respond to changes in need without changing the location of care. In other words, community-based escalation does not have to mean admission to hospital. Third sector contributions to community-based models of care have also been highlighted, especially from a flexible response perspective.

Effective multidisciplinary working lies at the heart of complex care management; yet in the past little support or training has been provided, either at pre-registration or post-graduate level (Lees *et al.* 2010) to support practitioners in working with other agencies within an MDT. Practitioners describe how they find themselves in a room with other professionals and are expected to function as an MDT, but with little support or structure to ensure that this approach is effective. In order to ensure a comprehensive approach to the management of those with complex care needs, work is underway to develop guidance and training and development materials on effective MDT working. Part of this work introduces the concept of MDT identity, exploring how best to capture the MDT as an organisational entity, and proposes outcome indicators to support measuring the effectiveness of MDTs.

Projected demographic changes over the coming decade, along with the move towards community-based care wherever possible, is likely to lead to a higher proportion of complex hospital discharge arrangements. This will place additional demands upon health and social care practitioners to maintain independence and avoiding higher levels of dependency. Development work is being undertaken with the regulatory agencies to identify those areas with low levels of delay, seeking to identify their key features and approach in order to support continuous improvement.

Finally, a Complex Care Forum has been established, to ensure that expert practitioners from health, social services and wider local government, third sector and independent sector organisations are able to link into the work of the Continuing NHS Healthcare National Programme and provide advice, expertise and guidance to support its work. Additionally, the forum is a route to ensure that actions undertaken on a national basis are fed through to operational practitioners in a timely manner. The expertise within the forum is used to develop and test out tools and service models that help to deliver a continuous improvement culture and a consistent and comprehensive approach across organisational boundaries. An example of work currently under development at the time of writing includes a 'Complex Care Review and Screening Tool'.

This work is still at an early stage of development. However, the move towards a proactive and structured approach to the identification, and management, of complexity will underpin service planning and ensure that Wales is better placed to manage the increasing demands on public services predicted to occur over the coming decade.

Bespoke support

The most effective form of bespoke support has been provided by using a blend of quantitative and qualitative information to help particular organisations understand their own care processes. Two examples are given below.

Collecting qualitative information

At ward level, it is clear from the pace at which ward teams work that staff have very little opportunity to reflect on the care they are delivering or on the experience of individual patients who have been on that ward.

Using a simple process of case note review, it is possible to clearly demonstrate the way in which the principles of good discharge planning have been applied at an individual patient level. The case notes are reviewed for specific markers that indicate active discharge planning, such as referrals to therapists and for social services. These are plotted as a timeline and can then provide the basis for discussion about how this contributes to the overall patient experience and discharge plan.

This process provides live qualitative feedback about the patients currently occupying the beds in a ward, and has found scope to make considerable improvements. Significant issues have been identified that have had to be raised at an executive level. Examining the patient episode gives organisations a clear indication of where there are weaknesses in their processes. Indeed, this approach has proved so powerful that it is being developed into a formal programme of support.

Collecting quantitative information

In Wales, the Emergency Department (ED) four-hour target needs to be achieved and monitored by the Health Boards. In order to assist organisations to achieve this target, it has been identified that patient flow throughout the Health Boards needs to be improved. A Patient Flow Development Programme has been designed, which incorporates a number of different practitioners and organisations. These include: bed managers, night nurse practitioners, on-call managers, on-call executives, discharge liaison nurses, community hospitals, and community resource teams.

This programme offers a series of workshops providing intensive support to frontline staff. It gives them the opportunity to discuss and propose new solutions to issues that hamper the flow of patients. The National Leadership and Innovation Agency for Healthcare (NLIAH) and the Delivery Support Unit (DSU) provide a blend of facilitation and coaching support to these staff that is pivotal to the flow of patients in hospital. The individual strands can be tailored to each Health Board and the outcomes are agreed in advance with the sponsoring manager and communicated and measured by the sponsoring executive director.

As a result of the programme, teams have been helped to understand how to use and interpret their own data, clarify and understand their roles, and develop consistency of bed management functions across Health Board acute sites. They have also been empowered to remedy certain issues that are within their own control – 'Just Do Its'. In the two weeks following the first workshop, one hospital achieved an average 8 % improvement in its Accident and Emergency reporting against the four-hour target, compared to the average for the previous two weeks.

Discharge liaison nurses

Since 2007, particular emphasis has been placed on the role and function of the discharge liaison nurse (see Chapter 10). This is because, as public expectations rise and individuals present with increasingly complex and diverse needs, traditional services and professions are less and less able to meet these needs in isolation.

Patients with less complicated healthcare needs are increasingly cared for in the community and have shorter hospital stays; therefore care planning for the remaining patients is bound to become increasingly complex. For this reason, ward-based nurses find managing the complexity of discharge for many patients on their wards very challenging.

Ward nurses are the lynchpins of effective care planning, of which the proactive management of discharge is a key component. The ward sister is ultimately responsible for ensuring that discharge happens in a timely way. A core level of knowledge and skills in relation to discharge planning is therefore essential to every ward nurse's role. However, the complexity of many patients' needs may often exceed the capacity and knowledge of ward-based nurses. To remedy gaps in knowledge, some of the discharge liaison nurses also have a responsibility to teach frontline staff, but this varies across Wales.

A wealth of knowledge and expertise exists throughout the country in relation to complex care and discharge planning. Each Health Board in Wales employs nurses whose role it is to support discharge in some way. Their title is often, but not always, 'Discharge Liaison Nurse' and their roles have been added to those of the traditional ward team. These nurses have extensive specialised knowledge and experience of complex care planning, and the health and social care policy and legislation that underpin it. They have often developed a wide network of contacts and relationships across health, social care and charitable and voluntary organisations. This makes them an invaluable source of information, education and advice for patients and their families, as well as for frontline staff, who may have little experience of dealing with complex issues and limited time to devote to coordinating and negotiating discharges.

A Discharge Liaison Forum, consisting of discharge liaison nurses from all organisations across Wales and facilitated by the Change Agent Team (CAT) in NLIAH, met several times a year to learn and share knowledge and experience. The work of the forum revealed that the discharge liaison nurse role in Wales was not well recognised or valued, with no standardised job description and much variation in their terms and conditions. Their work environment and position in the structure of NHS organisations varies across the country. There is no clearly defined professional or educational requirement for becoming a discharge liaison nurse, and once in post there is no structured career, or professional, educational development path for them to follow.

In 2010, the Royal College of Nursing in Wales (RCN Wales) became involved with the forum and provided a focus for the forum's agenda. Issues addressed included: defining the role of the discharge liaison nurse; examining the management of risk in relation to discharge practices; and outlining the professional development requirements for the role and links with universities. It was recognised that a specialist and/or advanced nurse in complex care planning and discharge management could make an even more significant contribution to the care planning and discharge process. However, it is also clear that the role needs to be carefully designed to be fit for purpose in the newly established Health Boards.

This work has also led in part to responsibility for discharge management being placed within the portfolios of the directors of nursing. The performance measures for nursing now feature a set of nursing metrics relating to hospital discharge. The RCN Wales, together with a group of discharge liaison nurses, has worked in collaboration with the Chief Nursing Officer for Wales. This will be supported by the development of a competency-based professional development and career framework to support complex care planning, in line with the Post-Registration Career Framework for Nurses in Wales.

Transforming care

Ward staff work in a busy and challenging environment, and this is a significant factor. Many wards report the challenge of working with limited numbers of staff, and express concern about the perceived increasing dependency of their patients. NHS Wales is tackling this complex issue with its Transforming Care (TC) initiative. The TC programme combines two other programmes, 'Releasing Time to Care' and 'Transforming Care at the Bedside', and is now embedded in the Welsh '1,000 Lives Plus' campaign.

Transforming Care is a modular programme, typically lasting two years. Year one of the programme is supported by a series of national events run by NLIAH. Then the second year of the programme aims to spread the learning and good practice achieved in year one throughout the organisation, with the support of facilitators.

The TC programme empowers nursing teams across Wales to make the necessary changes to improve the patient's experience by improving the safety and reliability of care. Whilst this work has focused on acute care, the programme has released nursing time and capacity to enable teams to re-focus their efforts back on care planning and ultimately the management of discharge.

Through the TC programme, wards and teams all over Wales have been able to quantify a number of significant improvements, such as:

- In one community hospital, direct care time has increased by 22%. The amount of time spent on handover has reduced by 50%. The time spent looking for equipment and consumables fell by 95% and in the last 12 months the ward has had no infection outbreak or any medication error.
- In a large secondary care hospital, direct care time on two of the participating wards increased by 38% and 29% respectively.
- A specialist tertiary hospital has been able to report 118 days without an instance of hospital-acquired MRSA infection, 116 days without a hospital-acquired CDif infection, and 245 days without a sharps incident.
- A ward at a district general hospital can report that no patient has developed a pressure sore there for over two and a half years.
- A ward in a mental health hospital has increased direct care time by 47%.

The next stage of the programme is to work with these teams to implement specific modules relating to discharge, which will lead to further changes and improvements.

Conclusion

In Wales, the approach has been to offer a blend of engagement, teaching and learning, as well as harnessing the knowledge and skills of staff, in order to advocate and implement good practice, support service and improve performance, and develop new ways of working. Work has been focused on closing the gap between 'what we think should happen for a patient' versus 'what actually happens'.

The work presented in this chapter has supported the ongoing and sustained reductions in delayed transfers of care in Wales. Work continues to further develop discharge management practices and improve patient flow by ensuring that frontline staff have access to the information, knowledge and support they need to make the necessary changes.

References

Chandler, L., Wyatt, M. and Roberts, I. (2010). Lost in Translation – reviewing the role of the discharge liaison nurse in Wales. *Journal of Health Service Management Research*. **23**: 1–4.

Lees, L., Price, D. & Andrews, A. (July 2010). Developing discharge practice through education: module development, delivery and outcomes. *Nurse Education Practice*. **10** (4), 210–15. Epub 27 October 2009

National Leadership and Innovation Agency for Healthcare (2008). *Passing the Baton: A Practical Guide to Discharge Planning*. www.wales.nhs.uk/sitesplus/829/page/36467

NHS Modernisation Agency (2004). *10 High Impact Changes for Service Improvement and Delivery: a guide for NHS leaders*.

Welsh Assembly Government and the National Leadership and Innovation Agency for Healthcare (2010). *10 High Impact Changes for Complex Care*. Continuing NHS Healthcare National Programme.

Welsh Assembly Government (2011). *Delayed Transfers of Care in Wales*. Cardiff: Welsh Government Publications Centre.

Chapter 8

Reforming discharge services in Scotland

Ros Moore, Deirdre McCormick and Graham Monteith,
with contributions from Fiona MacKenzie, Brian Slater and Margaret Whoriskey

In an attempt to provide a broad overview and direction of travel, this chapter briefly and selectively considers discharge planning and delayed discharges within a Scottish context. It begins with an overview of the political context and the delivery structures in the devolved administration in Scotland. This is followed by some definitions of discharge planning and delayed discharges. The chapter goes on to highlight some challenges that are driving and influencing discharge within NHS Scotland and to provide an overview of policy initiatives introduced between 1999 and 2011. A brief explanation of Community Health Partnerships, introduced as a mechanism for integrating health and social care in primary and community settings, is followed by some examples of ways in which whole systems support for change has been made available.

The chapter concludes with a single case example from an unexpected source, a brief reflection on the journey so far and a look ahead to future challenges.

Political context – Devolution

The establishment of the Scottish Parliament and the Scottish Executive (known since 2007 as the Scottish Government) is provided for in the Scotland Act (1998). The Act sets out those matters that are reserved to the UK Parliament and those deemed to be devolved. Matters relating to health and social care fall within the devolved category. (Exceptions include abortion, licensing of medicines and the regulation of some health professions.)

The Scottish Parliament was convened on 1 July 1999, a date that marks the transfer of powers, in devolved matters, from the Secretary of State Scotland and other UK ministers to Scottish ministers. Partnership has been a dominant theme at the heart of devolved Scottish health and social care service delivery (Greer 2004), and Scottish responses to tackling the challenge of delayed discharge have reflected this theme.

Delivery of healthcare in Scotland

Having rejected the internal market in favour of a single system approach in 2003, Scotland has relied on partnership, integration and cooperation to drive quality improvements, with a focus on shared outcomes and resource transfer to meet local needs. The responsibility for administering the NHS in Scotland falls on the Scottish Government Health Directorates (SGHD), whose other responsibilities include health policy, public health, performance management, service improvement and community care.

The devolved NHS in Scotland, NHS Scotland, is delivered primarily by 14 local area unified NHS Boards, organised by geography and known colloquially as 'territorial boards'. A total of 11 Boards serve the mainland, and three the islands. In addition, some clinical services that operate throughout Scotland are provided by 'special' NHS Health Boards. There are eight special boards, four of which provide clinical services. Examples include the Scottish Ambulance Service and NHS (Scottish Executive 2005a).

Devolution has meant that Scotland now sets its own health and social care agenda, establishes its own priorities and strategic direction, and develops its own policy, which the SGHD implements through NHS Boards. Each NHS Board sets its own priorities and develops strategies for implementation within the overarching context of a nationally set performance framework. Each NHS Board is directly accountable to ministers through an annual accountability review held in public.

Discharge planning in Scotland

As is the case elsewhere in the UK, admission to hospital in Scotland will normally be elective, and at the request of the patient's General Practitioner, for planned investigations or surgery. Alternatively, admission will happen as the result of a transfer from another NHS facility or as an emergency. The discharge planning process should begin as soon as practicable after admission and in case of planned admissions may begin prior to admission to hospital. Shepperd *et al.* (2010) provide the following basic definition of discharge planning: 'The development of an individualised discharge plan for a patient prior to leaving hospital for home'. Marks (1994) identifies several steps relating to the discharge planning process. These are:

- Preadmission assessment
- Case finding on admission
- Inpatient assessment and preparation of a discharge plan based on individual needs, for example a multidisciplinary assessment involving the patient and their family and communication between relevant professionals within the hospital
- Implementation of the discharge plan, which should be consistent with the assessment, requires documentation of the discharge process and finally monitoring.

In Scotland, a focus on discharge planning has led to initiatives such as the Planned Care Improvement Programme (2006), which supported the NHS to roll out and incorporate the good practice that existed in planned care, making the experience offered to some patients the norm for all. The issue of delayed discharges has been the driver behind this and many other initiatives of the last decade.

Delayed discharges – definitions and data

The Information Services Division (ISD), a division of NHS National Services Scotland, provides the following definitions of 'delayed discharge' and 'ready for discharge date' (Delayed Discharges Definitions and Data Recording Manual):

'A delayed discharge is experienced by a hospital inpatient who is clinically ready to move on to a more appropriate care setting but is prevented from doing so for various reasons. The next stage of care covers all appropriate destinations within and outwith the NHS (patient's home, nursing home, etc). The date on which the patient is clinically ready to move on to the next stage of care is the ready-for-discharge date which is determined by the consultant/GP responsible for the inpatient care in consultation with all agencies involved in planning the patient's discharge, both NHS and non-NHS (Multidisciplinary Team).'

In Scotland, 'delayed discharges' data has been collected and published nationally by the Information Services Division since September 2000, and since then quarterly, according to nationally agreed standard definitions. A report by Trevor Jones, Head of Department Scottish Executive Health Departments and Chief Executive of NHS Scotland, in March 2002 to the then Minister of Health and Social Care, outlined the scale of the problem (Jones 2002).

At that time, almost 10% of all NHS beds in Scotland were occupied by a patient whose discharge had been delayed. In addition, 300 patients had been waiting more than a year. In October 2001, numbers peaked and there were 3,138 patients waiting for discharge, an increase of 6.2% over the previous quarter. About 40% of these were in the acute sector. Of these patients, 2,191 were waiting longer than a six-week discharge-planning period, the common period within which all assessment and follow-on arrangements should be put in place.

The nature and scale of the challenge

The changing shape of Scotland's population

'The most important policy issue facing European Governments over the next 50 years is how to cope with ageing populations... For Scotland the future is now... its population is ageing faster and dying quicker than any other industrialised nation' *(Scottish Executive 2003a)*

The demographic changes facing Scotland are well documented, with the number of people in Scotland aged over 65 projected to be 21 % greater in 2016 than in 2006 and 63 % greater by 2031. For those over 75, the projected increases are 21 % and 83 % respectively (Scottish Government 2010a). Meanwhile, the number of people of working age has been falling significantly. This demographic shift will have a significant impact on the emergency bed numbers for older people, with an estimated doubling of emergency beds required by 2031, which will place significant additional demands on both health and social care services.

Remote and rural patients

One-fifth of Scotland's population live in rural areas. These areas are projected to show an especially strong demographic shift towards older age groups and a decline in younger, economically active age groups. This has implications for increased demand for healthcare for older people and for the recruitment of nursing and other staff required to provide this care (Scottish Executive 2005b, also known as the Kerr Report). Areas deemed 'remote and rural' account for a significant proportion of the country.

According to a government report, 'Delivering for Remote and Rural Health Care: The Final Report of the Remote and Rural Work Stream' (Scottish Government 2008a), rural patients' experience of care differs from that of urban patients, in that they often have to travel very large distances, using numerous modes of transport, sometimes in severe weather. This clearly has an impact for patients on their ease of access to services, and can also affect decisions about discharge and lead to discharges being delayed.

Changes in demography have a proportionately greater impact in remote and rural areas. The proportion of older people in need of care can be higher than the potential workforce available to provide it, thus making staff recruitment and retention more challenging. Meanwhile, clinicians need to have a wide breadth of expertise that is counter to the speciality-driven models that dominate the large Health Boards in Scotland's central belt.

The 'Scottish Effect'

Much has been written in the last ten years about the so-called 'Scottish Effect'. A report on the health of the people of Scotland (Scottish Executive 2005b) noted that, whilst Scotland's health was improving overall, it was doing less well than many of its neighbours and the differences in health between more and less affluent Scots were becoming more marked. Although the report emphasised the need to address the social determinants of health, it also raised the unanswered question of why, when matched with their English counterparts of comparable socio-economic status, Scots at that time were relatively less healthy over a range of indicators, from age-standardised mortality to specific disease outcomes. Dubbing this the 'Scottish Effect', the report recognised that, when it came to understanding determinants of health and disease, there must be other factors at work.

Since 2005, there have been a number of studies supporting the hypothesis of a 'Scottish Effect', including a report that focused on Glasgow where health improvement is particularly challenging (Scottish Government 2010b). Studies have found that, for the majority of outcomes investigated, socio-economic differences could explain the health differences between Greater Glasgow and Clyde and the rest of Scotland. However, there were four outcomes where the differences could not be explained in that way: anxiety, doctor-diagnosed heart attack, high GHQ score, and being overweight. The report concludes that the latter two could be explained by biological factors but the high prevalence of anxiety and doctor-diagnosed heart attack could not be explained and required more research.

Clearly, the 'Scottish Effect' leads to a raised demand for hospital services, and this has a big impact on the issue of hospital discharge. This unexplained phenomenon, which is still the subject of much research, has made it particularly important for Scotland to implement the improvements needed to ensure that patients can have access to hospital beds when they need them.

Access and availability

Additional factors contributing to delayed discharge, though not peculiar to Scotland, are numerous. These include: lack of widespread availability of home support, lack of care home places in all the required locations and lack of rehabilitation facilities, and waits for community care needs assessment.

An overview of some significant policy and legislative events, 1999–2011

Since Devolution in 1999, there have been a number of policy initiatives designed to improve discharge planning and tackle delayed discharges. For example, in 2000 a mandatory national data recording system for delayed discharge was launched, followed by the first ISD delayed discharge census. A learning network to share and disseminate 'good practice' was then established in 2001.

The 'Delayed Discharge Action Plan' was launched on 5 March 2002, by the Minister for Health and Community Care. It included a commitment to develop, implement and audit discharge policies and protocols. This was followed by a circular, which provided a model 'Framework for Productive Joint Hospital Discharge Protocols'. The basis for both documents was the Scottish Executive Circular, 'Community Care Needs for Frail Older People – Integrating Professional Assessments and Care Arrangements' (Scottish Executive 1998).

'Choice of Accommodation – Discharge from Hospital' (Scottish Executive 2003b) outlined how NHS Boards and local authorities should actively manage choice of care homes for people moving from hospital in a manner that minimises delays, and which is fair and consistent.

The White Paper 'Partnerships for Care' (Scottish Executive 2003c) led to the abolition of NHS Trusts and the establishment of Community Health Partnerships (CHPs). Further policy initiatives have included the introduction of free personal care, adults with incapacity legislation, national care standards and the single shared assessment.

Of particular note, a research review of discharge planning in Scotland (Hubbard *et al.* 2004) on what had worked in the opening few years of the Delayed Discharge Action Plan reported fairly inconclusive findings. The review highlighted the fact that, although there were a wide range of initiatives, it had been difficult to evaluate and monitor the success of these on their own. It suggested that a whole system approach was needed, but accepted that this remained largely an aspiration for most partnerships.

Most recently, the 'Healthcare Quality Strategy for NHS Scotland' (Scottish Government 2010c), which builds on 'Better Health Better Care' (Scottish Government 2007), outlines the government's ambition to deliver the highest-quality healthcare services to people in Scotland, through the combined effect of individual care experiences which are person-centred, clinically effective and safe. The aim is thus to ensure that NHS Scotland is recognised by the people of Scotland as amongst the best in the world.

The Quality Strategy will impact on all NHS Scotland's activities, including the targets against which performance is measured. Contained within the ambition to address wide-ranging issues of quality assurance is a specific aim: to make patients partners in their own care, to improve continuity of care, and to improve the personalisation of care and care planning. Successful implementation of the strategy by managers, doctors, nurses, allied health professionals and others should therefore have a significant impact on improving outcomes relating to discharge.

Sharing information for the benefit of patients is a key responsibility of NHS services in order to provide good-quality services. The 'eHealth Strategy' (Scottish Government 2008b) therefore aims to improve patient safety and effectiveness through the use of electronic information. The next 'eHealth Strategy for Scotland' is due to be published in 2011. Future developments are expected to address many of the issues highlighted in this chapter, and in particular to continue to support the shifting of the balance of care. They are likely to include a focus on improving information-sharing relating to long-term conditions, on improving self-management, on patient eHealth (which enables patients to engage with the NHS electronically), on improving mobile health telemetry (which allows remote measurement and reporting of information), on improving telehealth services (which enable consultations to take place remotely), and on improving the range and sophistication of telecare initiatives.

A mechanism for delivery – Community Health Partnerships

Achieving integration of care services was a key policy objective of Scotland's newly devolved government. Community Health Partnerships (CHPs) were therefore introduced in 2004 across NHS Scotland, as a mechanism for providing integrated health and social care in primary and community settings. CHPs were given flexibility, within statutory guidance, to develop to suit local circumstances and meet local needs. CHPs have created opportunities for NHS Scotland and its partners to work together to attempt to tackle health inequalities; to enhance anticipatory and preventative care; to shift resources to community settings to support patients at home; to provide a wider variety of services at local level, including the identification of more local diagnosis and treatment options; to enable appropriate discharge and rehabilitation; to reduce unnecessary referrals to specialist services; to manage demand and improve access (Scottish Executive 2005a). A range of CHP models have therefore been developed throughout Scotland.

In order to support CHPs to deliver effectively on this challenging agenda, it was recognised that they would require a range of dedicated resources and greater decision-making flexibility. In 2009, an Integrated Resource Framework (IRF) was developed jointly by the Scottish Government, NHS Scotland and the Convention of Scottish Local Authorities (COSLA), through the National Shifting the Balance Delivery Group (a Scottish Government group set up to address the delivery of this agenda). This was to help partners be clearer about the cost and quality implications of local decision-making, in response to the shared strategic objective to shift the balance of care by working in a more integrated way both within the NHS and across health and social care.

At the same time, the aim was to collect evidence that partnerships could use to help reduce inappropriate variation in practice and outcomes for patients and service users. The primary objective of the programme was to enable partners to make investment choices that were informed by a comprehensive understanding of current resource and activity patterns, across the whole health and social care system at locality/CHP level. Three simple questions underpinned the development of the IRF. They were:

1. How are we using our resources?
2. What are our resources achieving?
3. How can we plan and invest our resources in a different, more effective way, to support shifts in the balance of care?

Answering these questions helped support planning and the investment strategies required to cope with future demographic challenges.

There are numerous other examples of improvement support programmes, which have impacted on the discharge from hospital and delayed discharge agenda. Three of these are briefly described below.

Planned Care Improvement Programme

This was a programme, established in 2006, which set out to support NHS Boards in Scotland to achieve the following:

- Improvement to referral and diagnostic pathways
- Day surgery (rather than inpatient surgery) as the norm
- Working towards active management of admissions to hospital
- Working towards active management of discharge and length of stay
- Working towards active management of follow-up.

An overriding aim was to encourage whole system change in the way NHS Boards planned care.

Long Term Conditions Collaborative (LTCC)

Scotland is not alone in facing the challenges of an ageing population and the growing burden of chronic disease. These factors are common to almost all advanced industrial societies. There are many good local examples of care or integrated case management approaches delivering holistic care and real benefits to those with long-term conditions. The Scottish Government has set out to make such approaches more consistent and widespread across Scotland and to balance this professional care, on the basis of need, with enhanced support for self-management.

The Long Term Conditions Collaborative was developed primarily to support NHS Scotland and their partners in delivering a number of Health Improvement, Efficiency, Access and Treatment (HEAT) targets, relating to admissions and attendances at ED, and to deliver sustainable improvements in the quality of healthcare experience. (HEAT targets are a core set of ministerial objectives, targets and measures for the NHS, and they are set for a three-year period.)

The three-year national programme (2007–8 to 2010–11) engaged all 14 territorial NHS Boards and developed work streams on self-care, specialist care and complex care. There was specific emphasis on clinical systems improvement to improve access, reliability, safety and patient experience. A regional management infrastructure has supported the use of technical and behavioural management tools and techniques. These support teams have worked closely with other improvement programme teams, such as the Mental Health Collaborative (established in 2008 to support mental health service improvement) and 18 weeks Referral to Treatment Time programmes and others.

The Joint Improvement Team (JIT)

The Joint Improvement Team (JIT) was established by the Scottish Executive in late 2004, to work directly with local health and social care partnerships across Scotland. A rationale for this development was the recognition that achieving effective partnership working was a crucial element underpinning the design, development and delivery of all personalised health and social care services that work for patients.

The JIT has supported the implementation of a number of initiatives designed to tackle delayed discharge: care home placement improvements; hospital at home; rapid response; early supported discharge teams; rehabilitation; out-of-hours assessment; equipment and adaptation; and improvements in care pathways.

Most importantly, the JIT has been working with partnerships to help them sustain the 'zero standard'. This is the agreed position whereby no patient is inappropriately delayed in hospital for longer than the agreed six-week discharge planning period.

The JIT has assembled a team of experts who are available to work with partnerships. In addition, this team is working with Scottish Government officials to understand the reasons behind the most complex cases and to consider where the faults are that can lead to overly long delays relating to implementation of the Adults with Incapacity (Scotland) Act (2007).

Impact of policy initiatives – the numbers

As highlighted earlier, in October 2001 there were 3,138 patients waiting for discharge, an increase of 6.2% over the previous three months. Of these patients, 2,191 were waiting longer than six weeks, the period during which all assessment and discharge planning arrangements are usually put in place.

In response to these figures, a range of policy guidance and implementation activity was introduced, some of which has been highlighted earlier in this chapter. This was backed by additional funding and ambitious targets, with the objective of having no patients inappropriately delayed in hospital for longer than six weeks. Although this zero standard was achieved at certain points in 2008, 2009 and 2010, the most recently available data from January 2011 census showed it had since risen. The January 2011 census showed there were 169 patients delayed over six weeks, with a total delayed of 790. However, these latest figures still represent a 75% reduction overall, and a 92% decrease for delayed discharges falling outside the six-week period.

These upward trends in the reported figures can be partly attributed to the impact of the current economic climate on the availability of local authority care. There are, however, some interesting exceptions to this trend. For example, two of the 14 NHS Territorial Boards had no patients delayed beyond the six-week discharge planning period at the January 2011 census, Furthermore in 15 (of the 32) Scottish local authority areas there were no patients delayed beyond the six-week discharge planning period at the January 2011 census. This was also the case at the October 2010 census and at the January 2010 census.

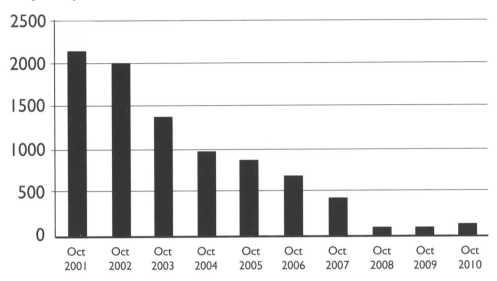

Figure 8.1 Graph showing delayed discharges waiting longer than the six-week discharge planning period, October 2001–October 2010

Further analysis

The first of the following tables shows the numbers of patients, from October 2001 to October 2010, experiencing delayed discharge. The second table gives the principal reasons for delay for the 168 patients delayed longer than six weeks in January 2011. Further information, including a breakdown into individual NHS Board activity for tackling delayed discharges and data, is given on the ISD website: http://www.isdscotland.org/isd/2359.html

Whilst analysis of this data is encouraging, demonstrating improvements in the number of delayed discharges, it is important to note that these figures do not include patients with extremely complex needs. These patients, whose delays have been affected by the implementation of the Adults with Incapacity Act (Scotland) 2007, are recorded and reported separately in the census publication and are excluded from the zero standard.

Table 8.1 Numbers of patients experiencing delayed discharge, from October 2001 to October 2010

Census date	Number
October 2001	2,162
October 2002	2,009
October 2003	1,377
October 2004	968
October 2005	875
October 2006	679
October 2007	425
October 2008	89
October 2009	92
October 2010	126

Table 8.2 Principal reasons for delay for the 168 patients delayed longer than six weeks in January 2011

Reason	Number	Percentage of total
Awaiting place availability in a care home	63	37.5%
Awaiting funding for a care home placement	51	30.4%
Waiting to go home	22	13.1%
Community care assessment reasons	21	12.5%
Waiting for 'other reasons'	10	6.0%
Waiting for healthcare assessment/arrangement reasons	1	0.6%

There have been many attempts to look beyond the data to gain a better understanding of cause-and-effect relationships. For instance, the Planned Care Improvement Programme (an 18-month Scottish Executive initiative commenced in 2006) showed clear evidence that concentrating on the relatively small group of patients with a length of stay longer than 28 days yielded a smaller system benefit than concentrating on the high-volume groups of patients.

This programme also highlighted one of the main causes of capacity blocks as the variation in timing of discharge of patients from hospital. It had been assumed that the inter-relationships between elective and emergency admission patterns were the cause of major variation in patient journeys, but closer analysis revealed that the greatest variation was in the number of discharges.

Accordingly, efforts were made to ensure that attempts to reduce variation started with the discharge process and not the admission process. Variation in discharge process leads to variation in length of stay, and it was emphasised that discharge should start at the point of admission. This is supported in both planned and unplanned care and remains a key component of any improvement process within the confines of capacity and flow.

Other related improvements

The increased focus on timely discharges from hospital has changed a mindset that previously accepted delayed discharges as an integral and inevitable part of hospital care. It has also brought with it a desire to address a range of related issues that impact both on improving the quality of patient care and on generating increased bed capacity.

We know that in some specialities it is possible to shorten admissions or even avoid admissions entirely, just through adopting different models of care. These alternative, community care models enable clinicians to treat and care for patients in non-hospital settings. Care at Home and Hospital at Home are two models that fall into this category. (The developing work on re-ablement in Scotland, which focuses on care at home, is also beginning to show improvements in relation to facilitating timely discharge.)

One commonly used term to describe these models is 'intermediate care', which can be defined as: 'Those services that do not require the resources of a general hospital but are beyond the scope of the traditional primary care team' (Oxford and Anglia Intermediate Care Project 1997).

They include:

- Intermediate care, which substitutes for elements of hospital care (substitution care)
- Intermediate care, which integrates a variety of services for people whose healthcare needs are complex and in transition (complex care)

There are a number of health settings in which new Care at Home or Hospital at Home models have been successfully delivered in the past decade. One example in Scotland can be found in the work of a small, award-winning team (the Fife Intensive Therapy Team or FITT), working within NHS Fife. This team, which won the Mental Welfare

Commission Award Principles into Practice in 2009, provides an intensive outreach service for young people with severe mental health problems. In order to understand the hospital-based context for the team's operations, it is important to note that in Scotland inpatient care for young people's mental health is delivered regionally by three inpatient units, with a modest total of 42 beds. (This is accurate at the time of writing, though there are plans in place to increase capacity to 48 beds.)

In an evaluation of the Fife Intensive Therapy Team outcomes, Simpson *et al.* (2010, p. 217) describe the new models of care arising from concerns about psychiatric inpatient provision for adolescents across the UK. This has resulted in the development of alternatives to traditional inpatient care and treatment, and the development of new models of intensive home- and community-based care. An essential element is that each nurse within the team operates with a caseload of around five. Simpson *et al.* argue that:

> 'flexible, responsive and adaptive interventions ensure that packages of care on offer reflect the level and nature of the assessed need. Interventions are community or home-based, and include an important component of identifying, labelling and building on the strengths of the family to enable them to continue to have the skills, confidence and stamina necessary for them to provide an appropriate level of care and support at home.'

With other NHS Boards developing similar models, it has been possible to avoid some admissions and, most importantly, shorten others. Initial findings suggest that there is a significant reduction in the average length of stay in hospital and that this reduction is occurring rapidly, that bed occupancy levels have reduced, and that access to inpatient care has improved.

Whilst this is a success story taken from a single sub-specialty, there are numerous examples of intermediate care that are achieving similar benefits for patients and for service commissioners. During 2010 the Scottish Government supported five intermediate care demonstrator programmes and supported the shared learning relating to these programmes (Joint Improvement Team, NHS Scotland).

Conclusion

This chapter has provided a Scottish perspective on post-Devolution efforts to address the issue of timely discharge from hospital. The chapter has given a brief insight into the broader context within which the NHS and their partners are currently operating. It has also provided examples of ways in which the Scottish Government monitors and supports policy implementation, and the efforts required to achieve the necessary changes and improvements.

Following a rejection of the internal market in favour of a single system approach in 2003, Scotland has relied on partnership, integration and cooperation to drive quality improvements. In addition, it has become increasingly clear that solving what at first seems like a single problem, delayed discharge, must involve whole system approaches to changing all aspects of the patient journey.

The implementation of the 'Healthcare Quality Strategy for NHS Scotland' (Scottish Government 2010c), designed to provide a whole systems approach to quality assurance, will have a key role to play in continuing the progress that has been made. The key priorities set by the Scottish Government for health will require targeted efforts to realise the wider vision of more integrated care and the use of information to promote better, more efficient and safer care for patients.

In Scotland, the context within which care is delivered has been subject to evolution rather than revolution. The next stage of this journey is certain to see greater-than-ever functional integration between health and social care services. Functional integration could contribute greatly to smoother transitions and the reduction of delays but could also bring further challenges.

Economic constraints, particularly those that are starting to affect services currently being run by local authorities, will be a significant factor. Meanwhile, shifting demographics are expected to contribute to a continued increase in the demand for beds and for care, making it more important than ever that patients are discharged on time, and that models combining improved care with alternatives to hospital are developed and implemented.

References

Delayed Discharges Definitions and Data Recording Manual (2010). http://www.isdscotland.org/isd/2359.html

Greer, S.L. (2004). 'How Devolution has led to Four Different Models for the NHS'. The Constitution Unit, School of Public Policy, UCL.

Hubbard, G., Huby, G., Wyke, S. & Themess-Huber, M. (2004). *Research Review on Tackling Delayed Discharge*. Edinburgh: Scottish Government.

Joint Improvement Team, NHS Scotland.

http://www.jitscotland.org.uk/action-areas/intermediate-care/

Jones, T. (March 2002). 'Delayed discharge in Scotland'. Report. Edinburgh: Scottish Executive. http://www.show.scot.nhs.uk/sehd/publications/dc20020305delaydisch.pdf

Marks, L. (1994). *Seamless care or patchwork quilt? Discharging patients from acute hospital care*. London: King's Fund Institute.

The Oxford and Anglia Intermediate Care Project (1997). Oxford and Anglia NHS Region.

Scottish Executive (1998). 'Community Care Needs of Frail Older People – Integrating Professional Assessments and Care Arrangements'. Edinburgh: Scottish Government.

Scottish Executive (2003a). 'The Scottish Report – Scotland the Grave?' Edinburgh: Scottish Government.

Scottish Executive (2003b). 'Choice of Accommodation – Discharge from Hospital'. Edinburgh: Scottish Government.

Scottish Executive (2003c). 'Partnerships for Care'. White Paper. Edinburgh: Scottish Government.

Scottish Executive (2005a). 'Building a Health Service Fit for the Future'. Edinburgh: Scottish Government.

Scottish Executive (2005b). 'Health in Scotland 2004'. Edinburgh: Scottish Government.

Scottish Government (2007). 'Better Health Better Care Action Plan'. Edinburgh: Scottish Government.

Scottish Government (2008a). 'Delivering for Remote and Rural Health Care: The final Report of the Remote and Rural Work Stream'. Edinburgh: Scottish Government.

Scottish Government (2008b). 'eHealth Strategy 2008–2011'. Edinburgh: Scottish Government.

Scottish Government (2010a). 'Reshaping Care for Older People – A Programme for Change 2011–2021'. Edinburgh: Scottish Government.

Scottish Government (2010b). 'The Scottish Health Survey: Topic Report: the Glasgow Effect'. Edinburgh: Scottish Government.

Scottish Government (2010c). 'The Healthcare Quality Strategy for NHS Scotland'. Edinburgh: Scottish Government.

Shepperd, S., McClaran, J., Phillips, C.O., Lannin, N.A., Clemson, L.M., McCluskey, A., Cameron, I.D. & Barras, S.L. (2010). *Discharge planning from hospital to home*. Cochrane Database of Systematic Reviews 2010, Issue 1. Art. No.: CD000313. DOI: 10.1002/14651858.CD000313.pub3

Simpson, W., Cowie, L., Wilkinson, L., Lock, N. & Monteith, G. (2010). The Effectiveness of a Community Intensive Therapy Team on Young People's Mental Health Outcomes. *Child and Adolescent Mental Health*. **15** (4), 217–23.

Section 3

Multi-professional discharge practice considerations

Chapter 9

Effective discharge of those with complex care needs
Sian Wade

This chapter focuses on issues related to the effective hospital discharge of individuals with complex care needs, and some of the challenges faced by those involved. Services need to be coordinated effectively in order to ensure a smooth transfer of care to the patient's home or a new setting, thus helping to bridge the gap between hospital and place of discharge (Shepperd *et al.* 2004).

A central tenet of the delivery of care to patients when in hospital is to treat their medical condition promptly so as to enable them to return home, for their own well-being. Alongside this, there is the need to minimise the patient's length of stay, and avoid unplanned readmission. Avoiding readmission has become imperative, with a reduction in bed capacity and the need to prevent patients getting a hospital-acquired infection or illness. Timely discharge planning has thus become a routine feature of healthcare systems.

Defining complex care

Patients deemed to have complex care needs tend to be those who have multiple health and care needs, requiring a set of complex interventions, often involving a range of services. Among the patients that tend to fit into this category are:

- Frail older people, often with many different care needs related to multiple health-related problems and frailty
- Patients who are terminally ill with palliative care needs, or who are at the end of life, who often have a range of complex care needs; this group of patients has become more prominent with an increased focus on end-of-life care pathways and the Gold Standard Framework, focusing on choice regarding place of death (DH 2008)

- Those with long-term conditions such as heart failure, chronic obstructive airways disease and diabetes
- Patients recovering from amputation with challenging wound care needs, or those requiring other complex care interventions

Social factors behind the need for complex discharges

Today's increased life expectancy and improved healthcare means that people with lifelong or ongoing health problems have a much greater chance of surviving and living longer. As such, they are more likely to have complex care needs. It is estimated that 17.5 million people in the UK have some form of long-term condition, i.e. about six out of ten adults (DH 2005a), or 30% of the population. Nearly half of these people have more than one condition, and the percentage of those over 65 years old with a long-term condition is expected to double by 2030 (DH 2005a).

The World Health Organisation (WHO) has estimated that long-term conditions will be the leading cause of disability by 2020. Further analysis shows that 80% of the time, energy and resources of healthcare staff and care services tend to be invested in 20 to 30% of the population – those with complex care needs (CSIP 2004/5, DH 2005a). Hence there has been a growing emphasis on finding ways to meet the needs of this client group (DH 2005a, 2005b, 2006).

The social context in which people are ageing or developing complex care needs today has changed a great deal. Lasslett (1989) and Stearns (1976) both assert that families are no less caring today than in the past, and this still appears to stand. However, the patterns of modern family life can present a real challenge in terms of providing support and care. There are smaller and much more complex extended family and social networks, described by Bengston *et al.* (1990) as 'beanpole families'. Increasingly, siblings and partners involved in helping to provide care are themselves ageing or disabled. In addition, people are increasingly moving away from where their parents live (both nationally and globally) in search of work. This has led to disparate far-flung networks that challenge the ability of those involved to provide extensive or effective care. Changing patterns in marriage, divorce and relationships can also weaken family ties and reduce ability or commitment to care for elderly or disabled relatives, quite apart from the daily demands of work, often involving significant responsibilities. All these factors combine to present a major challenge for health and social care professionals, who are planning complex discharges.

Recognising the moral imperative

It has never been so vital to ensure that the needs of individuals with complex care requirements are effectively and efficiently addressed within health and social care settings or services (DH 2005a). From a political perspective, it is crucial to meet these needs, especially in view of the reduction in beds, issues involving effective capacity management and use of resources (DH 2005a), along with the enormous debts incurred by the NHS in recent years (Internurse.com 2007).

Similarly, from the patient's and carer's perspective, it is crucially important to ensure that patients are cared for by the right staff, with the right skills, at the right time. Even more vital, however, from a quality of life viewpoint, is the moral and ethical imperative of ensuring that those with complex care needs get the best possible care within the constraints and resources available and that this care takes place wherever possible in the community (Annells 2004, Hainsworth 2005, Sargent 2006, DH 2005a, DH 2006). This has become a growing concern, with the global and national recession and significant cuts in health and social services funding and other services at present, along with current and proposed government policies and plans (Carers UK 2010).

There are additional challenges related to the increasing demand for formal carers. For instance, recruiting staff to fill vacancies has become a problem in some areas. In urban and inner-city locations, this may be due to issues of safety and staff feeling vulnerable, while in rural areas it may be that those groups of people who would be most likely to take on this kind of work have moved away due to cost-of-living issues as discussed by Isobella Aboderin (2004) in her article 'Modernisation and ageing theory revisited'.

Trends in hospital discharge

Traditionally, discharge has been associated with 'going home from hospital'. For some years, there was a move towards patients receiving only their acute care in district general hospitals, where the focus was less on discharge and more on assessment, treatment and intervention for those with complex needs. These individuals were then transferred on to less acute settings or services, such as specialist or rehabilitation wards, intermediate or transitional care wards or other settings where their ongoing care needs could be met. This meant that discharge planning was often deferred until the patient reached this service, increasing the overall length of stay. The essence of timely discharge is that: while patients can be moved from an acute to a rehabilitation setting, this move must include the discharge plan (with contemporaneous information) moving with the patient.

In recent years there seems to have been an increasing trend for patients to be discharged directly home, to be supported by a range of community-based services such as intermediate care or integrated community care services and rehabilitation in the home. Other models of care have also developed, such as those involving community matrons and virtual wards (Lewis 2007). Here, the patient is cared for in the community, by a team of community-based staff. Each patient has a managed, individualised, pre-planned treatment plan agreed for when a crisis arises, so as to try to prevent admission to hospital where appropriate, working alongside traditional community services.

In some areas, it seems that community bed settings are closing and bed numbers reducing, whilst the development of extra care housing facilities for independent living is becoming more popular (CSIP 2008/2010). Where there are transitional and intermediate care beds, patients will almost certainly need to meet specific criteria to be eligible for transfer to such settings. There will also need to be evidence that satisfactory discharge planning is progressing.

Challenges of the discharge process for patients with complex needs

Ideally, planning for discharge should form an integral part of the holistic care plan at an early stage of an admission, when an estimated date of discharge needs to be decided (Lees & Holmes 2005). Patients with complex care needs require a 'social diagnosis' of need, prior to discharge. Failure to do this may mean that it is very difficult to evaluate need accurately (Bowling & Betts 1984, McKenna et al. 2000). This is significant, since these patients are likely to need a greater level of after-care following discharge than they did before (Bowling & Betts 1984, Victor & Vetter 1988).

Planning for this client group usually occurs within a wider context, involving multiple, ongoing and underlying health and social care needs. Care arrangements must therefore be put in place before successful transfer or discharge to another service or home can occur (Bull & Kane 1996), along with the necessary equipment and other requirements. Failure to achieve this can lead to a failed discharge, with the patient going home and then needing to be readmitted soon after, with the associated distress to the patient and increased pressure on beds. Alternatively, staff in the community may find themselves in a difficult situation, whereby they are pulled away from other patient care to try to organise the required care and equipment at very short notice. A social diagnosis is just as important in this group as a medical diagnosis.

Delaying a discharge from hospital can also have consequences that may be lasting and sometimes even fatal (Annells 2004). This is perhaps particularly true in the case of older people, where the health of the patient may be precarious and severely challenged, due to compromised functional reserve and an increased risk of iatrogenesis (Illich 1975), hospital-acquired infection (Gould 2002) and/or age-related de-training. In such cases, patients may actually regress, particularly in terms of mobility and functional abilities (Wade 2004). Alternatively in the case of a terminally ill patient reaching the end-of-life stage, a delayed discharge may mean that they are unable to go home to die and instead die in a hospital ward. This may not comply with their wishes, even in settings where the Liverpool pathway is in use to try to assist a swift transfer home (see Chapter 21).

Individuals with complex care needs are also more likely to suffer the vagaries of bed management and multiple moves to other wards. This is because they take longer to recover and because they may need to wait for ongoing care in other settings or services. Once their acute or specialist care needs are resolved, it is these individuals who are most likely to be moved to make way for new admissions. Changes can lead to disorientation and regression in individuals with complex needs, even where there is no cognitive impairment (see Case study 1 below). Moving such patients can also challenge the ability of staff to remain truly person-centred, as they try to get to know the complex care needs of these individuals. Staff may also lose track of care arrangements and the progress being made towards discharge. Thus moves may generally be counter-productive, as these patients often have quite specific needs and flourish with staff they know well.

Case study 1: Rose

Rose Smith had severe arthritis and had been coping at home, with a carer coming in twice a day to help her with personal care and to shop and prepare her meals. She managed quite well, using a commode by her chair, which she could just transfer onto by herself, once up.

One Friday evening, her carer arrived to find her very confused and disorientated. It was late at night, and, feeling she could not leave her alone in this state, the carer dialled 999. On admission, it became evident that Rose had a urinary tract infection (UTI) and she needed antibiotics, but at this stage she was unable to administer these safely herself. There was no way of accessing intermediate care services at this time so she was admitted to the Medical Assessment Unit (MAU). The next day being a Saturday, the intermediate care service was unable to facilitate her transfer home so she spent a further 15 hours in bed on the MAU, before being transferred to a medical unit, where she remained in bed overnight.

The next day, due to a bed crisis, Rose was identified as a suitable patient to move to a surgical bed and she remained in bed. Rose declined to get up and, since rehab was not the focus of the nurses' work on this ward, they did not realise how important it was to encourage her to do so. The Monday was a bank holiday and Rose remained in bed. On Tuesday her bed was needed for surgery and a bed was found for her, back on a medical ward.

By this time Rose appeared to have a severe infection. She was also beginning to develop a pressure sore, despite efforts to prevent this. She was now unable to weight-bear and had been found to have Type 2 diabetes so she needed to stay in for further assessment and stabilisation. She was placed on the referral list for the elderly care rehab ward in the acute hospital, but there was no bed.

After two months and several episodes of deterioration, including two falls, together with several bed moves, a bed became available in the rehab ward and Rose was transferred. By this time she had deteriorated in many ways, including her memory and mental state, and it now seemed that the main consideration was whether she needed residential or nursing care!

For a successful discharge, a team and whole systems approach (involving the effective co-ordination of all health and social care services) is necessary. This responsibility often falls upon ward-based staff and is a central element of their role. Whilst planning at this early stage is good practice, it is perhaps more easily said than done – especially if the patient is acutely ill and/or their condition is very unstable. Families may find it difficult to engage in such discussions, and indeed it may be difficult to establish what the actual care needs are likely to be at such an early stage. The following list outlines key considerations when staff are planning the discharge of patients with complex needs.

Key considerations for successful complex discharge planning

- It should begin as soon as possible.
- Patients and carers/family should be at the centre of planning, with a clear picture of what they hope to achieve as the outcome – and any challenges identified.
- There should be comprehensive assessment, reassessments and documentation of events/key stages of the discharge plan.
- Referrals required and overall multidisciplinary goals should be identified.
- Each discipline should be clear about their input, the intervention, and the time required for these goals to be achieved. A predicted date of discharge based on these should be agreed – this will be estimated and may need to be re-estimated throughout the stay.
- A named member of the multidisciplinary team should take responsibility for coordinating discharge planning (Annells 2004).
- Any barriers to achieving the goals should be clearly identified and reported, as appropriate, to assist with making good any shortfall.

- Where transfers to other settings are envisaged, planning, training and arrangements should not be delayed.
- There needs to be effective coordination and constant review and modification, where there is a change in circumstances. This should include a reporting system to ensure that any difficulties are noted and responsibility for acting on these is allocated.
- Where appropriate, written information should be provided about lifestyle, medication, diet and medical symptoms, etc.
- Where funding is required, a funding application should be instigated as soon as needs can be identified.

Principles of effective discharge of those with complex care needs

Discharge planning is very much a process, rather than a single event. It is therefore a stage in the patient's care that requires a period of preparation and which has definite consequences. It cannot be examined in isolation from what has gone before or from what follows afterwards, when the patient leaves the hospital, as emphasised by Booth & Davis (1991) and Armitage (1981, p. 386). As such, it can be linked to the concept of successful aftercare, which can be regarded as 'counteracting or making good any deficiencies in an individual's ability to care for themselves' (New South Wales Health Department 2001).

For patients with complex care needs to be effectively discharged, the key principles are that the discharge should:

- Be timely, if quality of life is to be promoted and use of resources is to be effective and maximised
- Occur within a global context that is likely to involve multiple, ongoing and underlying health and social care needs, such that care arrangements, which form a key component in the continuity of community care, are in place before transfer or discharge to another service or home can occur
- Involve a whole systems approach
- Place the individual at the centre of the discharge process, promoting continuity of care through adequate information and communication flows between patients, carers and services, so as to ensure optimum outcomes for individual patients

For a successful discharge to occur, staff need to have grasped the key principles and to have developed a comprehensive understanding of the processes involved in planning and preparing for transfer or discharge of care (McKenna *et al.* 2000). This can often be challenging. This process can be effectively displayed diagrammatically as a flow chart, and Jewell (1993) provides a useful example of this, which has been adapted below.

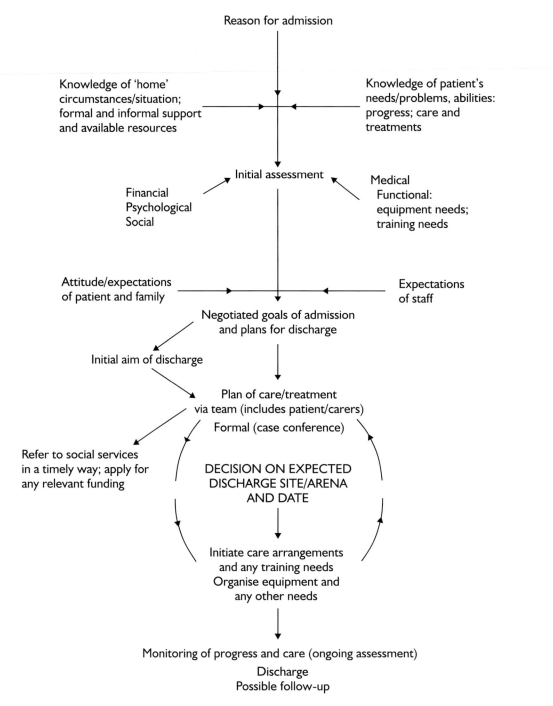

Figure 9.1 The discharge process

Care pathways

Care pathways have a very valuable part to play in relation to the patient's journey through hospital, but they do tend to be disease-focused (Ellis & Johnson 1997, Middleton & Roberts 2000). The potential of care pathways in helping patients with more complex needs, particularly where multiple pathology is present, is perhaps less clear and staff working in this field may have little exposure to using them, perhaps because of their specificity.

Wade (2004) argues, however, that much can be learnt from the principles of care pathways that is of relevance to this group of patients. Pathways help to ensure that care is organised, timely and focused, using evidence-based practice, providing the clinical record, and enhancing the identification of variances and risks (Oliver 2006). The requirement for multidisciplinary collaboration also aids timely involvement and continuous review of care. The introduction of end-of-life care pathways such as the Supportive Care Pathway or Liverpool Care Pathway (see Chapter 21), for patients with palliative care needs and other complex care needs, who have a life-limiting condition, are good examples of care pathways that can aid effective discharge (DH 2008, Marie Curie Palliative Care institute 2005).

Person-centred partnership working, where patient involvement is valued, should be part of the inherent culture of any service caring for clients with complex needs (Wade 2004). This aids agreement in reaching collaborative goals that are meaningful for patients and their discharge care needs, while supporting the value of effective multidisciplinary, inter-disciplinary or trans-disciplinary working (Moroney & Knowles 2006).

Involving patients in collaborative goal planning may be problematic, and this can impede opportunities to negotiate appropriate outcomes with them (Clark & Dyer 1998, Tripp & Caan 1999). Victor *et al.* (1993) found that patients and their carers remained peripheral to the transfer/discharge process, as did Tripp & Caan (1999), while Waterworth & Luker (1990) found that patients were often reluctant to become involved in decisions about their care. Strategies such as Supportive Care Pathways, along with a more consumer-orientated culture, have enhanced the focus on the involvement of patients and relatives; but it still seems that discharge discussions and planning can occur without such involvement.

The theory of constraints

Delays and their impact in the acute sector

The pathway of patient care can be greatly enhanced by looking at the processes and systems involved, so as to ensure patients' timely management and care whilst in hospital. The theory of constraints, as described by Shefter (2006), which is, in effect, a systems approach to improvement, has proved helpful throughout different services and settings. By identifying the constraints that hinder patients' progress on their pathway of care, strategies to overcome these constraints can be sought, with the aim of reducing the length of patient stay.

There are a number of possible reasons for delays. With a limited number of therapists, social workers and other specialists working in the acute sector, priorities need to be decided. In essence, attention is often given to those who are acutely ill, or those who, with some intervention, can be speedily discharged. Waiting for a patient to be seen by a particular specialist can be problematic, whilst waiting for results of investigations can be a cause of further delay. The organisation of ongoing investigations may depend on the results of earlier investigations, and can therefore contribute to increasing lengths of stay and perceived delays. As already discussed (see Case study 1), moving patients around or to other wards can also be very disruptive for them.

Using the theory of constraints as a strategy

The theory of constraints provides one way of addressing some of the constraints identified in delaying discharge. Systems based on this theory have been adopted in hospitals in the UK. They are computerised and are founded on the principle of looking forward and anticipating care needs. They are intended to be transparent for all members of the multidisciplinary team (MDT) to see, thus ensuring that important aspects of planning are not missed.

The various MDT members identify goals that the patient needs to achieve before they can reach their destination. These include any equipment and services or training needs that will be required. By recording the estimated time required to achieve the goals, and that required to obtain equipment or to set up services, the estimated date of discharge can be reached. The identified timescale is then divided into green, amber and red. As time passes, the situation may move from green through to red, with green being a 'safe' zone and red indicating 'danger' with regard to exceeding the planned length of stay and estimated date of discharge.

The patient will start in green, where they are well within the planned timescale for their predicted date of discharge. They may then move into amber, which acts as a warning signal that they are moving towards the date when they should be discharged. If they enter red, they have already exceeded or almost exceeded the estimated date of discharge. Thus, moving from green to red provides an alarm system, which is meant to trigger more concerted action to progress plans, or highlight the need to identify the constraints or barriers that are causing the delays. Progress needs to be reviewed daily; and where delays are identified, strategies can be put in place to expedite the progress – for example, involving higher management, to access funding for special equipment or services that may be needed.

The introduction of discharge coordinators

In many hospitals the introduction or growth of discharge coordinators has emphasised the importance of progressing effective discharging (Dinsdale 2002). In some ways it seems a shame that this service is needed, as it can lead to ward nursing staff losing their discharge skills. The advantages, however, are that these specialist staff can develop expertise concerning the services available and establish good working relationships with partnership agencies and parties. They can also help to provide some continuity of care for patients when they are moved between wards.

In addition, because the focus of their work is solely on discharge planning, they can spend all their time on this activity, especially when there are time-consuming and complex issues to address. These may include organising equipment or services, such as oxygen delivery, or indeed coordinating training needs for community staff, such as the use of a particular piece of equipment or giving IV therapy or Vac therapy. This is not to imply that community staff lack these skills. But, with the increasing complexity of technology now available, patients may have very individual technological requirements that community staff are unfamiliar with. Dealing with this type of complex discharge would challenge ward staff who are trying to meet a multitude of needs for patients on the wards with minimal staffing levels. (See Chapter 10 for more on the role of discharge coordinators.)

Community matrons

As mentioned earlier, the UK has introduced models of care designed to better manage those with chronic conditions and illnesses. Originally derived from the Evercare model in the USA, the overarching purpose is to optimise the health and well-being of ageing, vulnerable and chronically ill individuals (DH 2005a).

At the heart of the clinical delivery model is a personal care manager or nurse practitioner known as the community matron. The community matron helps individuals with complex needs to manage their conditions, and any impending crises, with a view to preventing admission where possible. Matrons can work very effectively with staff in other services. For instance, if a patient on their caseload is admitted, they can visit and work with the hospital staff to expedite the timely discharge of the patient. Having individualised, managed care plans may enable patients to go home within parameters that hospital staff would not normally accept as reasonable. For example, a patient may have a reading outside the normal accepted oxygen saturation rates, but for specific reasons it might still be possible for that patient to return to their home, with the necessary support in place. As discussed earlier, in some areas virtual wards are being developed to aid this, and community matrons play a pivotal role in these (Lewis 2007).

Additional mechanisms to enhance timely care and transfer of care

With growing bed and capacity problems, the imperative to move patients on has helped to stimulate the introduction of strategies such as daily early-morning consultant ward rounds, progress chasers, clinical site practitioners and tracking teams. The introduction of Gerontology Multidisciplinary Out-reach Teams, from specialist services, with whom peer trust is established, can also be immensely helpful (Harwood *et al.* 2002, Robinson & Street 2004). These staff can assess the probable trajectory of care needs of many complex discharge and transfer patients, and make appropriate referrals and arrangements at an early stage. They also assist in dealing with difficulties concerning transport, poor communication and swift patient transfers to a discharge lounge. This enables patients to be transferred/discharged without further assessment or delay as soon as they are ready and able to be moved.

The need for social services assessment or for continuing care funding should also be initiated at this stage – if appropriate – so that issues around funding have been addressed by the time the patient is ready to be transferred. One of the challenges here is that social services require the patient to be medically stable before they will assess them. However, because many of those within the category of complex care needs have fragile health, this can fluctuate. Thus, if assessment is not undertaken as soon as the patient is stable then the individual may regress or catch an infection (as exemplified in Case study 1). Similarly, a patient may be assessed as not qualifying for continuing care funding, consequently delaying their discharge; and whilst they wait, they may deteriorate. All being well, this should not be an issue for those at the very end of life, who qualify for fast-track continuing care funding, providing the level of care they need can be funded within the designated budget. But for those patients not at the end of life, achieving a successful discharge requires tenacity and sustained attention to detail throughout the patient's stay.

Teamwork and communication

Effective communication and coordination are essential to expedite efficient discharge planning (Payne *et al.* 2002), although this may not be easy to achieve (McKenna *et al.* 2000, Wade 2004, Moroney & Knowles 2006), due to time pressure and varying demands on staff. Similarly, effective teamwork, involving assessment, anticipatory, holistic, multi-agency working and communication, is vital in achieving satisfactory discharge of those with complex needs.

There are a number of organisational activities that provide ways of monitoring and reviewing progress and plans for discharge. These are:

- The organisation of care in the setting/ward
- Effective and easily accessible records
- Well-managed handovers (including electronic handover systems)
- Well-run ward rounds, with a nurse in attendance
- Well-run multidisciplinary discharge planning meetings and timely referrals
- Early communication with community staff at the outset, as they often know many of the patients with complex needs and their home circumstances and unique needs
- Patient boards or electronic boards to summarise key stages and document progress
- Involvement of a discharge coordinator or complex discharge planning nurse

The organisation of care in the setting/ward

Continuity of care

Continuity helps to promote effective discharge, as staff start to recognise the complex needs of individual patients and to understand and appreciate subtle changes, or comments they might make, that might otherwise go unnoticed. Staff get to know the best way for care to be given, and develop an understanding of any behaviour or communication difficulties that the patient may have.

Patients also benefit from familiarity and are more likely to build up a trusting relationship with staff they know, sometimes disclosing important information related to their care or discharge needs at a time when they feel comfortable and confident about doing so. In this context, however, it is important to be clear about who is responsible for the patient, and ensure that information is recorded and highlighted for this person.

It is important to ensure that continuity of care is achieved in the best possible way. This is not always easy in the modern NHS, where many services have to be available 24 hours a day, seven days a week, and where there are part-time workers and family-friendly employment policies.

Well-run ward rounds

Within medical settings, ward rounds are another important activity. They should always include as key elements: reviewing/confirming the expected discharge date, interventions still needed, social circumstances, and progress with discharge (Lees 2010). It is important for the ward round to involve a nurse who is looking after the patient and knows them as well as possible. This may well mean running ward rounds by teams, so that nurses can change as their team of patients are seen. It may be a bit inconvenient for the doctors, but having a key person present is surely more important.

Effective and easily accessible records

Collaborative, multidisciplinary records should maximise effective communication, as they help to save time, and avoid repetition, gaps in information and discrepancies (Hunt 1999). In hospitals, a single set of records has become the format for recording key MDT members' notes. Somewhere, in a very prominent position, there needs to be a place to enter the expected date of discharge, which can of course be changed. It is also important to have a designated area to document details of discharge records. This should include free text multidisciplinary pages, where conversations with patients, family and health professionals can be recorded. It should also include summaries of discussions from meetings. Unfortunately, lack of time is often cited as a reason for not documenting everything contemporaneously, but these records must be maintained, and must also be timely and monitored to account for events during time off.

Multidisciplinary discharge planning meetings

In settings or services where individuals have complex care needs, it is vital to hold multidisciplinary discharge planning meetings, and it is essential that these are conducted in an effective manner. The next section outlines how this can be achieved.

It is often difficult to find a time when all the team members are able to attend, due to other care duties/clinics/meetings. If a key member is not able to attend, this can sometimes interfere with ongoing plans, unless the person has provided adequate details of the patient's progress and concerns. Moroney & Knowles (2006) argue, however, that it is still better to go ahead with the meeting. A good time for many team members may not be a good time for nursing staff to attend, and yet the nurses are key members and central to coordination. Also, if a meeting is held at the end of the day, especially at the end of the week, this may make it harder to progress actions. None of these concerns is insurmountable. They are indeed an inevitable part of clinical life, and merely emphasise the importance of having a system in place to ensure that careful records are kept of progress and of actions that need to be taken.

What to cover in a multidisciplinary discharge planning meeting

First, the purpose of the meeting and expectations of what needs to be achieved should be made clear.

For each patient presented, there needs to be agreement about:

- The expected outcome (where and what level of care)
- The overall goal and individual goals and plan of care (to achieve the goals) from each member involved

- The expected/predicted date of discharge, or goals to be achieved before discharge is agreed so as to estimate predicted date of discharge
- What actions need to be undertaken to achieve discharge on this date, highlighting any significant blocks
- Who is, or needs to be, involved in this

Each discipline has to be clear about what needs to be achieved from their perspective if this outcome is to be achieved. The social worker should always be present at the meetings – and all contact details of 'area workers' should be available.

A review of possible barriers or constraints?

- These need to be identified and recorded
- Discussion should take place about what can be done to overcome them and how
- Individual needs to be identified and responsibility taken for addressing and resolving these, with a date by which it is expected that each one should be resolved
- The name of the person responsible for each action should be recorded, with a requirement to ensure that feedback is given on progress at the next meeting or sooner, as appropriate
- If no immediate solution can be found, the appropriate person to inform about this needs to be identified (e.g. the Director of Operations, Social Services or Chief Executive) and someone charged to undertake this, as action may be required at a higher level

Case conferences

If a case is very complex, it may be necessary to set up a case conference. This will require the presence of key people, such as community staff and relatives/carers. Where possible and appropriate, the patient should most certainly be present. Again, the purpose of such a meeting needs to be made clear and it needs to be well chaired. The outcomes of case conferences must be carefully recorded, as they address complex issues. They also provide a useful audit trail, and enable individual responsibility to be apportioned. An identified action plan, with a timescale for each aspect, is equally crucial.

Important considerations affecting complex discharges

Issues of time

There are several key challenges facing staff when they are trying to achieve a timely and effective discharge. A commonly identified concern is lack of time. There is no doubt that time is at a premium for healthcare staff, due to increasing patient dependency and increasing demands on their time, against a background of cuts in staffing and freezing of vacancies. Increasing fears of possible litigation and the need to make sure they 'cover their backs' both add to the pressure on staff. Well-organised care systems can help to ease these pressures if the documentation is focused and useful – and not too lengthy and onerous to complete.

The working practices and referral timescales of social services can be a challenge, and this is set to get worse, with the substantial reductions in funding that are now being made, as reported in the press in many areas. These financial pressures mean that hard decisions have to be made about how referrals are prioritised, which can lead to significant delays. Even when funding has been found, discharge may be delayed, due to difficulties in finding the care that is required – this is especially so where 'double-ups' (involving two carers or more) are involved. Waiting for continuing care assessments and decisions about funding can be another challenge, whilst the issue of patients or their carers finding ways to avoid or refuse discharge creates further challenges.

Illness trajectory/pathway and timescale

As discussed earlier, for goals to be set and a predicted date of discharge established, a good understanding is needed of the pathway of care, the trajectory and likely timescale of an individual's illness and the anticipated length of time they will require medical care in hospital. This may not be so easy for those who are frail and have complex needs, as their condition may fluctuate and they may be vulnerable to additional problems when unwell and/or have multiple needs. However, practitioners experienced in the field often have a general timescale in mind. This should act as a starting point, before identifying any constraints envisaged in arranging discharge or where intensive care needs are anticipated. Reassessment of the activities – in line with the discharge date – will be required, most importantly to inform their relatives and family of changes and the reasons for them.

Risk assessments

Risk assessment will be high on the agenda when making decisions about patients with complex care needs who are going back to their own homes. It is always necessary to undertake appropriate risk assessments, and in some situations it may involve taking some risk, with the possibility that the discharge may not be successful (Wade 2004). Whilst the individual has rights in terms of taking risks for themselves, these cannot be considered in isolation, for their own risks may impose risks on others. For example, a cooking pan accidentally catching fire in the kitchen may well create danger for others if the person is living in shared accommodation such as sheltered housing.

Where others are providing care or support, their safety must also be considered, and again a risk assessment may be required (Campbell 2001). Psychological risks also need to be considered, for example where a relative is required, or is offering, to give extensive help and has little or no support and little or no relief (not uncommon in contemporary health and social care scenarios). It is important to remember that all carers are eligible for their own carer's assessment (Carers (Recognition of Services) Act, DH 2000) and to have any benefits clarified and followed up.

Thus practitioners need to take many important decisions in relation to risk-taking. This is 'part and parcel' of successful rehabilitation and needs to be addressed in a recognised way that forms part of the clinical governance agenda. Decisions related to risk-taking are among many other decisions that often need to be made, and their importance should not be under-estimated. However, practitioners are perhaps becoming more risk-averse because of fear of litigation.

Home visits – pros and cons

Waiting for home visits can be problematic, especially as their effectiveness has been questioned (Bore 1994). Clark & Dyer (1998, p. 38) acknowledge that the patient is often in a state of anxiety on these occasions, and that the episodic nature of home visits means that the occupational therapist has little opportunity to monitor or evaluate them. Most areas now have established criteria that must be met to justify a home visit. But whatever the situation, when a home visit is deemed necessary, it needs to be timely and be arranged in a way that does not delay the progress of discharge. Involving community staff, who may already know the patient or who may need to be involved in the future, prior to discharge, may aid in planning these home visits and organising the most appropriate equipment, possibly saving time and money.

A home to go to?

Major delays in discharge can occur when a patient is homeless, becomes homeless, or needs adaptations to their home as a result of their changing care needs. In the past, there seemed to be only limited cooperation between health and housing services. This does seem to have improved in recent years, although there are still problems. There is often a need for considerable financial assessment, along with needs assessment. When re-housing is required, there may be long delays before appropriate housing becomes available. And if there are care needs, it may not be possible to set up care arrangements until the locality is known, causing further delay. When adaptations are required, there are often issues concerning who owns the property, and there may be delays in getting planning permission before work can even start.

Partnership working

While plans for discharge continue, care needs to be constantly evaluated and revised. It is important to communicate with the individual patient as far as they are able, as well as their family and friends, and any professionals and organisations involved in their care, to try to ensure that anything untoward has been anticipated and that plans seem acceptable (Johnson *et al.* 2003).

Where support is needed, it should be discussed and planned with those who will provide it, whilst also respecting and involving the patient. In this way, any concerns can be aired at an early stage and taken into account in planning, so helping to avoid delays. The required support may involve accessing funding or equipment (see Case study 2 below). Time spent on interventions to address these concerns is time very well spent.

Case study 2: Joe

Joe was a 78-year-old man who lived fairly independently in an upstairs flat. He sustained a stroke and it was evident at a fairly early stage that this would leave some significant left-sided weakness. This was likely to impede his mobility and almost certainly challenge his ability to climb stairs.

Joe was adamant that he wished to return home and so it was essential that plans were instigated at an early stage to discuss the various alternatives to enable Joe to fulfil his wishes. It was clear from the beginning that Joe would probably have residual disability and that changes would be necessary to adapt his flat.

It is true that, at this stage, the full impact of Joe's needs was not yet clear. Nevertheless, acknowledging the likely issues and being open and honest with Joe was important so that plans could be set in motion.

Discharge refusal

Many hospitals across the UK have experienced problems when patients (or relatives on behalf of patients) have refused to go home or be transferred to another setting. They may find different ways of delaying or preventing discharge, such as changing their mind about a care home once a place becomes available. Resolving delayed transfer of care is both a national and local priority.

From a legal perspective, once a person has been assessed as fit for discharge or transfer, it could be argued that they are trespassing, for there is no right to medical treatment. Article 8 of the European Convention on Human Rights requires that each individual's rights and those of their family are respected. An individual may allege that transfer of care violates their rights under Article 8. However, consideration needs to be given to another person's equivalent Article 8 rights – to a bed, in this case. It would be a breach of Article 2, the right to life, if a patient who no longer requires medical treatment refuses to be transferred. This would deprive another patient of medical treatment, which could adversely affect that patient's condition and prognosis (DH 2003).

Patients can use complaints procedures to delay discharge and this can eventually lead to a judicial review. It is therefore imperative that Trusts and staff are very explicit with patients and families about what they can reasonably expect from their stay in hospital, being clear about plans and dates for discharge and recording all discussions. If patients and their relatives are given appropriate verbal and written information throughout their contact with health professionals, then their expectations should be realistic and reasonable. If, through the Direction of Choice (LAC (92) 27, LAC (93) 18, and LAC (2004) 20), which recognises the importance of patient choice, a place is not available in the desired care home, alternative accommodation should be offered and means-tested. If a patient is eligible for social services funding and refuses the transfer of care option, they effectively adopt the status of a self-funder and become responsible for making their own arrangements. If the patient is a self-funder, efforts should be made to assist them in finding alternative accommodation.

Resolution of such issues requires stakeholders across healthcare and social care agencies to collaborate closely, and most Trusts now have agreed inter-agency standards and policies to address these issues satisfactorily – although the process does take time (OHA/OSS 2002). Where there are any concerns regarding impending problems, these need to be highlighted and referred to a higher level so that appropriate action can be instigated when appropriate.

Self-discharge

At the other end of the spectrum, staff can face real challenges when a patient who is not fit to be discharged, or who may be unsafe at home, or for whom care arrangements have not been finalised, elects to discharge themselves. If they are assessed as having capacity then there is a limit to what staff can do to prevent them going, apart from ensuring that the patient signs a self-discharge form. Staff can decline to arrange transport but if the patient is able to find their own transport, there may be little they can do to stop them. It could be argued that if they have the capacity to do this, the individual has capacity to manage at home. But in reality this may not be the case and their premature return may cause real problems for family, neighbours or community staff, which may lead to readmission or emergency care having to be put in place.

In an audit by Lees & Dyer (2008), it was found that high-risk patients do self-discharge. One major factor leading to self-discharge is that the 'patient feels better' and simply wants to go home, without being aware of all the issues/risks involved. Patients should always be counselled by a doctor prior to discharge; and in some cases they do then change their mind about self-discharge. Careful documentation of discussions with the patient is required.

Finalising discharge arrangements

Most settings and services have a checklist that is completed as discharge arrangements are made. The list usually includes the date when the arrangements are made and by whom, as well as a final checklist for the day of discharge. For patients with complex care needs, significant areas that need to be addressed include:

- The availability of the house key if no one will be there to welcome them, or organising a key safe at the home
- The availability of suitable clothing to go home in
- Clarity about transport and how this has been booked to tie in with care arrangements once home, if these are required
- Ensuring all after-care arrangements are in place and ready to start when the patient is home
- Provision of adequate support for lay carers, such as respite care/sitting, day/night care, counselling/emotional support

With the current challenges involving transport from hospitals, there needs to be a firm agreement that these patients will not be sent home late if there is a chance that they will arrive after the carer has been asked to visit. Most team members are familiar with these requirements, but it is still vital to complete the checklists. They act as a form of communication, and also provide a means of auditing or checking back if problems do arise (Lees 2010). There has been a significantly increased focus on checklists since the advent of the 'Ready to go?' (DH 2010) policy. This is advocated as one of the ten steps to successful discharge. In some cases, hospitals are including this on their array of ward metrics (standards) and regular feedback is provided for staff.

Conclusion

Effective and timely discharge of individuals is clearly important if their quality of life is to be promoted and if effective use of resources is to be maximised. It is evident that achieving this for those who are frail or who have complex and often fluctuating care needs is fraught with challenges. This is particularly true within large and unwieldy healthcare systems and social care services that are facing budgetary constraints, working alongside private or voluntary agencies. An increased focus on a whole systems approach, on better management of the processes involved, on effective mechanisms and a wider range of services to better address patients' needs, can provide a more robust infrastructure. If managed well, this infrastructure can enhance effective discharges. However, this is not to underestimate the demands made on staff involved in organising complex discharges, particularly as they often work under excessive and relentless pressure. Ensuring that staff are adequately prepared and experienced in using the skills required to deal with these complex discharges will aid them in their work.

References

Aboderin, I. (2004). Modernisation and ageing theory revisited: current explanations of recent developing world and historical western shifts in material family support for older people. *Ageing and Society.* **24**, 29–50.

Annells, M. (2004). Discharge from hospital: crocodile-infested water. *Journal of Clinical Nursing.* **13**, 537–538.

Armitage, S. (1981). Negotiating the discharge of medical patients. *Journal of Advanced Nursing.* **6**, 385–389.

Bengston, V.L., Rosenthal, C. & Burton, L.M. (1990). Families and Ageing: diversity and heterogeneity, in Binstock, R. & George, L. (eds), *Handbook of Ageing and the Social Sciences* (3rd edition). New York: Academic Press.

Booth, J. & Davis, C. (1991). Happy to be home? *Professional Nurse.* (March), 330–332.

Bore, J. (1994). Occupational therapy home visits; a satisfactory service? *British Journal of Occupational Therapy.* **57** (3), 85–89.

Bowling, A. & Betts, G. (1984). Communicating on discharge. *Nursing Times.* **80** (32), 31–32.

Bull, M.G. & Kane, R.L. (1996). Gaps in discharge planning. *Journal of Applied Gerontology.* **15** (4), 486–500.

Campbell, R. (2001). Predictors of caregiver burden over a three-month period following hospitalization of the patient. PhD dissertation, Digital Dissertations, University of Pennsylvania, PA, USA.

Carers UK (2010). 'New Plans for Carers' (2010). Caring October 2010. http://www.carersuk.org

Clark, H. & Dyer, S. (1998). Equipped for home from hospital. *Health Care in Later Life.* **3** (1), 36–45.

CSIP (2004/5). *Planning for Discharge. Health and Social Care Change Agent Team.* http://www.cat.csip.org.uk

CSIP (2008/2010). Extra Care Housing. http://www.ICN.CSIP.ORG.UK/housing/index.cfm?pid=716

Department of Health (1990). 'The NHS and Community Care Act'. London: HMSO.

Department of Health (2000). 'Carers (Recognition and Services) Act'. London: HMSO.

Department of Health (2003). 'Discharge from hospital: pathway, process and practice'. London: HMSO.

Department of Health (2005a). 'Supporting People with Long-Term Conditions: An NHS and Social Care Model to Support Local Innovation and Integration'. London: HMSO.

Department of Health (2005b). 'The National Service Framework for Long-Term Conditions'. London: HMSO.

Department of Health (2006). 'Our health, our say: a new direction for community services'. London: HMSO.

Department of Health (2008). 'End of Life Strategy – promoting high quality care for all adults at the end of life'. NHS 2008, 1–174. http://www.endoflifecareforadults.nhs.uk/eolc/DHELE. Strategy, July 2008.

Department of Health (2010). 'Ready to go? Planning the discharge and the transfer of patients from hospital and intermediate care'. London: HMSO.

Dinsdale, P. (2002). Call for radical overhaul of hospital discharge plans. *Nursing Standard.* **16**, 6.

Ellis, B.W. & Johnson, S. (1997). A clinical view of pathways of care in disease management. *International Journal of Health Care Quality Assurance.* **10** (2), 61–66.

Gould, D. (2002). Health-related infection and hand hygiene. *Nursing Times.* **98** (38), 48–51.

Hainsworth, T. (2005). A new model of care for people with long-term conditions. *Nursing Times.* **101** (3), 27–29.

Harwood, R., Kempson, R., Burke, N. & Morrant, J. (2002). Specialist nurses evaluate elderly in-patients referred to a department of geriatric medicine. *Age and Ageing.* **31**, 401–404.

Hudson, B. (2000). Inter-agency collaboration: a sceptical view, in Brechin, A., Brown, H. & Eby, M.A. (eds). *Critical Practice in Health and Social Care.* Milton Keynes: Open University Press.

Hunt, M. (1999). Multidisciplinary case notes: an audit. *Professional Nurse*. **14** (10), 701–703.

Illich, I. (1975). *Medical Nemesis*. London: Marion Boyars Ltd.

Internurse.com (2007). Cuts to District Nursing Hit Social Services – News – Independent Nurse 2007. http://www.internurse.com

Jewell, S. (1993). Discovery of the discharge process: a study of patients discharged from a care unit for elderly people. *Journal of Advanced Nursing*. **18**, 1288.

Johnson, A., Sandford, J. & Tyndall, J., (2003). Written and verbal information versus information only for patients being discharged from acute hospital settings to home. Cochrane Review, in The Cochrane Library 4. Chichester: John Wiley and Sons.

LAC (92) 27: National Assistance Act 1948 (Choice Accommodation Direction 1992).

LAC (93) 18 National Assistance Act 1948 (Choice of Accommodation) (Amendment) (England) Directions 1993 amendments to the Statutory Direction Of Choice.

LAC (2004) 20: Guidance on National Assistance Act 1948 (Choice of Accommodation) Directions 1992 and National Assistance (Residential Accommodation) (Additional Payments and Assessment of Resources) (Amendment) (England) Regulations 2001.

Lasslett, P. (1989). *A Fresh Map of Life*. London: Weidenfeld & Nicolson.

Lees, L. & Dyer, P. (2008). Why patients self discharge. *Nursing Management*. **15** (2), 22–26.

Lees, L. (2010). Exploring the principles of Best Practice discharge to ensure patient involvement. *Nursing Times*. **106** (25), 10–4.

Lees, L. & Holmes, K. (2005). Estimating a date of discharge at ward level: a pilot study. *Nursing Standard*. **19** (17), 40–43.

Lees L. & Emmerson, K. (2006). Identifying discharge practice training needs. *Nursing Standard*. **20** (29), 47–51.

Lees, L., Allen, G. & O'Brien, D. (2006). Using post-take ward rounds to facilitate simple discharge. *Nursing Times*. **102** (18), 28–30.

Lewis, G. (2007). Virtual Wards – real nursing. *Nursing Standard*. **21** (43), 64.

The Marie Curie Palliative Care Institute (2005). Care Pathways for the Dying. www.mcp cil.org.uk/files/LCP HOSPITAL VERSION

McKenna, H., Keeny, S., Glenn, A. & Gordon, P. (2000). Discharge planning: an exploratory study. *Journal of Clinical Nursing*. **9**, 594–601.

Middleton, S. & Roberts, A. (2000). *Integrated Care Pathways: A Practical Approach to Implementation*. Oxford: Butterworth-Heinemann.

Moroney, N. & Knowles, C. (2006). Innovation and teamwork: introducing multidisciplinary team Social Service (May 2002).

New South Wales Health Department (2001). Shared responsibility for patient care between hospitals and the community – an effective discharge policy. Australia: NSW Health Department.

Oliver, S. (2006). Benefits of patient pathways in rheumatoid arthritis care. *Nursing Times*. **102** (16), 28–31.

Oxford Health Authority and Oxfordshire Social Service (May 2002). Oxfordshire Acute and Community Hospitals Transfer of Care (Discharge) Inter Agency Standards. Oxfordshire: Oxford Health Authority and Oxfordshire Social Service.

Penhale, B. (1997). Towards effective discharge planning. *Health Care in Later Life*. **2** (1), 46–55.

Payne, S., Kerr, C., Hawker, S., Hardey, M. & Powell, J. (2002). The communication of information about older people between health and social care practitioners. *Age and Ageing*. **31**, 107.

Robinson, A. & Street, A. (2004). Improving networks between acute care and an aged care assessment team. *Journal of Clinical Nursing*. **13**, 486–496.

Rout, A., Ashby, S. & Maslin-Prothero, S. (2011). A literature review of interprofessional working and intermediate care in the U.K. *Journal of Clinical Nursing*. **20** (5–6) 775–783.

Sargent, P. & Boaden, R. (2006). Implementing the role of the community matron. *Nursing Times*. **102** (13), 23–24.

Shefter, S.M. (2006). Workflow technology: the new frontier. How to overcome the barriers and join the future. *Lippincott's Case Management*. **11** (1), 25–34 (Jan-Feb).

Shepperd, S., Parkes, J., McClaran, J. & Phillips, C. (2004). Discharge planning from hospital. *The Cochrane Database of Systematic Reviews*. Issue 1, CD000313. DOI.

Stearns, P.N. (1976). *Old Age in European Society*. New York: Holmes & Meir.

Tripp, I. & Caan, W. (1999). Is post-rehabilitation discharge of older people successful? *British Journal of Therapy and Rehabilitation*. **6** (10), 500–504.

Victor, C. & Vetter, N.J. (1988). Preparing the elderly for discharge home: a neglected aspect of care. *Age and Ageing*. **17**, 155–163.

Victor, C.R., Young, E., Hudson, M. & Wallace, P. (1993). 'Whose responsibility is it anyway?' Hospital admission and discharge of older people in an inner-London District Health Authority. *Journal of Advanced Nursing*. **18**, 1297–1304.

Wade, S. (2004). *Intermediate Care of Older People*. London: Whurr Publishers Ltd.

Waterworth, S. & Luker, K. (1990). Reluctant collaborators: do patients want to be involved in decisions concerning their care? *Journal of Advanced Nursing*. **15**, 971–976.

Weick, K.E. & Quinne, R.E. (1999). Organisational change and development. *Annual Review of Psychology*. **50** (1), 361–386.

Werret, J., Helm, R. & Carnell, R. (2001). The primary and secondary care interface: the educational needs of nursing staff for the provision of seamless care. *Journal of Advanced Nursing*. **34** (5), 629–638.

Chapter 10

An exploration of discharge coordinator roles

Liz Lees and Marie MacKenzie

Discharge coordinators were originally introduced in hospitals to improve the quality of discharge planning. The role is not new, but the way in which it is being adopted and integrated into clinical areas is changing. Discharge coordinators are now being introduced in the NHS in England and Wales in a variety of guises, and their role is relatively unsupported compared to other new roles, either nationally or locally. As the name suggests, their primary function is to coordinate the patient's discharge, improving liaison and communication between members of the multidisciplinary team (Shepperd *et al.* 2004).

There is a huge need to represent patients and carers, and guide them through the complexities of choice involved in planning for discharge from hospital. Equally there is a need to support the multidisciplinary team in the clinical area, to ensure that there is a central point of contact and continuity in the busy ward environment. The concept of discharge coordination therefore requires exploration, to identify its essential requirements and enable better understanding.

This chapter aims to:

- Provide a thorough explanation of the discharge coordination role
- Describe the core elements of the discharge coordinator role
- Differentiate between simple and complex discharge coordination roles
- Analyse ambiguity in discharge planning roles and associated job titles
- Make recommendations for those considering establishing such a role

Policy context

A noteworthy, inspiring guidance document, namely *Freedom to Practise*, combined case examples of patient care from the point of referral to the point of discharge with explanations of what nurses and allied health professionals are allowed and able to do within their Codes of Practice; it also included mechanisms to facilitate nurse leadership in the discharge processes (DH & RCN 2003). Moving the focus away from traditionally bureaucratic processes, which often seem distanced from the reality of everyday clinical practice, the radical approach of *Freedom to Practise* provided a quantum leap of tangible support for healthcare professionals dealing with hospital discharge.

A second strand of policy, reiterated in several policy documents, recommends developing key named individuals to act as discharge coordinators at ward level (modules 4a and 4b of www.dischargetraining.doh.gov.uk). Some may argue this is not a new concept and may have its roots outside the realm of discharge planning, in systems of ward organisation, leadership at the ward level and management. Whatever its origin, the policy is meant to provide members of the multidisciplinary team (MDT) and other agencies with a named person whose responsibility it is to liaise between them and coordinate the discharge plan (DH 2003).

Defining a discharge coordinator's role

A discharge coordinator is a person who has the designated responsibility of ensuring that the core aspects of the patient's discharge plan are in place in a timely manner and that the discharge process is started before admission (in elective cases), or as soon as the patient is medically stable (in emergency cases). A discharge coordinator usually liaises with the patient, family, carers and staff. A great deal of their time may be spent in managing the carers' and family's expectations as an 'advocate, negotiator and conflict resolution manager' (Chandler *et al.* 2010). Discharge coordinators are kept fully informed on all aspects of the patient's progress up to the point of discharge. They also often (but not always) follow up the patient after discharge. For example, NHS patients in receipt of continuing care are now followed up by community nurse liaison coordinators, rather than discharge coordinators who are based in hospitals. This change has been made in order to facilitate continuity of care and to enable those working in hospital settings to concentrate on their acute workload (DH 2009).

Yet the discharge coordinator's role cannot be a guaranteed role within every ward establishment, and elements of the role can vary tremendously from one clinical area to another. There is no single definition (Chandler *et al.* 2010). For instance, the role is sometimes designed with bespoke elements to suit the needs of a particular clinical area or pathway of care. Discharge coordinators themselves also make the role their own, which may mean that they anticipate and respond to the needs within their clinical environment and the team they work alongside. The decision to employ a discharge coordinator lies solely with the individual ward manager of a clinical area. However, this lack of consistency makes it notoriously difficult to extrapolate and measure patient and organisational outcomes, because not every ward has a discharge coordinator.

Evolution of the discharge coordinator's role – complex discharges

Discharge coordinators for complex patient discharges have been in existence for many years (Peters *et al.* 1997). Throughout the 1990s, coordinators were usually employed as part of a central hospital service called a discharge liaison team, whose primary function was to expedite predominantly complex discharges. Complex discharges were regarded as those where patients required the services of health and social care professionals in order to facilitate discharge from hospital to home, probably on a long-term basis with continuing healthcare needs (DH 2009). In addition, these complex discharge coordinators often interfaced with social work teams to collaborate on patient assessments, providing a unified health and social care perspective to guide decision-making (Holliman *et al.* 2003). This model of working meant that discharge planning communications from a ward were centralised through the discharge coordinators, who in turn managed the entire pathway of care.

The roles of social worker and nurse in discharge planning are entirely complementary; social workers understand the financial elements of patient assessment and counselling. Moreover, with the increasing complexity of social situations, including late divorce, homelessness, family members living at a distance from each other, and the rising incidence of dementia, social workers are trained to help with decisions regarding care and the wider social perspectives in such cases (see Chapter 9). Nurses provide information on the patients' nursing/medical status and actively teach patients about feeding tubes, skin care, medications, oxygen, dressings, and so on, which will enable nursing care to be continued after discharge.

This role continues today, albeit with attendant NHS policy differences aimed at securing funding, declaring fitness to discharge and referral to the correct Community Trust or Primary Care Trust (Sergeant *et al.* 2007). Additionally, with the increasing focus on end-of-life care, discharge coordinators are starting to specialise in this area in order to manage the transition from hospital to home smoothly and rapidly (DH 2008). (For more on this subject, see Chapter 21.)

The success (or otherwise) of the complex discharge coordinator role could be measured by the number of patients who are readmitted because the care arranged may not have been adequate for their needs (care failure) or measured by the number of 'changes' to a care package, post discharge. Changes to a care package do not always mean an increase in care. Some families simply cannot cope with a bombardment of carers in the home after discharge; as a consequence they may choose to cancel care arrangements. This may also lead to a care failure but for reasons other than inadequate care. In this case it may be inappropriate care that is the primary cause of readmission (see Chapter 9 on social diagnosis). However, it has been suggested that data of this specific nature is not collected in sufficient detail to pinpoint such issues.

With the introduction of a vast array of other new roles, the emphasis has shifted from expanding the traditional discharge coordinator role in acute hospitals, to Primary Care Trusts taking shared responsibility for expediting the patient's discharge (DH 2005). For example, the concept of 'pulling patients out of hospital' to reduce the length of inpatient stay and 'reducing inappropriate admissions' were the key drivers for the development of new community roles. Community matrons and other community-based healthcare staff provide a vital link between multi-professional clinical planning and the services/resources available to turn the plans into reality.

The key areas of expertise required for these roles are:

1. Taking responsibility for the whole process of discharge (not just individual tasks)
2. Ensuring a safe discharge
3. Working inextricably with the MDT
4. Being able to navigate a way around services to expedite discharge
5. Understanding community services and making links
6. Generating one's own workload and prioritising this
7. Being able to act as a patient's advocate
8. Being a resource and conduit for staff needing information
9. Providing informal teaching and cascading of information
10. Giving in-depth assessment of patients' healthcare needs
11. Continuing the development of one's own specialist knowledge
12. Providing equipment needed after discharge

Evolution of the discharge coordinator role – simple discharges

At the same time as the discharge coordinator's role has been developed for complex discharges, there has been gargantuan change in the way simple patient discharges are managed at ward level (DH 2004, 2010). The role is different from that of a complex discharge coordinator and may be undertaken by an experienced member of the administrative team and not necessarily a registered practitioner (nurse). An administrative (non-registered) coordinator of simple discharges will be able to handle communication tasks, thus releasing registered nursing time to care for patients.

Simple discharge coordinators carry out the following types of functions:

- Purposeful selection of patients to transfer to inpatient wards (to ensure patients' suitability against criteria from the accepting ward)
- Coordinating the patient's transport and medications for discharge
- Arranging transfer of the patient to a discharge lounge.
- Liaising with family and carers – updating them regarding MDT meetings
- Attending daily capacity (bed) meetings to report on expected bed capacity
- Liaising with nurses, doctors and MDT
- Carrying out simple discharge tasks consistently
- Inputting data systems to report bed capacity
- Requesting an assessment from social care (upon instruction from registered nurse)

(Systems and process have been developed to give a hospital-wide view of the daily discharges at ward level. The simple discharge coordinator is therefore usually responsible for communication of this from ward to Board level – at least in the submission of patient discharge figures (those that have been projected, those that have been determined and those that are delayed).)

This list is by no means exhaustive but the common trend is to improve communications at ward level and expedite discharge.

Sharing the role – a few words of caution

A registered nurse carrying out a discharge coordinator's role often develops his or her expertise on the job, and there is no programme of formal or recognised training. In some instances, the role is allocated to several nurses in the ward team, depending on their experience and ability to undertake it. The individual allocation of a nurse takes place on a daily basis. There is undoubtedly some overlap with the role of a non-registered discharge coordinator, but registered discharge coordinators are distinctive in that they are able to carry out nursing assessments and risk assessments, and coordinate nursing care – ready for discharge of the patient.

While this may sound like a sensible way to organise the coordination of patient discharge, it can only succeed if there are sufficient nurses on the ward rota to undertake the role. If there are not enough staff to carry it out, the role may not be in operation every day. Senior nurses are responsible for determining the vision for the ward team. If the coordinator's role is not valued or understood, wards may not choose to recruit them. However, if the coordinator role were to be planned as part of workforce changes and patient outcomes, the role could consequently be integrated into all ward areas.

Distinguishing between registered and non-registered roles

Discharge coordination is a generally accepted term that is used to describe the activities encompassed in instigating, organising and actively expediting a patient's discharge from hospital. The term 'discharge coordinator' is often used interchangeably with 'discharge liaison nurse'; this can create the illusion that their roles are synonymous. However, this is not the case and the distinction must be made clear.

A discharge coordinator may not always be a registered practitioner. If they are not registered, they will only concentrate on tasks that are primarily of a simple coordination nature and do not involve nursing or financial assessments. Conversely, if the discharge coordinator is a registered nurse, they may be allowed to carry out registered nurse functions but will not have taken on a role where the sole focus is discharge planning. Discharge will be one part of a wider role in the clinical environment where they work.

A discharge liaison nurse will be a registered practitioner (usually an experienced nurse) and their role will involve comprehensive and complex patient assessments, financial assessment and holistic care planning, to the point of handover to community teams for post-discharge care. They will specialise in this role to the extent that they may not be a member of a ward team – and may even have responsibility for complex discharges across a group of wards.

Overlaps, interfaces, similarities and confusion

There are often overlaps and interfaces in different roles, which can cause confusion. The list of discharge coordinator responsibilities at the end of this chapter illustrates this point perfectly. For example, while most are simple tasks, there are simple and complex tasks on the same list (see Appendix 1, p. 165. It may be advantageous for the patient to accept the role overlaps, for instance, when complex care packages require simple activities to be completed in order to expedite discharge from hospital. Nevertheless, it must be remembered that in person-centred care patients and relatives will not want to engage with several different discharge coordinators, social workers and ward staff members, as this will prove laborious, confusing and indeed counterproductive (Cox 1996). In fact, if too many professionals are involved it may well serve to delay a patient's discharge from hospital.

A deeper exploration of the discharge coordinator's role

In order to gain a deeper understanding of the various roles, ten semi-structured interviews were undertaken between June and September 2010. These interviews covered a range of roles, using a survey instrument. The instrument had eight sections, which included: demographics, core elements, simple and complex role descriptors, the model of communication and team working, advanced level descriptors and perceived benefits of the role. Of the ten semi-structured interviews, seven different job titles were revealed. These are listed below:

- Discharge Liaison Nurse/Sister
- Communication Nurse
- Clinical Nurse Specialist for Discharge Planning
- Complex Discharge Planning Sister
- Community Liaison Sister
- Discharge Planning Nurse
- Ward Discharge Coordinator (x3)

The NHS pay bands ranged from Band 2 to Band 7. The Band 2 post was predominantly an administrative role, carrying out simple coordination tasks, and was not involved in patient assessment. The Band 7 post was a registered nurse, undertaking comprehensive and complex discharges, with a remit interfacing hospital and community. In such cases, the respective differences in the roles were quantified by the levels of responsibility and the differences between non-registered and registered practitioners.

The areas of greatest ambiguity were perhaps in the middle-range posts, in Bands 3, 4 and 5, where the most role overlap was evident. It is not necessarily the case that a Band 5 coordinator will be a registered practitioner. Experience, and the ability to navigate the intricacies of referrals, assessments, documentation and knowledge in the area, can make this almost a niche role for administrative staff. In these clinical areas, there was also tension evident within the team, and confusion regarding levels of responsibility. For example, feedback from interviews indicated that there were difficulties for non-registered staff when it came to having the required level of authority to influence issues regarding discharge practice at ward level.

Hours of work

Seven out of the ten posts were full-time, with flexible working arrangements to suit the clinical areas where they were aligned. Some worked family-friendly hours, starting later in the day. The three part-time roles ranged from 22.5 hours to 30 hours per week.

Four of the ten posts were included in the shift numbers and were also expected to carry a caseload of patients and coordinate the ward. The remaining six posts were not included in the shift numbers, allowing these members of staff to concentrate on expediting discharges and releasing capacity in a timely manner. Only one of the posts had a job description for the role of coordinator.

Core elements of the roles

A literature search was undertaken to identify commonly occurring themes that would assist the definition of core elements or functions of discharge coordinator roles. These were divided into three key areas (whilst accepting that there would be a degree of overlap), namely:

1. Bed management
2. Bed coordination
3. Bed administration

These three key areas were further analysed to identify activities within each one (see table below).

Bed management	Attend bed meetings, gather audit data on discharge times and numbers of discharges, coordinate capacity, report to general manager, update estimated discharge dates
Bed coordination	Make clinical decision on who to admit, arrange transfers to discharge lounge, liaise for shift on behalf of ward team
Bed administration	Update electronic systems, arrange declaration of beds, escalate issues

The above table represents bed coordination as a micro-function in an organisational context. However, it must be remembered that coordination is a function that links together key roles or people responsible for capacity within an organisation, for the greater good of the patients.

The discharge coordinator's role was further explored using a concept analysis tool (Walker & Avant 1995), to understand why such roles might be introduced, what it is they critically need to possess to succeed, and finally what it is an organisation hopes to achieve from them.

A conceptual analysis of the role

Using a concept analysis, the discharge coordinator role can be analysed from three perspectives: antecedents, critical attributes and consequences, as summarised below.

Concept analysis framework

Antecedents:

- The need to expedite discharges from hospital
- The need to improve communication
- The need to align responsibility for coordination

Critical attributes:

- A discharge process
- Focused time to carry out the functions within the process
- Good communication and assessment skills
- A good knowledge of the referral mechanisms and access to services
- Well networked within the MDT

Consequences:

- Improved quality of discharge from hospital
- Patient-centred care and patient advocacy
- Reduction in length of stay (by comparison to matched wards without a coordinator)
- Leadership and coordination of discharge from hospital

Adapted from Walker & Avant (1995).

Future career opportunities

Finally, during the interview process coordinators were asked about their future career aspirations. It was acknowledged by nearly all of the junior registered nurses that the role was useful to 'gain experience of discharge planning' and to 'understand how organisational processes work', both of which were also cited as good for advancing through the clinical career bandings. There was, however, little conversation regarding career progression or a career pathway from registered nurses already undertaking such a role as a specialist post, such as discharge liaison nurses. Inevitably, once in these posts, it seems that discharge liaison nurses needing further development may not be well linked into a pathway that builds upon their existing knowledge and skills. It has been suggested that many opportunities exist to extend the scope of the role, particularly in the rapid discharge of patients, in taking on a role in the protection of vulnerable patients, and in caring for those with dementia who need additional assistance in their discharge planning.

Those coordinators undertaking a role in a non-registered capacity, while feeling valued as team members, expressed concerns regarding the lack of structure to enable them to change roles, let alone advance their roles. Their discussion focused mainly on 'needing support to get processes right on the ward' and wanting 'to be involved in plans regarding discharge planning'. The future for support worker roles is potentially bright, with abundant opportunities, given the financial constraints that exist in the NHS and the move towards giving support workers more prominent roles in supporting registered staff.

Pros and cons

Discharge coordination posts expertly serve the needs of individual clinical areas. However, it could be argued that an isolated discharge role can be detrimental to patient care, especially at times of annual leave or sickness, when no one else on the team may have the knowledge or skills needed to discharge patients, causing a potential halt in discharges from that area. In addition, such roles must be supported to keep abreast of new policies. They must ensure that they remain on course and avoid falling prey to changing agendas at ward level.

There is a difficult balance to be struck between the two options: employing a discharge coordinator to pragmatically get the job done, while risking the de-skilling of ward nurses; or sharing the responsibility of discharge planning across the team in order to retain and share the skills, despite the risk of a loss of focus on discharge at times when other aspects of care take priority.

Recommendations for the establishment of discharge coordinator roles

Firstly, discharge coordinator roles should be part of the organisational business plan and be transferable from one clinical area to another. However, bespoke roles that have been established to fit a process or pathway in a specific clinical area may not have transferability across an organisation. If the post-holder leaves the role, it may not be possible to find a replacement person with the same skill set. Job descriptions should therefore be reviewed, to ensure that they include core skills and responsibilities that align with organisational needs. Individual areas should be discouraged from creating their own job descriptions. A better solution would be for the Personnel/Human Resources Department to carry out this function and then only minor variations should be needed at ward level before the role can be introduced.

Alignment with NHS or other quality frameworks such as Commissioning for Quality and Innovation (CQUIN) can also be very helpful. Coordinators with responsibility for monitoring the progress of patients when they go back into the community are in a prime position to engage with initiatives to reduce the readmission rates for those patients at risk of readmission within 28 days. To some extent, discharge coordinators are already involved with actively preventing readmissions – but data demonstrating input and outcome from such activity may not be collated. This is where an 'invest to save' approach could be considered, implemented and evaluated.

To justify investment, discharge coordinator roles should be established to aim for a reduction in the length of stay (outcomes) and an increase in the quality of discharge. Discharge coordinators will need to remain highly focused on expediting discharges from hospital. Discharge outcomes could be set at: achieving discharge earlier in the day; achieving a determined volume of discharges each day; ensuring beds are freed within a specific timeframe, from point of 'fitness to discharge' within an hour, for example.

Discharge coordinators should also be given the task of stimulating a predicted, estimated length of stay for patients: promoting amongst the ward team (but not necessarily setting) an agreed estimated date of discharge (EDD); and assisting in the planning required to ensure safe and effective discharge achievement of the date. To this end, variances could also be measured.

Discharge coordinators must be integrated within a fully functioning MDT: a discharge coordinator role must work in a trans-disciplinary manner (across members of the team), to ensure transparency in communications. In cases where the coordinator attends the MDT meetings as part of their role, this must be accepted by all team members and the functions of the coordinator need to be clear.

Finally, a discharge coordinator should not be employed to speed up discharges without due respect for the processes with which they work and the people with whom they co-exist.

Appendix I

WARD DISCHARGE COORDINATORS

Responsible for:

- Attending patient discharge reviews every morning
- Update the discharge capacity system by 11 am, 3 pm
- Instigating Sections 2 and 5 (UK – community health assessments to be completed by senior nurse)
- Identifying patient's functional and social needs on admission (following nurse assessment)
- Completing the social history document
- Informing the patient at this time that you are discussing their discharge arrangements and informing them of their estimated date of discharge
- Filing social history document
- Escalating potential barriers to discharge to the ward coordinator/manager or matron on a daily basis; if potential problems are identified on completion of the social history document, they are to be escalated at this time – not when the patient is medically fit
- Attending the board round – by the ward whiteboard and giving discharge updates with medical team and ward coordinator at 12 noon and 4 pm
- Mini-handover after each bay, following ward round with coordinator if you do not attend the round
- Being responsible for clearly identifying patients who can go to discharge lounge on the day of discharge
- Ensuring that tablets to take out (TTOs) and external prescriptions FPIOs are completed 24 hours prior to discharge and ready by 11 am on the day of discharge
- Ensuring that transport is booked for AM discharge on the day of discharge or

asking relatives to collect patients by 11 am on the day of discharge
- Being responsible for notifying relatives of discharge date and time
- Completing the discharge checklist (first two sections), then clipping it to TTO for nurse to complete
- Ensuring that a social worker is allocated to patients after Section 2 is completed and generating a Section 5 when appropriate
- Being available at visiting time to give feedback to relatives and plan discharge
- Liaising with MDT as necessary during shift

References

Chandler, L., Wyatt, M. & Roberts, I. (2010). Lost in Translation – reviewing the role of the discharge liaison nurse in Wales. *Journal of Health Service Management Research.* **23** (1), 1–4.

Cox, C.B. (1996). Discharge planning for dementia patients: factors influencing caregiver decisions and satisfaction. *Health and Social Work.* **21**, 97–104.

Department of Health & Royal College of Nursing (2003). *Freedom to practise: dispelling the myths.* London: HMSO.

Department of Health (2003). 'Discharge from hospital: pathway, process and practice'. London: HMSO.

Department of Health (2004). 'Achieving "simple" timely discharge from hospital: a multidisciplinary toolkit'. London: HMSO.

Department of Health (2005). 'Case management [competencies] framework for the care of people with long-term conditions'. London: HMSO.

Department of Health (2008). 'End of life care strategy: promoting high quality care for all adults at the end of life'. London: HMSO.

Department of Health (2009). 'The National Framework for NHS continuing healthcare and NHS-funded nursing care'. London: HMSO.

Department of Health (2010). 'Ready to go? Planning the discharge and transfer of patients from hospital and intermediate care'. Quarry House, Leeds: Department of Health.

Holliman, D., Dziegielewski, S.F. & Teare, R. (2003). Differences and similarities between social work and nurse discharge planners. *Health and Social Work.* **28** (3), 224–231.

Peters, P., Fleuren, M. & Wijkel, D. (1997). The quality of the discharge planning process: the effect of a liaison nurse. *International Journal for Quality in Health Care.* **9** (4), 283–287.

Sargent, P., Pickard, S., Sheaff, R. & Boaden, R. (2007). Patient and carer perceptions of case management for long term care. *Health and Social Care in the Community.* **15** (6), 511–519.

Shepperd, S., McClaran, J., Phillips, C.O., Lannin, N.A., Clemson, L.M., McCluskey, A., Cameron, I.D. & Barras, S.L. (2010). 'Discharge planning from hospital to home'. Cochrane Database of Systematic Reviews 2010, Issue 1. Art. No.: CD000313. DOI: 10.1002/14651858. CD000313.pub3

Walker, L., & Avant, K. (1995). *Strategies for Theory Construction in Nursing.* Norwalk, CT: Appleton & Lange.

Chapter 11

Occupational therapists and collaborative working

Jo Brady

This chapter highlights the significance of occupational therapists (OTs) and nurses working in partnership with the multidisciplinary team (MDT) to achieve seamless discharge planning from an acute hospital setting. It addresses the role of the OT and the way OTs work, and links all this together within a patient-centred approach to hospital discharge.

Setting the scene

Effective discharge planning should commence as soon as a person is admitted to hospital, (or earlier, if there has been an opportunity to attend a preadmission clinic). Discharge plans should be reviewed seven days a week, throughout the hospital stay.

In January 2003, the Department of Health issued 'Discharge from hospital: pathway, process and practice' to assist the MDT with discharge planning. Fundamental to its approach is the idea that 'discharge from hospital is a process, not an isolated event'. As part of this process, assessment may be required to determine the level of care and support needed to support safe discharge from hospital. How this information is gathered will vary according to local policy at individual hospitals. However, it is the shared responsibility of all members of the MDT who are involved in the patient's care. This team may include occupational therapists, physiotherapists, social workers, nurses and speech therapists, among others.

The role of the OT and assessment for discharge planning

The role of the OT will be presented in this chapter, to promote a wider knowledge and understanding of the principles, concepts and application of occupational therapy. Underpinning all discharge planning is accurate information gathering, good communication, effective liaison and consideration of more than one professional perspective. These aspects will be demonstrated and supported by case examples to highlight how a holistic, multi-professional approach can increase confidence and support safe timely discharges.

The unique aim of occupational therapy is to assess the complex physical, psychological, cognitive and social needs of individuals in order to support them, to maximise their potential, and help them lead healthy and fulfilling lives by improving their function. The specialised problem-solving skills of OTs mean that they can deliver rapid assessment and maintain a patient-focused holistic approach.

Occupational therapy aims to enable and empower people to be competent and confident in their daily lives, to promote their well-being and minimise the effects of dysfunction and environmental barriers. In order to achieve these aims, OTs (in partnership with patients) use everyday tasks therapeutically to achieve meaningful goals that are relevant to patients' daily lives.

Many activities of daily living are so familiar that they are 'taken for granted'. Function could be described as the activity of being occupied mentally and/or physically. Being 'occupied' in this way is necessary to our very existence, but this type of activity may not be consciously recognised, and can therefore be 'taken for granted'. Functional status is the vital marker that determines how a patient is discharged. At this point, the OT and the nursing team collaborate closely to address any concerns that are influencing discharge planning. Effective communication with the wider MDT helps to achieve a safe and coordinated discharge from hospital.

What is occupational therapy?

- What is it?
- Why is it important
- How does it work?
- And what role does the OT have in supporting discharge planning?

The OT role is to assist patients to gain or regain functional independence in all possible aspects of daily activity. Essentially, the OT should adopt a holistic, person-centred, problem solving-approach, viewing 'purposeful .... activities as a means of restoring health, function and quality of life' (Hagedorn 2000, p. 6). Such activities are 'as necessary as food and drink' (Miller & Walker 1993, cited in Hagedorn 2000, p. 6).

In the 2004 Department of Health document, 'Achieving timely "simple" discharge from hospital: A toolkit for the multi-disciplinary team', it is suggested that: 'At least 80% of patients discharged from hospital can be classified as simple discharges: they are discharged to their own home and have simple ongoing health care needs which can be met without complex planning.'

Whether they are involved in 'simple' or 'complex' discharge planning, OTs often act as the 'hub of the wheel'. Standing with the patient and alongside nurses, the OT has a pivotal role in networking, coordinating and liaising with many and varied personnel. The complexity of the discharge plan depends on the patient's circumstances and discharge planning needs, and the relative complexity of the discharge ultimately dictates the level of involvement of the MDT. The table below illustrates the wide range of people with whom a hospital OT regularly communicates in order to facilitate discharge.

The OT network for discharge planning (Adapted from Turner *et al.* 1996)

Patient				
Family	**Friends**	**Neighbours**	**Carers**	
WARD	ALLIED HEALTH PROFESSIONALS	COMMUNITY	RESOURCES	AGENCIES
Medical team – consultant	OTs	Social service OT	Equipment stores	Voluntary, cultural or religious
Nurses	OT technicians	Community OT & physiotherapist	Equipment suppliers and manufacturers	services, e.g. Focus or RNIB
Healthcare assistants	Physiotherapist Discharge liaison nurse	GP	Wheelchair assessment centre	Employment services
Ward clerks	Speech therapist	District nurse	Functional assessment centre	City housing department
	Dietician	Social worker	Specialist assessment teams	
	Chiropodist	Community psychiatric nurse		
	Psychologist	Assertive case managers		
	Continuing care nurses	Intermediate care		
	Psycho-geriatrician	Home care services		
	Interpreters	Residential services		
	Social work, – hospital and community	Wardens		

Inevitably, there is some overlap between disciplines but, in liaising with such a broad range of individuals on behalf of the patient, the OT and nurses both play a central role in coordinating and driving forward the discharge plan. J.A. Mattison, writing in

1929 (cited in Trombly 1995, p. 10) described the OT as '(providing) every opportunity for the coordination of all hospital efforts toward returning the patient to community life and economic usefulness'. This description still captures the importance and value of the OT's relationship with nurses, in the facilitation of discharge planning. In other words, no single professional is individually responsible for facilitating discharge; it always requires liaison and teamwork.

In an acute hospital setting, liaison with the nursing team and medics is of major importance in establishing a patient's medical status, their likely prognosis and their anticipated length of stay. Collaborative working will achieve seamless, safe, successful discharges and reduce the risk of readmission.

Of equal importance to the success (or otherwise) of the discharge planning process is liaison with the patient's significant others. These include family, friends, neighbours and carers, who can make vital contributions towards meeting the patient's needs and wishes (Turner *et al.* 1996).

Problem-solving and patient function

A problem-solving approach facilitates personal independence and autonomy, enabling the focus of intervention to be the individual person. Fundamental to its efficacy is the assessment of functional activity and the evaluation of the outcome, using activity analysis.

Activity is central to the philosophy of occupational therapy. To gain an understanding of the true nature, value and application of occupational therapy in the discharge planning process, it is therefore necessary to understand the concept of activity analysis.

Activities of daily living have been referred to as people being engaged 'in doing simple things' (Hagedorn 2000, p. 3). That which is 'simple' is defined as 'easily understood or done; presenting no difficulty; consisting of or involving only one element or operation' (Allen 1990). However, being able to perform many activities of daily living requires a very complex interaction of skills and abilities.

A fundamental principle of occupational therapy is to bridge the gap between dysfunction and function. This requires an understanding of the inherent qualities of each activity. It will then be possible to restructure the activity so that the patient can accomplish it.

In the hospital setting, where time and resources are limited, the OT will use an activity that encompasses a wide range of performance components, yet is familiar and non-threatening, such as making a hot drink. As demonstrated in the table below, the most routine of tasks requires a complex interaction of mind and body performance components, clearly consisting of more than one element or operation. Perhaps such activities would be better described as 'commonplace' or 'routine and habitual' because describing them as 'simple' can devalue their use, meaning and worth.

Making a hot drink – activity analysis

(Adapted from AOTA 1994, Turner *et al.* 1996)

Performance area	Making tea
Performance task analysis	1 Enter kitchen 2 Assemble necessary items 3 Fill kettle 4 Prepare mug 5 Make tea 6 Drink tea

Performance components
Performance demands

Motor	Sensory	Cognitive	Perceptual	Emotional	Social
Mobility Standing balance/tolerance Muscle strength Exercise tolerance Energy levels/oxygen Gross movements of upper body – bending, stretching, reaching – core stability Gross movements of upper limbs – shoulder ab/adduction, rotation, forearm pronation/supination Fine movements upper limb – wrist + hand, grip ability and strength, joint flexion/extension Hand to mouth coordination Sip + swallow	Proprioception Coordination – esp. hand/eye Visual / tactile – in unison + separately Degrees of touch, temperature + pressure Body awareness Sensation of movement Hearing Smell Taste Thirst satisfied	Motivation (thirst) Social – knowledge of activity and where it occurs Decision making Judgement Memory and knowledge Logical and sequential thought Organisational skills Safety awareness Maintaining attention + concentration	Visual/tactile – temperature Figure ground discrimination Form constancy Praxis Gnosis Object recognition Depth perception Appreciation of form + colour Stereognosis	Gratification	Communication Interaction Social skills

Precisely because such activities are routine and commonplace, they are often taken for granted and not consciously acknowledged. However, in addressing these complex performance components, OTs provide a commonsense, problem-solving approach. They can thus enable people to address limitations that compromise their ability to, for example, wash, dress, cook and generally interact with their environment. The value of routine and commonplace activities is certainly recognised and appreciated, when (as a consequence of physical or mental limitations) they can no longer be carried out.

The OT has to be able to identify the skills needed to perform an activity and have a thorough understanding of the activity itself. The patient takes an active role in the treatment process but it is the professional's knowledge and expertise in applying activity analysis that decide whether or not the outcome is a success. In essence, it is a collaborative, person-centred, problem-solving exercise.

Clearly, it is vital to raise awareness of the importance of evaluating functional performance in activities of daily living. Activity analysis has a significant role in assessing the impact of illness and disability (Kielhofner 1995). It can also provide information that is crucial for the discharge planning process.

Working in partnership: Nurses and occupational therapists – 'tailor-made' discharge planning

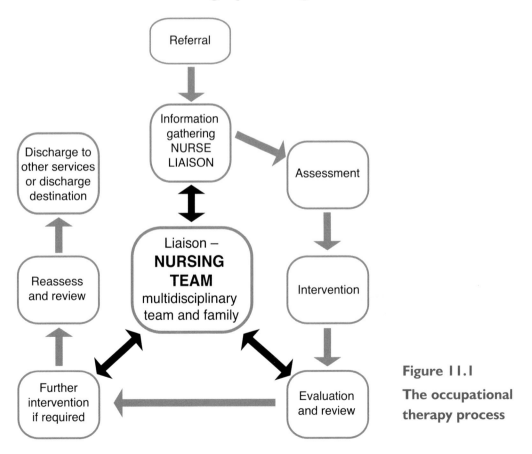

Figure 11.1

The occupational therapy process

Effective discharge planning should be multidisciplinary in nature, timely, proactive and patient-centred. It should take account of key factors such as the patient's usual living arrangements, and ensure that the patient's health and functional safety are not compromised after discharge.

To support the discharge planning process, as previously mentioned, the OT contributes an in-depth assessment. Liaison with the nursing team provides a discharge plan that is tailored to meet patient needs, uphold patient autonomy and advocate choice and partnership working in the therapeutic process (COT 2005). Figure 11.1 illustrates the OT process, highlighting the interaction with the nursing team. The following three examples illustrate the 'tailor-made' nature of OT intervention and nurse collaboration in patient-centred, needs-led discharge planning.

Rapid assessment and discharge

Jean is a 56-year-old lady admitted to hospital with exacerbation of coronary pulmonary obstructive disease (COPD). She lives with her husband, who is employed in the building trade, in a two-storey house. She is independent with personal hygiene but reports not managing well with 'domestic activities of daily living' due to breathlessness and decrease in energy levels.

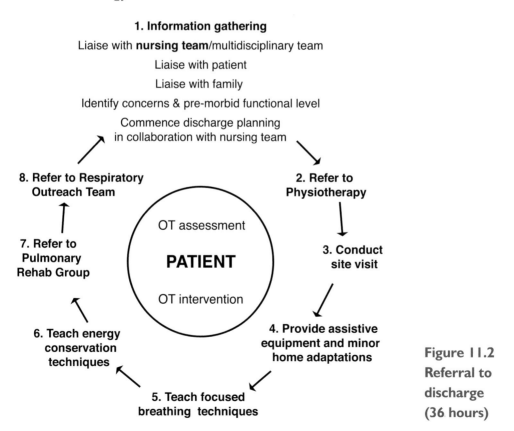

Figure 11.2
Referral to discharge (36 hours)

Short- to medium-term length of stay

Miriam is a 76-year-old lady admitted to hospital with increasing confusion and urinary frequency. She has a past medical history of arthritis, upper respiratory tract infection, multiple urinary tract infections and early-onset dementia. She lives alone in a house and her family visit regularly and complete shopping and heavy housework. Her family have raised concerns about her safety at home.

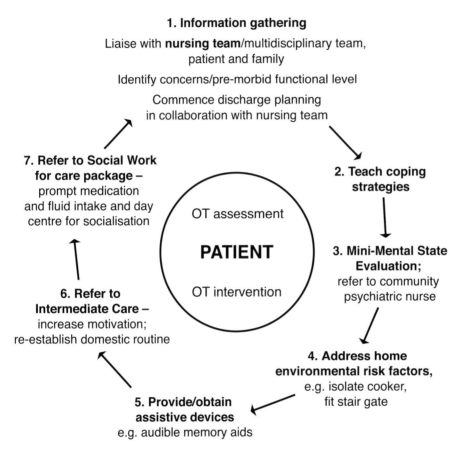

Figure 11.3 Referral to discharge, 2 weeks

In-patient rehabilitation

Peter is a 46-year-old male who has had a below-knee amputation. He lives with his wife in a two-storey house. He is a computer graphics designer (see Figure 11.4).

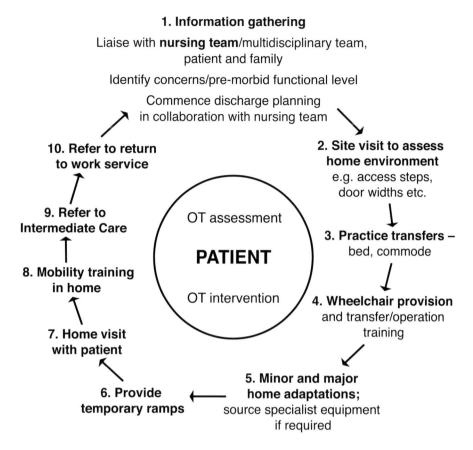

1. Information gathering
Liaise with **nursing team**/multidisciplinary team,
patient and family
Identify concerns/pre-morbid functional level
Commence discharge planning
in collaboration with nursing team

**10. Refer to return
to work service**

**2. Site visit to assess
home environment**
e.g. access steps,
door widths etc.

**9. Refer to
Intermediate Care**

OT assessment

PATIENT

OT intervention

3. Practice transfers –
bed, commode

**8. Mobility training
in home**

4. Wheelchair provision
and transfer/operation
training

**7. Home visit
with patient**

**6. Provide
temporary ramps**

**5. Minor and major
home adaptations;**
source specialist equipment
if required

Figure 11.4 Referral to discharge, 6 weeks

Discharge planning and OTs

Discharge planning has been defined as the systematic identification and organisation of services and support to assist patients to manage in the community post-discharge (Shepperd & Iliffe 2002). This definition indicates that health professionals, nurses, doctors and AHPs need to understand and interpret patients' and carers' needs from the perspectives of both the patient and the carer.

It also assumes that health professionals appreciate the patient's home environment and the social support available, as well as the patient's ability to regain their previous level of functional ability once they have left hospital. Most importantly, it assumes that health professionals know whether the patient's needs can be met within the community setting.

However, whilst discharge planning is a fundamental core skill for OTs, which is taught through a formal academic programme, this is not the case for all health professionals. Lees & Emmerson (2006) pointed out that formal discharge planning skills were absent from the pre-registration education syllabus. Generally, the nurse's repertoire of discharge planning skills is enhanced by learning 'on the job'. Whilst this may be viewed as a negative, it should be remembered that there is much value and relevance in experiential learning. All in all, it is through team-working, mutual respect and understanding of each other's roles, in conjunction with collaborative planning, that experience will be gained and learning achieved.

From an OT perspective, case management includes assessment (of the patient and their environment), evaluation, activity analysis, problem-solving and risk management, which are all fundamental core skills for an OT (Hagedorn 1997). Using their clinical judgement, expert knowledge of risk assessment and case management skills, OTs provide a valuable resource, to effectively support nurse-led discharges.

Reviewing the literature, it is clear that an exhaustive amount has been written about hospital discharge. The Department of Health has produced numerous guidelines, workbooks and initiatives on the subject. These documents have established that in order to effect a good, safe, discharge, planning should commence soon after admission, in the case of emergency or non-planned admission, and at pre-assessment clinics for planned admissions. 'Ready to go?' (DH 2010) highlights the fact that the patient and their carers should be involved in the process.

What occurs during discharge planning can have a major impact on the patient's experience of being in hospital and their eventual return home. Delays in discharging patients back to their home environment can have a negative effect on long-term outcomes. These include loss of confidence, loss of independence, loss of autonomy and the risk of hospital-acquired infections (House of Commons Health Committee 2002).

Clearly, we need to adopt a patient-centred approach, focusing on the needs of individual patients and their carers, so that they can play a meaningful role in the discharge process. This will reduce the risk of readmission to hospital and, importantly, premature entry into residential care. The NHS Institute for Innovation and Improvement's Releasing Time to Care productive ward series includes in their programme a helpful module on admission and discharge planning (see www.institute. nhs.uk/productive).

Achieving a patient-centred discharge approach

Deeming someone medically/socially/functionally fit is complex and multi-dimensional. The three perspectives are very briefly summarised below, to demonstrate their value and the need to interlink these considerations in the discharge planning process.

Lack of medical fitness can be described as a pathological state represented by deviation from 'normal' parameters of the body. The medical model conceptualises being healthy as the 'absence of disease' and as 'functional fitness' (Jones 1994).

Historically, decisions about health and disease were once regarded by doctors as matters for them alone. Patients had a passive role. Having been told what was the matter with them (and sometimes not even that!), their only task was to obey whatever instructions the doctor thought fit to issue. Most modern definitions of health continue to be based on the notion that when medical symptoms have been addressed or resolved the person is medically fit.

Disease (meaning 'dis-ease') is a term that evolved from its original meaning of 'a state of being not at ease' to describe a biomedical reductionist view of the body.

For an OT, the concept of functional fitness goes far beyond 'an absence of disease'. Occupational therapy is not solely concerned with the biological and physiological processes of the body. It also encompasses psychological, environmental and social influences.

Functional fitness is of significant importance in achieving a successful discharge and can mean different things in different situations. An OT deals with the everyday activities that are performed without conscious thought or effort, such as getting in or out of bed, washing your face, or preparing a meal. It is only when these activities cannot be performed that we notice we were doing them at all. They are the unnoticed foundation stones of everyday living.

For example, a broken arm will significantly compromise a person's ability to wash and dress, feed themselves or attend to toilet hygiene. Arthritis in knees and hips will compromise mobility. So how does an individual access their kitchen to prepare meals or reach the only toilet, which is upstairs. Hence, although an individual may be deemed medically fit for discharge they may not be functionally fit. In other words, they may have lost the ability to address personal care or domestic routines.

It has been identified that being functionally fit and an individual's perceptions of their functional fitness are heavily influenced by 'social status, values and norms, which are also influenced by roles and environmental factors' (Turner 1996, p. 104).

Social fitness depends on the patient's perspectives, i.e. their way of seeing, knowing and doing, and will be dominated by their cultural and social influences. These societal and cultural influences are also inextricably bound up with, and reinforce, different values, motivations and behaviours (Jones 1994).

Social fitness may also partly depend on material factors that may be outside an individual's control, such as damp housing, poor diet, reduced mobility or lack of formal or informal support. Some experts have long since said that 'the support of family and other social systems are most important in enhancing the capacity of (patients) to function in their daily lives' (Kielhofner 1992, p. 7).

The multidisciplinary team generally encompasses a patient-centred approach to varying degrees. However, as previously discussed, the key principle of using activity analysis to evaluate the impact of illness/disability on function within the patient's environmental context is unique to OT. By working together, with understanding of each other's perspectives and philosophies, OTs and nurses can enhance the patient experience by achieving timely and appropriate discharge planning.

Two case examples (see below) will illustrate the importance of connecting the medical, functional and social perspectives.

Case study 1: Mr G.

Mr G., aged 70, lives alone in a house. He was previously independent with mobility, personal and domestic activities of daily living. He has no relatives but a neighbour gets the heavy shopping weekly. Following a collapse at home and being found by his neighbour, Mr G. was admitted to hospital and diagnosed as having experienced a stroke. On admission, Mr G. presented with right side weakness, poor mobility and slurred speech.

Within four days, Mr G. reported to nursing staff that he was washing independently, mobilising independently around the ward and speech was almost back to normal. All medical aspects had been addressed so discharge was planned forthwith. However, a nurse mentioned to the ward OT that she had observed Mr G. wearing his shirt back to front and trying to comb his hair with the tube of toothpaste. Consequently, the nurse requested a full OT assessment.

Following OT assessment, it was determined that although Mr G. had appeared outwardly to regain his previous level of function, it was severely compromised due to his perceptual processing ability being affected. When moved from the ward setting (where demands on functional ability are few) to the OT Assessment Unit, Mr G. was no longer able to perform basic personal care and domestic tasks appropriately and safely. He was unable to recognise items of clothing and how he should dress; he had lost his ability to name objects and know their function; he was unable to sequence a task and tended to perseverate an action (e.g. repeatedly wash his face and nothing else). He also required prompting to initiate and maintain an activity.

All of the above would significantly affect Mr G.'s functional safety at home. Mr G. did, however, demonstrate capacity to make his own decisions and expressed a wish to return home.

Very close liaison occurred between Mr G., his neighbour, a social worker and the OT to establish an appropriate care package, as well as consultation with

Intermediate Care for ongoing rehabilitation at home. Once all plans were established and in place, Mr G. was discharged home.

If Mr G had been discharged when 'medically fit' there would have been a high risk of an accident occurring, perhaps as a consequence of washing the electric kettle in the sink or switching on the gas cooker and not lighting it. In addressing medical, functional and social perspectives together, the risk of readmission was reduced and a safe, successful discharge was achieved.

Case study 2: Mr A.

Mr A., aged 75, living alone since his wife died four months ago, has been admitted to hospital six times in the last ten weeks with diarrhoea and vomiting. No particular medical cause has been identified. Following resolution of the episode, the patient is discharged home, having only seen medical staff.

A seventh admission occurs nine days later for the same complaint. A nurse, concerned that he may not be coping at home although he presents as physically and functionally independent whilst on the ward, discusses the patient with the ward OT. Following a thorough OT assessment, it is discovered that the patient's wife provided all support for cooking and shopping; the patient has limited cooking skills and poor awareness of food hygiene; his fridge has not worked properly for the last three months and, for financial and functional reasons, he is not able to buy a new one.

Using clinical reasoning and problem-solving skills, the OT surmises that the diarrhoea and vomiting are inevitable consequences of eating less than thoroughly cooked and potentially contaminated food,

OT recommendations:

A referral to be made to Social Work for financial advice and assistance to purchase a fridge and establish support for shopping.

The patient to be found a transitional care bed until a fridge is purchased.

Clearly, if patients' functional and social needs are not addressed, they are likely to be at high risk of readmission. They may also require more serious and more costly medical intervention as a consequence of potentially avoidable accidents or worsening of medical conditions.

It is evident that all three perspectives have key roles to play in the patient's journey from admission to discharge. Failure to recognise or acknowledge the value of complementary approaches can give rise to misunderstanding, miscommunication and conflict. However, cultural, situational and political factors can sometimes exacerbate already difficult circumstances. Some cultures 'may encourage the maintenance of the sick role and the acceptance of how sick people perform' (Sumsion 1999, p. 35). This can and does lead to 'knee-jerk' responses to relatives' persistent and sometimes unrealistic requests. The resultant pressure can lead to MDT communication dissolving, confusion and contradictions arising, and discharges being delayed unnecessarily.

Patients and relatives may also have unrealistic expectations of the hospital experience and anticipated length of stay. We must remember that, for the elderly population, hospital care has changed out of all recognition. For instance, many individuals still use the term 'convalescence' when health professionals are referring to Intermediate Care rehabilitation and getting patients home as soon as possible. With effective communication, involving the patient and their families in the early stages of discharge planning can help allay anxiety and offer reassurance. (See table on page 181 opposite.)

All members of the MDT must maintain a balance between professional perspectives, government directives and the realities of discharge planning. The team members must trust and respect each other's professional skills, expertise and judgement.

Whilst we have to be flexible to meet the needs of the patient, the table below demonstrates that we must approach discharge planning 'at a level that facilitates the resolution of problems rather than adding to them' (Sumsion 1999, p. 34). In this way, we can support the patient in achieving a personally acceptable lifestyle within their particular cultural and social environment. The key to achieving a consensus on discharge planning is for each MDT member to communicate proactively and concisely, as well as recognising the value of partnership and a whole systems approach in order to achieve positive discharge practices.

The way forward

This chapter has identified the focus of occupational therapy and explained how a better understanding of the OT's role can assist the nursing team in further developing their discharge facilitation skills. By pooling of resources emphasising the ethos of collaborative working, the nursing team can become valuable mediators. They form a vital link between the patient, the OT and other health professionals during the discharge planning process.

Nurses and OTs can achieve this by being allies in promoting 'joined-up thinking', the sharing of information, collaborative participation in learning and development training programmes, and above all by demonstrating ownership of, and commitment to, seamless discharge planning.

Nurses and occupational therapists: Working in partnership and achieving a positive discharge outcome through effective communication

76-year-old man. Unstable blood sugar levels. Wife and supportive family. Lives in first-floor flat (no lift). Family keen for discharge home. Son states care package being set up by community social worker and family will be assisting patient's wife until services in place. Medics have documented that the patient is medically fit for discharge the next day.

ACTION	OUTCOME
Scenario A Single patient record information taken at face value Transport and tablets to take out (TTOs) arranged Patient discharged home into care of family District nurses informed of discharge **Scenario B** Concerned re: patient transfer status – maximum assistance x 2 to achieve any transfers Patient referred to Physio and OT OT conducted thorough assessment and liaised with multidisciplinary team Social Work Dept contacted; advised that patient was not due a review for another 6 months and no existing care package was in place Met with family to gain pre-morbid functional status Required minimal assistance x 1 to transfer Wife provided all care – feeding, personal hygiene Warden-controlled ground-floor flat secured Discussed care package – family agreed to have one morning call per day to assist patient's wife as other family members work full time Social Work referral made Intermediate Care rehab bed agreed to by family on behalf of patient – referral made	**Scenario A** Next day post-discharge district nurse attended to administer insulin Found patient had slept in chair as wife unable to transfer patient into bed or onto the commode Patient readmitted to hospital. **Scenario B** Patient transferred to Intermediate Care Care package established Move to ground floor flat achieved All functional and social needs addressed Readmission risk avoided

Multi-professional discharge practice considerations

To recap, the golden rules are:

- Start planning discharge on or before admission
- Establish whether the patient has simple or complex needs (see table below)
- Inform the patient, family or carers of the estimated discharge date
- Note any existing care packages and ensure that Social Work partners are involved early in the planning
- Record contact numbers of relatives or carers
- Discuss keys, clothing and transport home
- Check whether the patient requires blister/medipacks for discharge medication
- Keep the patient and family members informed of discharge plans daily

Types of discharge – from complex to simple

Discharge type	Presenting needs	Possible discharge requirements	Possible multidisciplinary involvement
Complex discharge	Full assistance required with activities of daily living (ADLs), e.g washing and dressing, toileting, etc. All care bed/hoist Assistance x 1–2 to transfer Elderly, living alone or with dependent relative Social services support Sensory deficits Psychiatric history – agitated, wandering Carer crisis Family dispute re: discharge destination Recurrent falls Multiple presentations at hospital	Residential/Nursing home placement Continuing care assessment Large care package Best interest meeting Specialist equipment/home adaptations Medication	Nursing staff Occupational therapist Social worker Physiotherapist Complex discharge nurse District nurses Psychiatric liaison Pharmacist

	Mobile with aids Requires minimal assistance with ADLs Living with family Living with dependent spouse Lives alone independently	Re-start existing care package Commence small care package Re-start/refer to district nurses Housing issues Medication	Nursing staff Social worker Occupational therapist Physiotherapist Pharmacist Intermediate care Housing department
	Independent with ADLs Independent mobile Lives with family Lives with spouse Lives alone Needs domestic assistance	Small care package Supported discharge Rehabilitation Medications	Nursing staff Social worker Occupational therapist Physiotherapist Pharmacist Intermediate care
Simple discharge	Independent with ADLs Independently mobile Lives alone/with spouse	Outpatients appointment Medication	Nursing staff Pharmacist

Conclusion

It must be remembered that successful discharge planning can only be accomplished through collaborative working and effective communication with the patient, their family or carers. It is not what we do as individual professionals but how individual professionals do it as a team ('it's not what we do, it's the way that we do it').

References

Allen, R. E. (1990). *The Concise Oxford Dictionary.* Oxford: Oxford University Press.

American Occupational Therapy Association (1994). Uniform Terminology for Occupational Therapy. 3rd Ed. *The American Journal of Occupational Therapy.* 48 (11), 1047–1054.

College of Occupational Therapists (2005). *Code of Ethics and Professional Conduct.* London: College of Occupational Therapists Ltd.

Department of Health (2010). 'Ready to go? Planning the discharge and transfer of patients from hospital and intermediate care'. Quarry House, Leeds: Department of Health.

Hagedorn, R. (1997). *Foundations for Practice in Occupational Therapy.* UK: Churchill Livingstone.

Hagedorn, R. (2000). *Tools for Practice in Occupational Therapy*. UK: Churchill Livingstone.

House of Commons Health Committee (2002). *Delayed Discharges* (third report of session 2001–2002 HC, CM5645). London: HMSO.

Jones, L.J. (1994). *The Social Context of Health and Health Work*. UK: Palgrave Macmillan.

Kielhofner, G. (1992). *Conceptual Foundations of Occupational Therapy*. Maryland, USA: Williams & Wilkins.

Kielhofner, G. (1995). *A Model of Human Occupation*. 2nd Ed. Maryland, USA: Williams & Wilkins.

Lees, L. & Emmerson, K. (2006). Identifying discharge practice training needs. *Nursing Standard*. **20** (29), 47–51.

Mattison, J.A. (1929). *Occupational Therapy and Rehabilitation* (cited in Trombly 1995, p. 10).

Miller, R.J. & Walker, K.F. (eds) (1993). *Perspectives on Theory for the Practice of Occupational Therapy*. Aspen, USA: Gaithersburg.

Shepperd, S. & Iliffe, S. (2002). Hospital at home versus in patient care. *The Cochrane Library*. **2**, 81–82.

Sumsion, T. (ed) (1999). *Client-Centred Practice in Occupational Therapy*. UK: Churchill Livingstone.

Trombly, C.A. (1995). *Occupational Therapy for Physical Dysfunction*. 4th Ed. Maryland, USA: Williams & Wilkins.

Turner, A., Foster, M. & Johnson, S.E. (1996). *Occupational Therapy and Physical Dysfunction*. 4th Ed. USA: Churchill Livingstone.

Wilcock, A. A. (2001). *Occupation for Health, Vol 1, A Journey from Self Health to Prescription*. UK: British College of Occupational Therapists.

World Health Organisation (1986). *The Ottawa Charter for Health Promotion*. Canada: Health and Welfare Canada, Canadian Public Health Association.

www.dh.gov.uk (27 April 2006) Publications, Policy and Guidance.

Young, M.E. & Quinn, E. (1992). *Theories and Principles of Occupational Therapy*. UK: Churchill Livingstone.

Chapter 12

Medication considerations and discharge

Karen Richardson

The aim of this chapter is to highlight medication issues related to discharge from hospital. Information-gathering and communication about a patient's medication are considered, and common problems and barriers are discussed. The effects of non-medical prescribing, IT and hospital pharmacy services on timely discharge from hospital are also acknowledged. Two case studies illustrate the role of the pharmacist in medicines reconciliation and timely discharge.

In particular, this chapter discusses:

- The importance of medicines reconciliation on admission to hospital
- The value of effective communication between patients, pharmacists, nurses, doctors and other multidisciplinary team (MDT) members about medicines during the patient's hospital stay
- The significance of communicating medication changes to the patient and primary care team on discharge from hospital

Medication and discharge planning

A wide range of issues may impact greatly on the patient's life once discharged; not least of these is their medication. Few patients leave hospital without any medication. Surgical and manipulative procedures may require pain relief and/or antibiotics; while medical monitoring of a long-term condition may necessitate a change in a patient's drug therapy. A patient may have been found to be suffering from a previously undiagnosed disease and this will mean that new drugs will have been prescribed. The patient may have been admitted to hospital due to a medication side-effect or an adverse drug reaction, and this will result in dosage changes, or stopping or swapping of medications. For all these reasons, the process of managing medicines appropriately for a patient's needs is essential for effective discharge planning.

The importance of good communication

Various changes have been made in the NHS to provide a pharmacy service that is responsive to patients' needs during their stay in hospital. Hospital pharmacists need to work in partnership with doctors and nurses to effectively communicate information about medication changes that have occurred during a patient's hospital stay. Without effective communication, changes may be counterproductive. On discharge, the first point where communication can, and often does, fragment is between secondary and primary care.

Healthcare professionals should be aware of medication changes for patients they are responsible for, but the patient is sometimes left out of the loop. If this happens, serious confusion can arise, due to the patient's lack of knowledge and understanding, of medication schedules in general and changes to those schedules in particular. Solving this communication problem is vital, in order to ensure that effective treatments are used both in and out of hospital. Nurses are ideally placed to work with pharmacists, doctors and other prescribers to help the patient get the best from both formally prescribed and informally purchased medication.

Medication at admission, in hospital and at discharge

Drug treatments are often taken for granted, both by patients and by healthcare professionals. Involving the patient in management of their existing medication whilst in hospital is crucial to achieving timely discharge.

Obtaining an accurate drug history on admission (medicines reconciliation)

On admission, a full drug history should be obtained, to ensure that medicines prescribed on admission correspond to those that the patient was taking prior to admission. This should include everything that a patient ingests, inhales, injects, inserts or applies. Despite the difficulties that can be encountered in extracting all relevant information from the patient, the record should include the following items:

- Prescribed medication
- Purchased medication
- Herbal remedies
- Alternative therapies
- Illicit drug use

Healthcare staff also need to know about any allergies the patient may have, to particular drugs or foods.

All the above items can independently affect the patient's health and may also interact with each other. Such effects can be detrimental but on occasion may be beneficial. Issues that could arise might include:

- Not taking prescribed medication (will the patient admit this?)
- Using over-the-counter (OTC) medications that are similar to prescribed medications, such as paracetamol preparations
- Cardiovascular effects of illicit drugs, such as cocaine
- Not mentioning illicit drug use and herbal remedies (such as St John's Wort), many of which may interact with prescribed medication

The information-gathering role

Who is best placed to elicit this information? The answer may well be a combination of individuals with the appropriate knowledge base to detect potential and actual problems. In most cases, junior doctors will play a central role throughout the admission process and in documenting an initial drug history.

In 2007, the National Institute for Health and Clinical Excellence (NICE) and the National Patient Safety Agency (NPSA) produced guidance for medicines reconciliation on admission of adults to hospital (NICE & NPSA 2007). The guidance states that hospitals should have a policy in place for medicines reconciliation on admission and pharmacists should be involved as soon as possible after admission.

Medication errors commonly occur on admission to hospital. The NICE guidance quotes unintentional variance of 30–70 % between medicines taken prior to admission and prescriptions on admission. This could potentially lead to increased morbidity, mortality and economic cost, and underlines the importance of accurate medicines reconciliation on admission to hospital.

Nurses also play an important role in information-gathering about patients' medicines. Patients, relatives and carers may give other information throughout the hospital stay. A team approach is required to gather complete information on medicines, with the pharmacist having a pivotal role.

Some patients may not be able to provide a drug history on admission – for instance, a confused patient, a dementia patient, a patient for whom English is not the first language, or a patient who is very unwell on admission. In these situations, an alternative drug history source will be needed, such as a relative or carer, or the patient's GP. In cases where patients have been transferred from nursing or residential settings (including interim and intermediate care), the staff from these settings can also play a crucial part in providing an accurate drug history.

Whoever collects the drug history information, it is important to ensure that as much as possible is found out about how a patient takes their medication. The reality may differ significantly from the intention of the prescriber or from the information given to the patient by the dispensing pharmacist! Such differences may have a significant impact on the patient's health and can, indeed, contribute to admissions or to discharges that are not timely. Patients often use devices (known as compliance aids) to assist them with taking medication. These devices include monitored dosage systems, dosette boxes and blister packs. It is important for hospital staff to identify patients using these devices on admission, as this will also help to ensure a smoother discharge process.

Case study 1: Medicines reconciliation

An 89-year-old lady who usually lives alone is admitted to hospital late at night. She was found wandering in the street by neighbours. She is very confused and unable to give any kind of history, including a drug history. Nursing staff are unable to contact her family overnight. She is seen the following morning on the Elderly Care Admissions Unit by the pharmacist, who telephones her GP's surgery. The surgery tells the pharmacist that she has recently been prescribed fentanyl patch, 25 micrograms every 72 hours.

The pharmacist asks the named nurse if the patient is wearing a fentanyl patch. The nurse checks the patient and she is wearing a patch. The pharmacist informs the doctor and documents a drug history in the patient's notes. The fentanyl patch is removed from the patient and stopped, as it may be contributing to her confusion.

Nurse prescribing as part of the admission process

Nurses are the most frequent point of contact for patients on admission. Since 2002, the advent of supplementary and independent nurse prescribing has increased the number of nurses with more detailed pharmacological knowledge but these may not always be the nurses who admit the patient. If they were, prescribing on admission would be much simpler. It would no longer be necessary to attempt to contact the doctor to transcribe medication to the drug sheet. Medication could be prescribed immediately.

The introduction of nurse-led admission and discharge policies should provide an effective framework for transferring patients into and out of hospitals safely, sensitively and efficiently. Any nurse involved in such an initiative should have the skills, knowledge and experience to ensure that medication and other ongoing care continues appropriately. Nurse prescribers would be ideally placed to carry out such a role. Pharmacist prescribers could also carry out a similar role.

Using the patient's own medication while in hospital

Many hospitals allow the use of Patient's Own Drugs (PODs). These are sometimes called Patient's Own Medications (POMs), or they may have another acronym, specific to that institution. In the past, patients' medication was taken from them on admission and disposed of, causing significant wastage.

Nowadays, PODs schemes allow any medication brought into hospital to be kept in a locked cupboard by the patient's bed, provided that there is a safe system in place to facilitate this. PODs can then be used during the patient's stay and are available to be taken home, thus removing the need for that medication to be dispensed on discharge.

Medication on discharge

If communication and education about medication on admission is important, then communication and education about medication on discharge is equally vital. All parties involved in the further supply of drug therapies need to know what changes have been made to medication schedules during the patient's stay. They should also know why these changes have been made, so that the correct information can be communicated to the patient.

The drug supply difficulties that may arise on discharge are many and varied. Their significance may be interpreted differently by each individual involved, but they can all have a serious impact on the patient's experience of discharge. These are some of the problems that can occur:

- Delays in obtaining take-home medication: irritating for the patient and for hospital bed managers
- Lack of understanding of changes in medication: confusing for patient, carers, GP and pharmacists involved in administration and supply at home
- Delayed communication of new dosage schedules and new drugs to GP practice and community pharmacy responsible for supply: may result in incorrect medication (sometimes the drug regime that was in place before admission) being prescribed and supplied to the patient, thus causing more confusion and potential harm

If a patient usually has their medicines dispensed into a compliance aid (such as a blister pack), hospital pharmacies may not prepare these or may require a long notice period (e.g. 48 hours) to get one ready. If arrangements are made with a community pharmacy to prepare these, a similar notice period may be required. If this is not arranged in advance of the discharge, this will cause a delay on the day; or it will necessitate a longer stay while this is arranged. An assessment of the patient's ability to medicate during their stay will be necessary to avoid last-minute changes to the discharge plan.

Occupational therapists and social workers may also request these devices for patients who have carers coming into their homes to prompt medication-taking, but use of a compliance aid should always be for the benefit of the patient. It is also worth considering that a wide range of different compliance aids are available. However, not all medication can be dispensed into compliance aids (such as warfarin, and medicines to be taken when required).

Having an identified or named nurse responsible for patient discharge should help to resolve such problems. For example, the nurse will have developed a rapport with the patient (and carer/relatives) during their hospital stay and there will have been opportunities to discuss their drug therapy. Relatives and carers often play an important role in medication administration and compliance.

As with admissions, the ability of the nurse to write a take-home prescription or authorise such a supply should also speed up the process. In some hospitals, pharmacists are involved in transcribing (copying) or prescribing take-home medication. For most nurses, the simplest way of ensuring that any changes in medication happen correctly and without delay is to become adept at collaborating with professionals who work in the community such as GPs, pharmacists and community nurses. This will certainly help to prevent some of the problems that can occur after discharge. It could also reduce the number of drug related readmissions.

Independent nurse prescribers could prescribe take-home medication as part of their discharge role. They could also contact their colleagues in the community with the exact details at the point of discharge. Non-prescribers could liaise with independent pharmacist prescribers in either secondary or primary care to fulfil this function. This would ensure continuation of the correct medication. Hospitals will vary in the amount of medication they provide for patients on discharge but most will give between a two-week and one-month supply.

Case study 2: Medicines management on discharge

An 82-year-old lady who lives alone, with good support from her family, takes ten regular medicines, which she has dispensed into a blister pack by her local community pharmacy to assist her compliance. She has a history of stroke and some problems with short-term memory so she finds that the blister pack aids her compliance. Before using the pack, she was very confused with medication-taking, frequently taking double doses of some medicines and omitting others.

She is admitted to hospital after a fall caused by postural hypotension. Her bendroflumethiazide 2.5 mg in the morning is stopped and her amlodipine dose is reduced from 10 mg once daily to 5 mg once daily. A decision is made that she can go home after spending one night in hospital and a discharge letter is written by the junior doctor. The pharmacist advises nursing and medical staff that the patient usually uses a blister pack.

The pharmacist telephones the patient's usual community pharmacy and advises them of changes to medication. The pharmacist arranges for the FY2 doctor to write a FP10 prescription for the new amlodipine tablets and faxes a copy to the pharmacy. The community pharmacy agrees to make up a new blister pack for later that afternoon. Nursing staff arrange for a relative to take in the original FP10 prescription into the pharmacy and pick up the new blister pack. Nurses also ask the relative to remove old blister packs from the patient's house.

Political initiatives on medication and discharge planning

Three key policy areas have been selected for discussion here, with particular emphasis on how government policies positively or negatively impact upon the nurse's role and the effectiveness of patient discharge from hospital. Discharge planning continues to evolve rapidly and, in doing so, changes the interface with the pharmacist's role in both secondary and primary care settings.

Hospital pharmacy services

Hospital pharmacy departments tend to be open from 9 to 5 pm, Monday to Friday, with reduced opening hours and staffing at weekends. Some hospital pharmacies have introduced shift working to provide longer opening hours. Outside of opening hours, an on-call pharmacist is available but usually they are not on the hospital site; a few hospitals have an on-call resident pharmacist staying on the hospital site.

These working patterns impact on how much input pharmacists can have when patients are immediately admitted or discharged to or from hospital. Another factor is the difficulty in recruiting and retaining pharmacists in hospitals, particularly those at the entry-level 'Agenda for Change' pay bands. Inevitably, this staffing problem affects the ability of pharmacy departments to achieve medicines management objectives. A team approach, in which pharmacists communicate and work effectively with doctors, nurses and other members of the MDT (such as occupational therapists and social workers) will result in a smoother discharge process, regarding medications.

More positively, there is an increasing use of trained pharmacy technicians to perform tasks traditionally done by pharmacists. After appropriate training, pharmacy technicians can perform medicines reconciliation, assess suitability of PODs for re-use in hospital and assist with timely ordering of medicines for patients.

Pharmacy technicians can also reconcile take-home medication, a role currently performed in many hospitals by the nurse discharging the patient. In this way, pharmacy technicians can also free up nursing time, while still supporting other aspects of discharge from hospital.

Non-medical prescribing

Since the 1990s, nurses have been able to prescribe from a limited formulary as district nurses and health visitors. This has facilitated the supply of practical post-discharge necessities such as dressings, simple analgesia and laxatives. Extended independent and supplementary nurse prescribers have been in existence since 2002/3. Nurses are now able to prescribe from an increasingly extensive independent formulary for both minor ailments and more serious conditions. This situation is unlikely to remain static with other registered professionals also being trained to prescribe. Non-registered professionals, such as physician assistants, cannot yet prescribe. But as an integral part of specialist teams this will require consideration in the future. Prescribing is directly linked to care pathways, such as the Liverpool Care Pathway and so includes some palliative care drugs. This increases post-discharge prescribing scope but also increases the need for effective admission and discharge communication.

Supplementary prescribers, nurses and pharmacists and also, potentially, radiographers, physiotherapists and podiatrists, can prescribe for any condition within their competence, under strict criteria agreed between themselves and an independent prescriber (usually a doctor). Again, this has many benefits but requires full communication between all prescribers on admission and discharge.

Independent prescribing for suitably trained nurses and pharmacists was announced in April 2006. This policy allows qualified individuals to prescribe from the whole of the British National Formulary (BNF). This should remove the need for debate about the legality of transcribing a patient's medication onto hospital medication sheets on admission, as such individuals could prescribe them legally. They could also prescribe any take-home medication required.

Should suitably qualified staff members not be available to prescribe, Patient Group Directions (PGDs) could be set up to facilitate the continued supply of essential medication (RCN 2006). PGDs are not new; they have been in existence for some time and support clinical situations both in acute emergencies and upon discharge. This may also allow the supply of medication that would otherwise be unavailable in the community, such as IV solutions. However, having said this, the situation is constantly evolving, and this may not be the case for much longer.

Information technology (IT)

The introduction of nationwide NHS IT systems has been long awaited. When implemented, these IT systems will allow real-time access to patient records for accredited personnel. This will mean that a patient's prescribed medication record can be transmitted directly from their GP practice to the hospital ward on admission, and the reverse process can occur on discharge. Community pharmacies will ideally be included in the information loop to ensure continuation of correct medication schedules after discharge.

All these measures should mean that fewer medication errors occur. However, this will still depend on the right information going to the right people and also, to a large extent, on the patient. History-taking on admission will be able to focus more on the patient's knowledge and understanding of their medication, and any discrepancies will be noted and dealt with.

Post-discharge medication

There is little point in changing medication, or any other aspect of therapy, in hospital if the changes are not maintained when the patient returns home. Therefore it is vital that patients are fully aware of medication changes on discharge from hospital. The patient's GP should be informed as soon as possible. Any compliance aid the patient was using prior to admission should be considered, and arrangements to continue necessary compliance aids should be made, prior to discharge from hospital.

Community pharmacists, under the terms of their contracts, now undertake Medication Use Reviews (MURs) with their patients. Although any patient can request a review, as can healthcare professionals with the consent of the patient, they are especially useful for those individuals whose medication has changed or has become increasingly complex. Reports are made to the patient's GP and these should help discharge nurses ensure that dosage changes are monitored, and any problems with changes in medication are identified. Other ways of supporting patients at home might include telephone calls from the discharge nurse (Lees 2004). These would provide opportunities to ask questions, give reminders of dosage schedules and pick up on any problems encountered.

Concluding points:

In summary, nurses (in partnership with pharmacists) need to:

- Make sure they and the patient and/or their carers know what medication they were taking on admission and identify patients using compliance aids
- Liaise with pharmacy as soon as possible so that discharge medication arrives on the ward without delay

- Ensure that ward patient records are clear in case other nurses have to deal with queries post discharge
- Explain the medication changes that have happened during the hospital stay to the patient and/or carer
- Provide information about why and how to use the medication given on discharge
- Contact the patient's GP and community pharmacist to explain any medication changes made and to advise on the length of supply given on discharge

Note: This chapter has been adapted from Chapter 9, 'Discharge and medication' by Ross Groves, in *Nurse Facilitated Hospital Discharge* (M&K Update, 2007).

References

Department of Health. http://www.dh.gov.uk/en/Healthcare/Medicinespharmacyandindustry/Prescriptions/The Non-MedicalPrescribing Programme/index.htm

Lees, L. (2004). Improving the quality of patient discharge from emergency settings. *British Journal of Nursing.* **13** (7), 345–432.

National Institute for Health & Clinical Excellence & National Patient Safety Agency (2007). 'Technical patient safety solutions for medicines reconciliation on admission of adults to hospital'. NICE patient safety guidance 1. London: NICE.

Royal College of Nursing (2006). 'Patient Group Directions for Nurses'. London: RCN. www.rcn.org.uk/direct

Royal Pharmaceutical Society of Great Britain, The Guild of Hospital Pharmacists, The Pharmaceutical Services Negotiating Committee & The Primary Care Pharmacists Association (2006). 'Moving patients, moving medicines, moving safely. Guidance on discharge and transfer planning'. London.

Useful websites related to prescribing

www.dh.gov.uk
Search here for Department of Health publications, including health circulars and reports and for NHS Executive publications and information.

www.hmso.gov.uk/acts.htm
For Acts of Parliament and associated legislation, including Statutory Instruments.

www.nurse-prescriber.co.uk
Educational pages, forums, news and other resources available to healthcare professionals involved in prescribing and medicine management.

www.portal.nelm.nhs.uk/PGD/default.aspx
For a centrally maintained archive of approved group protocols for the supply and administration of medicines.

Chapter 13

Doctors, ward rounds, discharge and the interface with the multidisciplinary team
Mark Temple and Philip Dyer

Effective bed management is a key concern of all NHS acute trusts and length of stay is widely used to assess the efficiency of bed utilisation. With operational costs of a large acute medical ward having gone up to around £1 million per annum, reducing length of stay and increasing bed occupancy rates are seen as vital tools in balancing the books. However, increased bed occupancy rates are also associated with increased inefficiency; so effective bed utilisation is crucial to the successful functioning of a hospital. Inefficient bed utilisation, on the other hand, can completely undermine elective services and emergency care and will result in increased cost pressure on hospital.

For clinical staff, the effective coordination of discharge is a vital part of the hospital pathway for the individual patient. For the acute Trust as a whole to make available the resources and staff needed to maintain efficient service provision, effective (timely) delivery of patient discharge is equally important. These considerations make planning discharge in advance doubly vital. Patients, their carers and healthcare staff all need to be involved in discharge planning so that discharge proceeds on the planned day and time (Lees 2010).

Effective, timely discharge from hospital is at the core of an efficient NHS and has been the focus of a series of Department of Health publications promoting best practice. These include 'Achieving timely "simple" discharge from hospital – a toolkit for the multi-disciplinary team' (DH 2004) and 'Discharge planning: pathway, process and practice' (DH 2003). The former was aimed at the simple discharges and the latter is aimed at more complex discharges. The Department of Health also published 'Emergency care briefing: modernising discharge from hospital' (Lees, 2006). The aim of this paper was to provide all staff working in emergency care settings with information on the major challenges to discharge planning, key web-based links, references and simple suggestions to achieve best practice. Latterly, the Department of Health have published further guidance in the form of ten steps for discharge and transfer of patients from hospital (DH 2010a).

However, achieving changes to discharge practice that are safe, effective and consistent requires an understanding of the many facets of the discharge process. The risks of an ineffective or poorly coordinated discharge should be widely recognised. Elwyn and colleagues (2005) summed up the risks of adverse events and error during discharge by stating: 'Avoid hospitals if you can, but if you can't take additional care when leaving.'

The objective for every patient is to be discharged from acute hospital care as soon as the patient no longer requires this level of care. 'Timely discharge' thus means that the patient is discharged home or to a pre-existing place of care (such as a nursing home) as soon as they are clinically stable and fit for discharge.

Discharge decision-making – the doctor and the multidisciplinary team

Discharge from hospital should be planned and implemented by the multidisciplinary team (MDT). The team should include medical and nursing staff, allied health professionals (AHPs) and social workers. The more complex the discharge, the greater the number of team members that are likely to be involved and the greater the requirement for effective planning and communication between members of the team, the patient, carers and other agencies or staff. It must be remembered, however, that good communication between all health professionals is essential for any type of discharge. The timeliness of the discharge, the quality of the arrangements for care post-discharge, and the level of understanding of the patient and their carers throughout the discharge process all reflect the effectiveness of the MDT's working practices.

The MDT requires a clinical leader and this role is commonly filled by the consultant in charge of the patient's care. The consultant in charge is the member of the team with the clearest medico-legal responsibility for all aspects of the patient's care while in hospital. This responsibility is a major reason for the consultant conventionally assuming the role of team leader. However, the consultant may not be the team member with the best skills to coordinate arrangements for a complex discharge. In designated nurse- or therapist-led wards, the discharge process is led exclusively by non-medical staff.

Doctors have three crucial areas of involvement in the discharge process. These include:

- Conducting ward rounds
- Recording (medical) management plans in the case notes
- Participation in the MDT meetings

Ward rounds and clinical decision-making

Ward rounds have a pivotal role in delivering high-quality hospital-based care. Ward rounds should be multi-professional, enabling doctors and other healthcare professionals to develop an integrated plan of care. According to Manias & Street (2001), the goals of the ward round in both medical and surgical practice include:

- Enhancing the quality of care
- Improving communication
- Addressing patient concerns and problems
- Planning and evaluating treatment

Multi-professional training and education are also enhanced by the ward round. Little is known, however, about the origins of the ward round and its variations in practice. The ward round provides the opportunity for genuine multi-professional working. The benefits of multi-professional clinical practice are not confined to acute ward settings but are also enshrined in good practice initiatives such as the care programme approach or CPA (Easton & Oyebode 1996).

Medical and nursing trainees receive virtually no training in relation to the objectives of the ward round: how to participate in it; how it should be structured; and how to get the desired outcomes. Lees *et al.* (2006) listed key components of a good post-take ward round and these can be applied to encompass all types of ward rounds. These key components include:

- Information-gathering
- Engaging the medical team and MDT in the ward round discussions and decisions that arise
- Assimilation of information
- Teaching/educating all members of the MDT and patients
- Decision-making based on the information available
- Listening to and involving the patients in decisions about their care
- Giving verbal explanation of the decision to all members of the ward round, including patients
- Providing a written record of the decision (i.e. a management/discharge plan, preferably using some sort of pre-written proforma)
- Empowering nursing staff and other members of the MDT to implement agreed actions and problem-solve after the ward round is finished
- Reviewing progress of previous ward round decisions

All participating staff should be aware of the start time and likely duration of the ward round in advance. The agreed timing and duration of the round should take into account the likely nature and number of patients to be reviewed and the availability of the MDT.

Although medical and nursing staff are the core participants, for a variety of reasons ward rounds may be conducted solely by medical staff. Doctors commencing rounds at erratic times, without prior warning, provide little opportunity for other staff to attend. Limited nursing staff numbers on busy acute wards also prevent nurses from participating in several ward rounds per day, especially when these are conducted simultaneously on the same ward by different medical teams. The lack of multidisciplinary input in ward rounds has been noted in psychiatry (Rix & Sheppard 2003) but this is also common in both medicine and surgery.

In the context of a busy acute medical and surgical ward, routine participation in ward rounds by nurses requires leadership, a culture of prioritising multi-professional working and considerable consistent effort. The effectiveness of decision-making on 'doctors only' rounds depends on the information available from the case notes, or from the patient, and the quality of communication with other healthcare staff. Poor communication is a frequent problem and this may, at best, be a hurried handover of major decisions made to a ward nurse by the most junior member of the medical team at the end of a doctor's ward round. Doctors frequently fail to discuss discharge plans on rounds and the entry in the clinical notes relating to the round may bear little relation to the issues discussed (Lees & Holmes 2005).

'Doctors only' rounds disenfranchise other members of the MDT, who cannot share information with medical staff, or raise issues of concern or points that require clarification, or participate in treatment and discharge decisions. Patients report that they don't understand what is said by doctors on ward rounds, and rely on other members of the team to explain management and discharge decisions made on ward rounds (Lees & Holmes 2005). It has been shown that doctors rely on nurses to supplement information and provide extra detail about patient assessment during ward rounds (Manias & Street 2001).

During a multi-professional ward round, each member of the MDT should be aware of their role. The skill, experience and manner of the senior clinician, often a consultant, when conducting the round are critical in maintaining focus and optimal input from all participants. Pathak et al. (2000) observed the individual skills of 12 senior consultants with more than 10 years' experience in neurosurgical practice at three different university hospitals during their ward rounds. The ward rounds were reported to show evidence of good productivity and flexibility amongst 92% and 75% of the consultants respectively.

Pleasantness of the climate was reported to be above average on rounds conducted by just 50% of the consultants, with poor objectivity shown by 42% of consultants.

In addition, 42 % of the consultants were not consistently well understood. Only half of the consultants were reported to use words and phrases fitting the circumstances of the round; 42 % spoke unnecessarily between discussions and introduced the problems of the patient poorly to the MDT; and only 33 % managed to use humour effectively. Pathak *et al.* concluded that conducting ward rounds in neurosurgical practice needs a holistic approach, with motivation, planning, leadership skills and a structured curriculum to fulfil objectives. The range of these failings emphasises the variety of skills required by the consultant conducting the round. And it is likely that many of these failings are common to ward rounds wherever they occur.

One area of concern has been the tendency of the consultant in charge to dominate the MDT on ward rounds, resulting in an 'impotent' team. Gair (2001) observed team practice in a care of the elderly setting and reported a lower than expected level of medical dominance. Gair related this finding to the consultant's own views on the nature of rehabilitation, leading to a consensus among team members as to the purpose of geriatric assessment, and to a high level of team stability. He concluded that reducing the level of medical dominance encourages all team members to contribute, and thus enhances patient care.

More training for doctors in team skills was considered beneficial, including inter-professional training. Gair stressed the importance of the consultant avoiding monopolisation of the conversation and recommended inviting comments through questions. Encouraging participation through asking open questions, such as 'What does everyone think about what has been said?' or 'Can anyone add something more?' will lead towards a more inclusive ward round and at the same time test the strength of a point of view.

Teaching is an integral part of the consultant's role, and the expectation is that the consultant in charge should help to create a learning climate for the MDT during ward rounds. In *The Doctor as Teacher,* the General Medical Council states that 'all doctors have a professional obligation to contribute to the education and training of others' and that 'every doctor should be prepared to oversee the work of less experienced colleagues' (GMC 1999).

Interdisciplinary teaching rounds have been shown to promote more efficient patient care by providing an opportunity for enhanced communication among healthcare professionals (Felten *et al.* 1997). The consultant ward round is a setting where experiential learning occurs, which is highly valued by trainees. Talbot (2000) found the ward round to be a very useful teaching resource after a questionnaire sent to 500 senior house officers (SHOs) in North Trent. The trainees found the ward rounds particularly useful when learning professional attributes and skills but less useful for learning clinical science principles and management strategies. In relation to discharge planning, the ward round provides an important opportunity for senior staff to embed good discharge practice as a core responsibility of junior medical and nursing staff.

Great potential exists within the hospital environment for shared learning and this may provide an extension to experiential and self-directed learning (Gibson & Campbell 2000). Reeves *et al.* (2000) undertook a pilot project for pre-registration house officers and newly qualified nurses to focus upon areas of the hospital service that could be improved, including discharge planning and intravenous drug administration. The participants were asked to work together to solve problems based on clinical scenarios. The study concluded that such sessions encouraged collaboration between members of the clinical team, for the benefit of patient care, and addressed some important clinical governance issues.

Kilminster *et al.* (2004) reported that patient-focused interprofessional workshops offer added value for pre-registration house officers, pharmacy students and student nurses who attended a series of workshops in Leeds. Participants emphasised the value of learning communication skills, both with other professionals and patients, and the development of increased awareness of other people's roles

A 1994 study showed that medical students learn from attending both outpatient clinics and ward rounds. The learning experience was reported to be better in the outpatient clinic. However, the students did not make full use of the learning potential of either (Davis & Dent 1994). Consultant psychiatrists surveyed about their ward rounds reported that these were largely a compromise between professional efficiency and patient satisfaction, with little mention made of any educational element (Hodgson *et al.* 2005).

Although ward rounds are recognised learning opportunities for medical students and junior doctors, there has, up to now, been little emphasis on acquiring the skills needed to conduct a successful ward round. However, the reform of postgraduate medical education embodied in the Modernising Medical Careers initiative ('Operational Framework for Foundation Training', DH 2005) has helped focus attention on neglected areas of junior doctor training.

An initiative in Worthing, relating to best practice on the post-take ward round, has been highlighted in the Modernising Medical policy. Here, Dr Gordon Caldwell has incorporated a standardised instant assessment and feedback process into the routine post-take ward round (Caldwell 2006). This has greatly improved the effectiveness of the post-take ward round and offers learning points and objectives for both trainee and trainer. The time invested in assessment of the ward round has yielded rewards, including quicker ward rounds. The time saved can then be used for more teaching or for increased communication with patients. For this mode of learning to be effective, the importance of including protected time for reflection (for both teachers and learners) needs to be emphasised.

Dr Caldwell's group has also developed a ward round checklist (Herring *et al.* 2011). The World Health Organisation has already recognised the potential of checklists, with the introduction of the surgical safety checklist to reduce morbidity and mortality (Hales *et al.* 2008). The Caldwell ward round checklist is called a 'considerative checklist' because it is used to record that a matter has been considered, and if necessary a decision has been made. The considerative checklist has encouraged high-quality documented evidence, safer medical care, and improved team working, communication with patients and team and patient satisfaction (Herring 2011).

The nurse's role in ward rounds

Where multidisciplinary ward rounds occur routinely, the criteria for discharge need to be clearly stated, together with the responsibility of MDT members to ensure that these criteria are met and the discharge implemented. Board rounds are used to update nurses between ward rounds and, if organised, form an essential routine daily check on discharge progress (Lees & Delpino 2007).

'SMART starts' have been introduced in some acute ward areas for the purpose of proactively planning patient discharge. Although this system is still in the early stages of implementation, the principle is to identify, in advance, three key patient groups in readiness for the ward round, namely: sick patients; patients likely to be fit to go home; and patients who will require transfer to another area within the hospital. Some 'SMART starts' are conducted with the input of an area matron to help resolve difficulties in the process or equipment that might otherwise occur. As yet, there has been no formal evaluation of the system and it is not always consistently applied. For this good discharge practice to become embedded and flourish consistently, decision-making skills (critical to the ward round process) and accountability need to be continually reinforced in the practice setting.

Decision-making is clearly fundamental to discharge planning, yet there appears to be some reluctance amongst nursing staff to take it on. It is uncertain whether this is because of competing clinical priorities, a feeling that medical staff should make decisions about discharge, or simply a reluctance to make key decisions about discharge. Decision-making requires confidence, and confidence is gained through knowledge and experience. The structure supporting nurses and their individual accountability is provided by the 2008 'Nursing and Midwifery Code of Professional Conduct: professional standards, performance and ethics', which states that 'You are personally accountable for your practice and any decisions to act or not act' (NMC 2008). This means that nurses are answerable for their actions and omissions, regardless of advice or directions from another professional.

Recording management and discharge plans

The ward round is the core clinical decision-making period for ward inpatients. Decisions need to be recorded in the patient's clinical record clearly, accurately and contemporaneously. However, the time available to record management plans in any one patient's case notes is restricted by the pressure to move the round on, to review the next patient. Recording decisions in the case notes is often delegated to the most junior doctor on the round. This doctor may have limited understanding of the importance of the decisions made. They may also have the least experience of recording salient points rapidly in case notes. A ward round checklist, as described by the Caldwell group, will help to ensure that all important points are checked and recorded in the notes (Herring *et al.* 2011).

In discharge planning terms, the effectiveness of the ward round depends on all members of the MDT having a clear understanding of the agreed discharge plan and their role in relation to it. The entry in the case notes informs all of the MDT members (not just those attending the ward round) about the plan and their role in delivering it. However, several steps are required to get the case note entry right (Lees & Holmes 2005). First, the discharge plan needs to be discussed on the round, then discharge decisions have to be made, and finally these decisions need to be summarised accurately and legibly in the case notes. Although this may sound simple in principle, maintaining high standards of clinical documentation is a persistent problem, despite the emphasis put on it by professional bodies and medical defence organisations. Fernando & Siriwardena (2001) found that junior doctors on a surgical ward round frequently failed to document the consultants' clinical findings and management decisions. In addition, information given to patients by consultants regarding clinical findings and treatment planned was recorded in a median of only 6% of consultations.

The use of a standardised proforma on ward rounds has been shown to improve documentation. Thompson *et al.* (2004) reviewed the impact of a proforma tailored record on the decisions made during a post-take ward round. The introduction of the proforma led to a significant improvement in the documentation of diagnosis, management plan, prophylaxis for deep vein thrombosis, and resuscitation status, all of which were felt to have a considerable impact on patient care. Doctors found this proforma straightforward, user-friendly and useful to clinical practice. Compliance was enhanced by its inclusion in the patient admission pack. Other health professionals, especially nurses, found it a useful reference document when they received a new patient on the ward.

Providing an estimated date of discharge (EDD)

Providing a clear estimated date of discharge (EDD) can be viewed as a critical summary of a careful multidisciplinary discharge planning process (Lees 2008). The objectives of discharge planning include providing the patient and carers with advance information on the timing of discharge and arrangements for post-discharge care and follow-up.

The Department of Health discharge 'toolkit' (DH, 2004, DH 2010a) recommends that the date of expected discharge should be estimated at the earliest opportunity after the patient's admission. However, to assess the EDD effectively, the diagnosis needs to be reasonably secure. Key assessments by the MDT have to be available and there needs to have been sufficient time to observe the patient's level of stability and response to treatment. In practice, the post-take ward round conducted by a consultant together with the rest of the MDT, within 12–24 hours of the patient's admission, often provides the first practical opportunity to determine the EDD (Lees et al. 2006).

Although the post-take ward round is the natural time for decisions to be made about the likely length of hospital stay, doctors seem reluctant to commit to an EDD (Lees 2008). In our experience, the clinical entries by medical staff on the post-take ward round focus on clinical findings, results of tests and likely diagnosis and planned further investigations. The estimated length of stay in hospital is frequently not considered by medical staff, despite this being a leading concern of patients and the major cost in relation to inpatient services.

Lees & Holmes (2005), in a survey of inpatients, highlighted patients' concerns about discharge and the fact that doctors are poor at providing this information.

It is not clear why doctors are often so reluctant to routinely provide information on EDD. This may relate to the unstructured nature of many consultant-led ward rounds, the lack of training on making rounds effective, the absence of multidisciplinary representation, or excessive focus by senior medical staff on the challenges of diagnosis and treatment rather than predicted time in hospital.

Some patients admitted as emergencies have complex discharge requirements. For instance, they may need multiple assessments by therapists and social workers, and this will make it difficult to give an EDD. However, there is a widespread reluctance to volunteer an EDD, even for patients on standard inpatient medical pathways. There is some evidence that doctors feel that providing an EDD exposes them to criticism, should the estimate turn out to be incorrect. Doctors say that the need to ensure that the patient and carers understand that this is only an estimate requires extra explanation by medical staff and repeated fine-tuning of the EDD on successive ward rounds (Lees & Holmes 2005).

Lees et al. (2006) introduced a simple summary discharge planning label for completion by doctors on the post-take ward round. A key element of this label was to prompt routine EDD for all patients admitted to an acute medical unit (AMU). An EDD had to be completed for all patients, with a simple tick box response for those predicted as 'same day' or 'discharge within 24 hours'. For patients with an EDD longer than 24 hours, the label prompted responses about key inpatient referrals or investigations required and the predicted admission pathway, e.g. transfer to general medical or specialist medical ward.

An audit of the first 50 labels used revealed that only six had an EDD entered. One of the initial reasons for the labels was to prompt and summarise decision-making when a nurse was unable to attend the post-take ward round. However, it was recognised that this acted at best as an aide mémoire, and the requirement for a nurse to join the ward round remains crucial. As a result of this audit, a colour-coded A4 sheet was designed, with prompts to medical staff to complete information on clinical findings, investigation results, diagnosis and management plan, in addition to the EDD. This post-take ward round record sheet is now used exclusively in the AMU. Since this work was completed, further audits have been undertaken, based on the information on the ward round record sheet within the clerking documentation used by consultants and their teams.

There is little evidence to help determine why the EDD is not routinely documented on consultants' ward rounds. However, some possible explanations include:

- Doctors dislike the uncertainty of stating an EDD and getting decisions wrong.
- The EDD is viewed as not having a significant impact on the patient's management plan or length of stay
- There is no strategy to manage consultants who continue to 'do their own thing', taking the view that 'Discharge of a patient will occur when I have finished with their care'

For EDD to become a routine part of clinical review of patients, doctors must feel that the decision is important in management of their patients (including their length of stay in hospital) and that the decision will be viewed by all staff as an important clinical objective for the benefit of the patient. (For more on EDD, see Chapter 27.)

Using electronic records to monitor progress towards discharge

The emphasis on optimising the use of bed capacity has led acute hospitals to explore discharge applications on their electronic patient records (EPR). Capturing timely data on EDD on the EPR, which are updated at least daily, can be used to estimate the bed capacity that will become available in the next 24–72 hours or more. This information can be augmented by incorporating standardised systems that allow ward staff to confirm discharge.

Our own Trust (Heart of England) uses a traffic light system to indicate both medical fitness for discharge and whether the discharge is same day (green), next day (amber) or delayed (red). Dedicated screens on the EPR can be used to summarise progress for each patient towards discharge. Outstanding interventions or assessments needed for that patient can also be viewed and updated remotely by all members of the MDT. The underlying principle is to look forward and project capacity requirements. These systems need to be refined further, to include estimated time of discharge. This will help to ensure that demand and capacity are well managed, as the cause of imbalance between the two, especially during weekdays, is often late discharge from the wards.

Implementing discharge

Implementing discharge seven days a week is critical to the safe operation of acute hospitals and the delivery of their emergency services. Discharge planning, which should have started from the initial consultant review, needs to ensure that as many patients as possible are discharged early in the day (ideally before 11 am). This will enable the hospital to maximise bed capacity available for emergency admissions, which peak in the afternoon and early evening.

All members of the MDT must be aware of their responsibilities in relation to discharge and, wherever possible, empowered to implement discharge. Once the decision to discharge has been made, and related documentation, actions and communication have been completed, it is vital that the planned discharge proceeds. Nursing staff therefore need to be confident about taking the lead role in ensuring that the patient leaves hospital promptly and safely. The ability to implement planned discharges out of hours, particularly at weekends and on bank holidays, independently of medical staff, is crucial.

In emergency care there has been much emphasis on criteria determining whether or not hospital admission is required. In recent years, increasing pressure on bed capacity and the priority given to promoting discharge have led to renewed interest in criteria-based discharge documents for certain acute medical conditions. These distil best practice guidelines into a series of logical steps applied by member(s) of staff to an individual patient, recording and prompting specific interventions.

Discharge bundles are now being used to guide safe discharge for specific acute illnesses. North West London Hospitals Trust has a series of bundles in use, including a COPD Discharge Bundle. The discharge bundle criteria are listed in a coloured peel-off section on an A4 sheet, which is stuck in the case notes. If the criteria are met, the completing nurse is then directed to a final 'safe discharge checklist'. The British Thoracic Society has evidence-based guidelines for discharge criteria for patients with community-acquired pneumonia, which can be easily applied by nursing staff (BTS 2004).

At weekends in acute hospitals, there can often be a dramatic drop in discharge. Wong *et al*. (2009) showed that weekend discharge rates of general medical patients were 50 % lower than reference weekday rates, with holiday Monday rates 65 % lower. Consultants have a crucial role in making (new) discharge decisions at weekends. Although this is routine on post-take discharge rounds, these rounds are confined to a review of patients admitted within the previous 12–24 hours. A major reason to increase seven-day working by senior medical staff is the recognition that patients may become medically fit for discharge over the weekend. They could then be discharged by a consultant-led team, which has been constituted to make this clinical decision and implement the discharge.

Discharge – the future

The process of discharging patients safely has never been more important than it is at present – in the context of a resource-constrained NHS, struggling to meet a relentlessly increasing demand for emergency medical care. Although discharge has previously been a relatively neglected aspect of healthcare, there is growing evidence that safe, timely discharge is moving to a central position in healthcare strategy.

In the UK, the coalition government, very early in its term, signalled a new emphasis on safe successful discharge as a key measure of quality of care in the revised 'NHS outcomes framework 2010/2011' (DH 2010b). This was reinforced by the introduction of a penalty aimed at reducing avoidable admissions within 30 days of hospital discharge. Hospitals re-admitting a patient within this period would not receive any further payment for the additional treatment.

This policy makes an explicit link between the quality of inpatient care, discharge and avoidance of readmission. The framework states:

> 'Making hospitals responsible for a patient's ongoing care after discharge will create more joined-up working between hospitals and community services and may be supported by the developments in re-ablement and post-discharge support. This will improve quality and performance and shift the focus to the outcome for the patient'
> *(DH 2010b).*

The policy is endorsed in the Government White Paper 'Equity and Excellence: Liberating the NHS' (DH 2010c), and is central to domain 3 of the 2011/12 NHS outcomes framework, 'helping people to recover from episodes of ill health or following injury' (DH 2010d). However, the indicator has been altered to emergency readmission within 28 days of discharge. It is also recognised that further work is needed on the interpretation of readmission rates and how these can best be used as a measure of recovery (DH 2010d).

Over the next decade, advances in information technology will continue to have a huge impact on the care of patients in hospital, their discharge, and the ability of health services to maintain health and treat illness in the community. Validated, evidence-based, clinical decision-making software tools offer the prospect of monitoring illness and level of dependency in the community, and matching this with clinical interventions, including admission to hospital. Application of similar tools to hospital inpatients will help standardise the quality of care and timing of discharge for in-patients, while maximising care in the community and minimising the use of secondary care resources.

The most profound impact of clinical decision-making software on the discharge process is likely to involve objective data generated on the clinical requirements for admission to, and remaining in, an acute hospital bed, according to severity of illness and response to treatment – in line with best practice care. This data, and the relentless pressure on healthcare resources, will undoubtedly drive strategy in the health economy to reduce the use of expensive inpatient care to a minimum. The NHS will need a new paradigm in creating alternatives to acute hospital care.

References

British Thoracic Society (2004 update). 'BTSS guidelines for the management of community acquired pneumonia in adults'. www.brit-thoracic.org/guidelines

Caldwell G. (2006). Real-time assessment and feedback of junior doctors improves clinical performance. *The Clinical Teacher*. **3**, 185–188.

Davis, M.H. & Dent, J.A. (May 1994). Comparison of student learning in the out-patient clinic and ward round. *Medical Education*. **28** (3), 208–212.

Department of Health (2000). 'The NHS Plan'. London: HMSO.

The Department of Health (2003). 'Discharge from Hospital: pathway, process and practice'. London: HMSO.

Department of Health (2004). 'Achieving timely "simple" discharge from hospital – A toolkit for the multi-disciplinary team'. London: HMSO.

Department of Health (2005). 'Operational framework for foundation training. Modernising Medical Careers'. www.mmc.nhs.uk

Department of Health (2010a) 'Ready to go? Planning the discharge and transfer of patients from hospital and intermediate care'. London: HMSO.

Department of Health (2010b). 'Revision of the operating framework for the NHS in England 2010/11'. www.dh.gov.uk/prod_consum_dh/groups/dh_digitalassets/@dh/@en/@ps/documents/digitalasset/dh_116860.pdf

Department of Health (2010c). 'Equity and Excellence: Liberating the NHS'. www.dh.gov.uk/prod_consum_dh/groups/dh_digitalassets/@dh/@en/@ps/documents/digitalasset/dh_117794.pdf

Department of Health (2010d). 'NHS outcomes framework 2011/2012. Technical details of indicators'. www.dh.gov.uk/prod_consum_dh/groups/dh_digitalassets/@dh/@en/@ps/documents/digitalasset/dh_122954.pdf

Easton, C. & Oyebode, F. (1996). Care management. Administrative demands of care programme approach. *British Medical Journal*. **312**, 1540.

Elwyn, G., Foster, A. & Freeman, G. (27 July 2005). 'Mind the gap: the risk of adverse events and errors during patient discharge'. www.saferheathcare.org.uk/IHI/Topics/DischargingPatients/WhatWeKnow/

Feachem, R.G.A., Sekhri, N.K. & White, K.L. (2002). Getting more for their dollar: a comparison of the NHS with California's Kaiser Permanente. *British Medical Journal.* **234**, 135–141.

Felten, S., Cady, N., Metzler, M.H & Burton, S. (1997). Implementation of collaborative practice through interdisciplinary rounds on a general surgery service. *Nursing Case Management.* **2** (3), 122–126.

Fernando, K.J. & Siriwardena, A.K. (2001). Standards of documentation of the surgeon-patient consultation in current surgical practice. *British Journal of Surgery.* **88**, 309–312.

Gair, G. (2001). Medical dominance in multidisciplinary teamwork: a case study of discharge decision-making in a geriatric assessment unit. *Journal of Nursing Management.* **9** (1), 3–11.

General Medical Council (1999). *The Doctor as Teacher.* GMC.

Gibson, D.R. & Campbell, R.M. (2000). The role of cooperative learning in the training of junior hospital doctors: a study of paediatric senior house officers. *Medical Teacher.* **22**, 297–300.

Hales, B., Terblanche, M., Fowler, R. & Siddald, W. (2008). Development of medical checklists for improved quality of patient care. *International Journal of Quality Health Care.* **20**, 22–30.

Herring, R., Desai, T. & Caldwell G. (2011). Quality and safety at the point of care: how long should a ward round take? *Clinical Medicine.* **11** (1), 20–22.

Hodgson, R., Jamal, A. & Gayathri, B. (2005). A survey of ward round practice. *Psychiatric Bulletin.* **29**, 171–173.

Kilminster, S., Hale, C. & Lascelles, M. (July 2004). Learning for real life: patient-focused interprofessional workshops offer added value. *Medical Education.* 38 (7), 717–726.

Lees, L. (2006). 'Emergency Care Briefing Paper: Modernising Discharge from Hospital'. National Electronic Library for Health. http://libraries.nelh.nhs.uk/emergency/viewResource.asp?uri=http%3A//libraries.nelh.nhs.uk/common/resources/%3Fid%3D63696&categoryID=1414

Lees, L. (2008). Estimating Patients' Discharge Dates: applied leadership. *Nursing Management.* **15** (3), 30–35.

Lees, L. (June 2010). Exploring the principles of best practice discharge to ensure patient involvement. *Nursing Times.* **106**, 25, 10–14.

Lees, L. & Holmes, C. (2005). Estimating date of discharge at ward level: a pilot study. *Nursing Standard.* **17**, 40–43.

Lees, L., Allen, G. & O'Brien, D. (2006). Using post-take ward rounds to facilitate simple discharge. *Nursing Times.* **102** (i8), 28–30.

Lees, L. & Delpino, R. (2007). Facilitating Timely Discharge from Hospital: Combining patient name boards and discharge planning information. www.nursingtimes.net

Manias, E. & Street, A. (2001). Nurse doctor interactions during critical care ward rounds. *Journal of Clinical Nursing.* **10**, 442–450.

NHS Confederation Briefing. (5 May 2006). 'Why we need fewer hospital beds'. www.lho.org.uk/download.aspx?urlid=10511&urlt=1

Nursing and Midwifery Council (2008). 'Code of Professional Conduct: Standards'. www.nmc-uk.org

Pathak, A., Pathak, N. & Kak, V. (2000). Ideal ward round making in neurosurgical practice. *Neurology India.* **48**, 216–22.

Reeves, S., Freeth, R. & Wood, D. (2000). A joint learning venture between new nurses and junior doctors. *Nursing Times.* **96** (38), 39–40.

Rix, S. & Sheppard, G. (2003). Acute wards: problems and solutions: Implementing real change in acute inpatient care – more than just bringing in the builders. *Psychiatric Bulletin.* **27**, 108–111.

Talbot, M. (2000). Professional modeling: a questionnaire study of junior doctors' attitudes to aspects of experiential learning on the hospital ward round. *Medical Education.* **34**, 312–315.

Thompson, A.G., Jacob, K. & Fulton, J. (2004). Do post-take ward round proformas improve communication and influence quality of patient care? *Postgraduate Medical Journal.* **80**, 675–676.

Wong, H., Wu, R.C. & Tomlinson, G. (2009). How much do operational processes affect hospital inpatient discharge rates? *Journal of Public Health.* **31** (4), 546–553.

Chapter 14

Patient involvement and patient perspectives on discharge
Jamie Emery

The aim of this chapter is to highlight the importance of involving both patients and, crucially, their carers in preparation for leaving hospital care. The chapter addresses key aspects of patient discharge, which can broadly be classified as communicating and listening to patients' and carers' views in the period leading up to discharge. It is written from the perspective of Patient Advocate Liaison Services (PALS) and therefore represents everyday discharge situations as they arise in practice. Solutions are suggested, using input from a team with considerable experience.

Frontline clinical staff face many challenges in discharging patients. The pressures on making beds available that exist in an acute hospital environment sometimes mean that the focus is more on achieving discharge than the process that is used to make discharge happen. In this sense, discharge becomes an event, rather than a process (Jewell 1993). Involving relatives with sometimes high expectations can sometimes be seen as a hindrance. Moreover, what staff believe they have communicated is not always the message that patients and carers receive.

The benefits of patient involvement have long been recognised. In today's NHS, particularly since the Darzi Review (Darzi 2008), and latterly under the new administration, the patient involvement movement has gathered pace. The introduction of the CQUIN payment framework (DH 2008) means that NHS organisations are now financially rewarded on the basis of how patients rate their experiences. Involvement in care, especially in communicating the discharge plan to the patient, is one of the standards by which organisations are assessed (DH 2008). This chapter will demonstrate how, by involving and speaking to patients and carers about the discharge and transfer planning process, we can make the process clearer and easier for patients, carers and ourselves.

Monitoring patient involvement in the discharge process

The Commissioning for Quality and Innovation (CQUIN) payment framework makes a proportion of providers' income conditional on quality and innovation within all NHS organisations. This means that national standard contracts require commissioners to make 1.5% of contract value for providers to earn.

'Goals should reflect local priorities which must be stretching and focused.

CQUIN goals are influenced by:

- Local & national priorities
- Commissioner/provider discussions
- Local clinical engagement
- Patient and public involvement

CQUIN helps to ensure that quality is part of the commissioner-provider discussion everywhere'

Department of Health, 2008.

For the last year, at the Heart of England NHS Foundation Trust, in Birmingham, we have routinely recruited existing Trust staff from non-clinical areas to go out to the bedsides across all of our wards. These staff have asked patients and carers 12 questions about their care, to gauge the quality of their experiences. This has taken a considerable effort, and shows that achieving genuine patient involvement is a huge challenge.

One of these questions is: 'Have staff talked to you about your discharge?' Patients can reply: 'yes', 'to some extent' or 'not at all', with each response weighted as 10, 5 or 0 respectively. A red/amber/green scale shows how each ward performs, depending on the responses of patients.

As an average, across all standards and since monitoring started, we have scored 84%. We score highest on respect and dignity, where we score 93% on average. For patients' experiences of discussing discharge, we score 54% (14% below our next lowest marker and 30% below our average). This demonstrates that our involvement of patients in their discharge from hospital remains a challenge.

Results for all standards are uploaded in real time to an internal website across the organisation. The results display a purely quantitative measure of how patients on each ward have perceived their care and the staff delivering care. Whilst the tool is quite a blunt instrument and a crude analysis of a hugely complex area, the online and real-time nature of the analysis has allowed us to arrive at baseline. This assessment allows performance tracking of nursing at Trust or site level, or down to individual wards.

When asking patients this question about discharge, staff are often met with puzzlement, as if it's expected that we won't talk about this until we absolutely have to. A typical response is, 'I've only been here two days.' However, if we don't talk to patients about discharge, we are ignoring one of the most important aspects of their stay with us. Feedback from patients and carers strongly suggests their preference is for this conversation to start from admission, and to continue for the duration of their stay.

Ward teams feel the data that has been collected from patients does not always reflect the nature of discussions that have actually taken place, and that professionals do speak with patients and carers about their discharge or transfer. A key point here is the patient's perception that we haven't talked about it, either *to* them or *with* them (there is a subtle difference), and this will be explored further in this chapter.

Staff could be supported in their efforts by documentation designed to accommodate contemporaneous discussions about discharge (Lees 2010). This would provide an ongoing commentary to all on progress towards discharge. It would also have the added benefit of providing a constant reminder to the team of how important going home (or elsewhere) is to patients and carers.

Complaints about discharge and why we receive them

In a large acute hospital, discharge is a theme that has always frequently come up in patient complaints. There also tend to be complaints about quality of care provided, staff behaviour and attitudes, but discharge can be relied upon to be in the top five themes that come up in complaints.

Complaints regarding the NHS often stem from poor communication or miscommunication issues. However, involving the patients in a person-centred care approach could vastly reduce complaints regarding discharge planning. It is often the case that ward teams feel that their communication has been consistent and informative. But if patients and carers are not involved as equal partners in the whole process, particularly around discharge, understandings become cloudy. And it needs to be remembered that patients' and carers' perceptions are their realities.

To be effective, communication and involvement needs to meet the expectations of both patients and carers. There are no hard and fast rules to this and every individual is different. Communication that has been well received in one instance cannot be applied to every situation, so genuine involvement is something that needs to be sought on a case-by-case basis. This very much depends on the self-awareness of staff and their ability to read individuals' behaviours and communication styles and preferences.

Nevertheless, there are general principles and examples of good practice that do apply in all cases. Indeed, when the majority of patients are discharged or transferred they are apparently satisfied. However, the number of actual complaints and, other softer intelligence suggest otherwise. Analysis shows that, from a patient's and carer's perspective, we need to be smarter about our relationships with them. Essentially, patients and carers need to become our collaborative associates.

Ineffective communication during the admission period raises anxieties. Around 80% of complaints tend to be made by relatives or carers, as opposed to patients themselves. This is certainly sometimes due to the capacity or the ability of the patient. But generally the relatives can be relied upon to say what the patient doesn't want to make a fuss about, perhaps fearing that recriminations may follow, should they 'have the cheek to complain'.

A vital component of any concern or complaint is a patient's or carer's understanding of what is happening, whether it involves discharge or any other aspect of their care. Emotions and feelings run high when people are admitted to hospital. The unfamiliarity of their surroundings and the forced break from their usual routines may alter patients' and carers' views and understanding of matters. We may feel that we have told them something and explained it in the best way possible. But the fact is that, often despite our best efforts, patients and carers don't always take on board what we may feel is explicit information. This all demonstrates why staff should work more closely with families and speak to them more about plans for discharging the patient.

How can we communicate better about discharge?

The well-known research conducted by Albert Mehrabian in the 1960s may help us with this issue (Mehrabian 2007). This research showed that 7% of verbal communication is understood, and that the vast majority of communication actually occurs through tone or body language. This is particularly true in the hospital setting, where patients' and carers' usual sensory perceptions are often altered by their surroundings. Four important elements are addressed below, with examples and solutions:

1. Involvement
2. Method of communication
3. Advance notification of discharge
4. Use of family members as advocates

1. Involvement

Actually asking patients or carers themselves what they want or need can have a profound effect on their experiences and make managing challenging situations far easier for us. The following case study, although not specifically related to discharge, illustrates this.

Case study 1

A regular user of hospital services, who is an elderly post-polio patient, and a wheelchair user with quite profound physical disabilities and respiratory complications, is interviewed. She is scathing about the countless contrary experiences of care she has had in the past, when she was 'done to'. However, when she was actually involved in her discharge planning, she was overjoyed and glowing in her praise for the nurse she encountered. In fact, she insisted that senior management should be made aware of this shining example. What the nurse actually did was quite simple. She merely asked: 'How would you like me to care for you?'

The nurse, as part of her assessment, went on to stress that the patient was the expert in her own care and that the nurse would be guided about how, specifically, care should be given. This was such a small thing for the nurse to consider but made a huge difference to our patient and her experience of hospital on this occasion. This shows that if we can routinely involve patients in our plans, including discharge, we can improve experiences and prevent complaints.

2. Method of communication

Letters are commonly issued to patients to explain discharge; and for more complex discharges, such letters may involve social services. However, staff dealing with discharge planning need to be aware that, whilst a letter may fulfil a requirement, and many patients or relatives will understand its content, the local adult reading age, particularly in more socially disadvantaged areas, is sometimes lower than you would expect it to be. Indeed, the average adult reading age in the UK is thought to be around 12 to 14 years, and it is claimed in some areas to be as low as 9.5 years (Plain Language Commission 2008). Readability tests can help us with this problem, but there is no substitute for actually asking patients and carers for their thoughts. This will give us some real insight into what different people actually understand by our communications.

Local demographics also need to be considered, when deciding whether a letter explains beyond doubt within the patient's or carer's understanding. When English is not the patient's first language, a family member can usually translate, but again the issue of local reading ages may come into play.

3. Advance notification

One of the main reasons for complaints about discharge is that, when the day comes, it is often a complete surprise to patients and carers. This is because, as far as they have understood, nobody has mentioned discharge until that point. Clearly, we need to be very explicit in the way we talk to relatives and carers about discharge. We also need to involve relatives and carers from day one – and set realistic expectations about what is right for the patient and when discharge is likely to be.

One quite simple way to instil this information in the minds of patients, and also to involve them, is to introduce the estimated date of discharge into ward areas (Lees 2008). (For more on this, see Chapter 27.) This strategy places a clear responsibility on frontline staff to update the expected date of discharge as and when plans inevitably change. However, in the act of doing so, an opportunity presents itself to have the discharge conversation with patients and carers.

Such a notice or communication also demonstrates another key point – that patients don't always feel they have permission to speak up and ask questions, for fear of being viewed as awkward or as 'causing a fuss'. In her book on the subject of 'Englishness', Dr Kate Fox talks at length about how not wanting to make a fuss is a typically English trait (Fox 2005) and this is absolutely how our patients, and often their relatives, feel.

If we are to truly involve our patients in discharge and ultimately improve their experiences, we have to address the fact that patients, and, to a lesser extent, relatives, are highly reluctant to ask questions because they don't want to be too much trouble. Being admitted to hospital is a frightening experience, heightening a patient's sense of vulnerability, in an already difficult situation. We therefore need to make it clear to patients that they absolutely have permission to ask questions and a right to be involved in the decisions that affect them.

Evidence from previous examples demonstrates that positive outcomes can be achieved with families and carers simply by involving them in the process, as opposed to the discharge being handled as an event.

4. Use of family members as advocates

Invitations to multidisciplinary team (MDT) meetings and case conferences can be a way of preventing concerns escalating, and of letting a family see the full extent of the multidisciplinary efforts involved in a patient's discharge.

Case study 2

In this case, it was assumed that the relatively young members of a family did not need or want to be involved in a patient's care or discharge. English was not the preferred language for other family members, so the patient's grand-daughter, who was intelligent and articulate, largely spoke on the family's behalf. The patient had dementia and the family had many concerns about how they were going to cope with caring for their relative at home. The issues were raised because the family had the impression that the clinical team expected to discharge the patient back home as previously, even though the dementia had become so acute that they could no longer cope.

Once it had been highlighted that the grand-daughter actually could liaise on the family's behalf and the nature of their concerns had been explained, the situation changed. The grand-daughter felt empowered to ask questions, whereas previously she had felt left out and sometimes belittled by the professionals who seemed to be making recommendations without listening to her family's worries.

As a result, a review from an appropriate medical professional was arranged, and discharge plans were altered. The family were involved and included in the process from that point on.

It is quite common for relatives to complain that they have not been advised of a discharge date or to question the decision to discharge, particularly when a patient is declared as medically fit for discharge. The implication, from a family perspective, is often that the hospital is ready to discharge the patient without considering any ongoing care needs. In one such case, a relative said: 'I am my mum's carer. She lives with me. I know her better than anybody but nobody would listen to any of my concerns and it was frustrating and upsetting.'

Nobody working in that MDT would have wanted to engender these feelings, yet this situation was a direct result of not speaking to family members about the discharge. The situation was then managed by simply inviting and involving the family with MDT meetings and giving them permission to contribute their opinions. This approach paved the way for a far less complicated and more amicable discharge.

When a doctor states that a patient is 'medically fit for discharge', it often throws families into blind panic, prompting anxious phone calls to PALS departments, to Chief Executives' secretaries, MPs' offices, and the local media. If only somebody explained to the patients and carers what this term actually means, in a way they could understand, we would avoid many of the complaints. And, more importantly, we would not cause so much anxiety and stress in the very people we are here to serve.

Patient and carer views of discharge

Hospital admission and subsequent discharge can often represent a step change in the personal circumstances of a patient's relatives. Their loved one may be going from being a spritely and active mother, father or spouse to a very different person with very different needs from the ones they had prior to their admission. This change in their relative is not expected and may, in large part, not be understood.

Case study 3

Recently, at the Heart of England Foundation Trust, we dealt with an elderly patient's daughter-in-law and son. The patient had fractured her neck of femur and underwent successful surgery. Despite the personal upheaval for this lady, she made a good recovery.

However, in the days following the operation, the available discharge options were not made clear. The relatives became increasingly anxious about her discharge, and it developed into a very difficult situation. This was exacerbated by some staff members assuming that the patient would be going to a residential placement and saying as much to her.

The family's plan was always to take the patient back to their home, to live in a purpose-built part of the house, in pleasant surroundings, receiving care from her family. This was the outcome the team were aiming towards, and there was no reason whey this was not possible. However, the family didn't always get this consistency of communication. On occasions, the patient was led to believe that the discharge back to her family's home would not be possible, and this caused her some upset.

This situation was dealt with simply by taking the time to listen to the family's wants, needs and anxieties. These were considered and assurance was given that the discharge to their home was not in any doubt. We then pressed ahead with making arrangements on this basis.

In complying with our duty to discharge to a safe place, we are often misunderstood by families. Most people leaving hospital don't need longer-term support. Some need support for several weeks and some will need it for the rest of their lives. From an acute perspective, we are transferring the patient to the best possible available environment for their ongoing care and rehabilitation. But from a relative's perspective, we may appear to be moving their relative to another place just to free up a bed. It often needs to be made clear that the patient's best needs are not being served in the acute hospital setting, and it can be particularly helpful to explain the risks involved for elderly patients simply by being in hospital.

Intermediate care settings now exist to allow for timely discharge from hospital and prevent premature admission to long-term residential care. These intermediate care facilities can provide a more appropriate environment for the right type of care to be provided, once a patient's medical needs for hospital admission are addressed. Alternatively, families may need information about options involved in discharging patients back to their home, promoting their independence and mobility by putting an appropriate care package in place.

In such a situation, you can involve a family a great deal and they may still not understand why discharge is appropriate. The point is that, if expectations and realities are clarified as early as possible, families are then not dealing with surprise, on top of all their other anxieties, when it comes to discharge day.

In the vast majority of cases, the NHS provides very high-quality care and some remarkable treatment to get patients to a stage where they can be discharged or transferred to a safe and appropriate setting. But it is the way we act during the period when the patient is a guest with us that often defines the discharge experience for all involved.

As an ancient (and very wise) Chinese proverb puts it: 'Tell me and I'll forget; show me and I may remember; involve me and I'll understand'.

References

Darzi, Professor/Department of Health (2008). 'High quality care for all: NHS Next Stage Review'. London: HMSO.

Department of Health (2008). 'Using the Commissioning for Quality and Innovation (CQUIN) payment framework'. London: HMSO.

Fox, Dr K. (2005). *Watching the English: The Hidden Rules of English Behaviour*. London: Hodder & Stoughton.

Lees, L. (2008). Estimating Patients' Discharge Dates: applied leadership. *Nursing Management*. **15** (3), 30–35.

Lees, L. (2010). An action research project: Improving the quality of nursing documentation on an Acute Medicine Unit. *Nursing Times*. 106 (37), 22–26.

Jewell, S. (1993). Discovery of the discharge process: a study of patients discharged from a care unit for elderly people. *Journal of Advanced Nursing*. 18, 1288.

Mehrabian, A. (2007). *Nonverbal Communication*. New Jersey, USA: Transaction Publishers.

Plain Language Commission (2008). Writing by numbers: are readability formulas to clarity what karaoke is to song? www.clearest.co.uk/files/WritingByNumbersKaraoke.pdf

Section 4

Education for discharge planning

Chapter 15

Developing educational opportunities to fit the future workforce

Ann Saxon

Current fundamental changes in the NHS are driving the need for practitioners to be knowledgeable, enterprising and innovative (DH 2010a) in order to improve patient safety and advance healthcare outcomes. Technology to support patient care is at the forefront of healthcare development in education, with particular emphasis on the safe discharge of patients.

The enhancement of teaching and learning has enabled practitioners to develop skilled, creative and innovative ways of delivering education. This chapter explores the opportunities for senior nurses in corporate positions and practitioners engaged in developing educational materials to promote better discharge planning practice and make the best use of the technology that is available to them.

Professional regulation

The Nursing and Midwifery Council (2010) has set out recommendations for an all-graduate nursing profession from September 2011; and educational establishments are in the process of redesigning their curricula to meet the new standards. Degree-level registration underpins the level of practice needed for the future and will enable nurses to work more closely with other professionals (NMC 2010). They suggest that programmes should be flexible (using a blended approach to learning) and offer a full range of learning modes, including the use of technology. The subject of technology-supported learning will be explored further in this chapter.

Learning means developing and enhancing change (Reece & Walker 2007, p. 59), not only through reflecting on our own lives, but also by enabling us to experience personal growth. Learning about discharge planning through innovative education gives practitioners an opportunity to engage in a collaborative approach to learning. It also allows them to apply their new skills in practice, whether as a student nurse or a registered practitioner.

Teaching is not only about designing educational packages. The teacher should not just be seen as a purveyor of knowledge (Reece & Walker 2007, p. 3) but also as a facilitator: a person who enables students to learn for themselves. Designing innovative educational material for effective discharge planning should create opportunities to enhance inter-professional working and increase learning by means of sharing experiences and becoming more self-directed as a learner.

The political perspective

The current political perspective has put discharge planning high on the agenda for all healthcare organisations. The Commission for Quality Innovation (CQUIN) set out a national framework for locally agreed quality improvement schemes (DH 2010). They have also set a national goal related to the personal needs of patients, which should be included in patient discharge plans. For example:

- Were patients informed of the side-effects of medication when going home?
- Were patients given a contact person if they were worried about anything when going home?

Local agreements are required on how best to collect and collate this information from all patients entering any service. Practitioners engaged in discharging patients should have the appropriate skills and knowledge to perform this role. Currently the Patient Advocacy Liaison Services are taking this on – by sending out letters in advance of elective admissions to advise patients on what questions they should ask. However, this can serve to disengage front-line practitioners in their duty to integrate this as part of their role if it is carried out by other members of the team.

The Healthcare Commission National Patient Survey (2004) identified delays in the day of discharge home from hospital as a key area where standards could be improved. This led to the 'Achieving timely "simple" discharge from hospital' toolkit for the multidisciplinary team being developed by the Department of Health in 2004. Further developments have been instigated to date.

The creation of any educational material for healthcare practitioners should be supported by current sociological, political, professional and personal knowledge of the factors influencing discharge planning, and the effects this has on patients and their carers who may need simple or complex packages of care. Some of the considerations can be seen in the following list.

Considerations in developing educational material for discharge planning

- Current policy: (national service frameworks, legislation, patient service agreements)
- Epidemiology: (chronic disease)
- Sociological perspective: (demographics, ageing population, disability, long-term conditions)
- Professional knowledge: (key skills, competency, role development, inter-professional working, leadership)

The pace of change in the NHS is relentless; and education must keep pace with the changes so that it can be pro-active, rather than reactive. Therefore, when designing any educational materials for healthcare practitioners, it is essential that all of the above factors are considered and implemented throughout.

The educational arena

Preparation for professional practice usually requires the learner to follow a particular syllabus to meet the required outcomes for a programme of learning laid down by a governing body such as the Nursing and Midwifery Council (NMC) or the Health Professions Council (HPC). As previously mentioned, in 2011 nursing will become an all-graduate profession in line with other allied health professions such as physiotherapy and occupational therapy. Other graduate professions have been supported by assistant practitioners for many years.

Nursing may well see a change in the required skills mix in the coming years. For instance, discharge planning needs a range of skills, from assessment and planning to referrals and booking of appointments. The awarding bodies for professional practice set minimum standards, which have to be explicitly laid out in any curriculum design. When developing new course material and educational packages, it is advisable to check the most up-to-date published standards. These can usually be found on the websites of the professional bodies – for example www.nmc.org.uk, or www.qaa.ac.uk

The Quality Assurance Agency for Higher Education (QAA) is the governing body that oversees the development of professional courses in higher education institutions (HEI). The QAA was established in 1997 to provide an integrated quality assurance service for UK higher education. They describe the level of achievement a student has to reach in order to gain an academic award, such as a degree. The QAA ensures that standards are similar across the UK. They review the standards of education by carrying out an educational audit. They have developed subject benchmark statements, which identify the expected outcomes of a particular degree in a range of subject areas.

Education for discharge planning

When designing any new courses, it is therefore advisable to match course content to the subject specialist benchmark statement. The statements are very generic and are not specific to areas of practice. For example, in relation to discharge planning, it would be necessary to use the broad categories provided below.

QAA Subject benchmark examples: Healthcare programmes

Subject specific benchmarks	Healthcare programmes
• Professional autonomy and accountability • Professional relationships • Personal and professional skills • Identification and assessment of health and social care needs	• Practice • Knowledge, understanding and skills that underpin the education and training of healthcare professionals

The QAA has also set up a code of practice, which has ten sections:

1. Postgraduate research programmes
2. Collaborative provision and flexible and distributed learning (including e-learning)
3. Students with disabilities
4. External examining
5. Academic appeals and student complaints on academic matters
6. Assessment of students
7. Programme approval, monitoring and review
8. Career education, information and guidance
9. Placement learning
10. Recruitment and admissions

www.qaa.ac.uk/aboutus/Pages/default.aspx

When designing new materials for programmes developing discharge planning skills, it is advisable to ensure that the course follows the code of practice in terms of quality, including, for example, the use of e-learning and other types of collaborative provision.

The use of e-learning

People often describe e-learning as 'a catalyst for change', because it cuts across institutional structures and impacts on all aspects of practice (Conole & Oliver 2007). Most educational organisations have a well-structured e-learning platform that engages learners in a range of activities such as:

- Assessments
- Blogs
- Study groups
- Learning materials

The use of e-learning materials should follow guidelines for students to ensure that they have been designed in the most effective way, encompassing recommendations from the Higher Education Funding Council Executive (HEFCE). It is also important to consider the special educational needs of particular students and the policy that is in place to support and protect learners with a disability (SENDA 2005).

In the government's White Paper 'The Future of Higher Education' (DfES, 2003) the HEFC was given the responsibility of ensuring that e-learning was embedded in a full and sustainable way.

They put forward three aspects for consideration when devising an e-learning strategy:
1. The need to implement use of the Internet and new technologies
2. New approaches to learning and teaching are emerging in response to diverse student and employer demand; this includes workplace learning and blended learning
3. Wholly Internet-based learning has recently captured the imagination because of the opportunities to explore exciting technological approaches and to provide global delivery (HEFC 2004)

www.hefc.ac.uk

According to a 2008 report from the Economist Intelligence Unit, online learning is gaining a firm foothold in universities around the world, and is seen as a key feature in providing education for those who may previously have been excluded (EIU 2008). It suggests that no generation is more at ease with technology than today's young people, who have grown up in an immersive computing environment. Most universities have to respond to globalisation, which has created an ever-expanding overseas market. This has also included making healthcare training and education available to those were previously unable to access them.

Other considerations when designing new courses

There are many influences from policy and practice that should be taken into consideration before embarking on new initiatives in designing courses for discharge planning practice. Evidence suggests (DH 2004, DH 2010a) that it is not only nurses who are involved in planning discharge for patients. Other health professionals may also be leading this process – for example, physiotherapists, occupational therapists, medical practitioners and social workers. It is important that an inter-professional approach is taken when planning any new course to ensure that the new skills being offered complement each other, rather than duplicating those of other professionals. This will mean that patients and carers have the benefit of a range of health professionals to optimise hospital discharge (DH 2010a).

There are many opportunities that can be embraced when developing new courses and methods of delivery, in order to ensure that courses meet the needs of twenty-first century practitioners. The next part of this chapter will explore the need to modernise healthcare education.

Modernising education

Modernising education has long been on the agenda of many professional groups, not only healthcare practitioners. Information for patients and carers is now widely available and their expectations of care are far higher than in previous times.

Access to the media has encouraged patients and carers to express their opinions of care more widely, especially since the introduction of Patient Advocacy Liaison Services (PALS), which have given them a way of voicing their concerns. Health professionals have had to respond to these comments in a constructive and pro-active way.

Age UK (2010) offers guidance in relation to discharge planning and the legal rights of patients. One way of responding to changes in healthcare and the expectations of patients is to develop a wide repertoire of skills that can be applied in practice. Developing new skills in discharge planning could be one way of matching expectations to needs that have been expressed by patients. Bradshaw (1972) put forward a taxonomy that has been used to explore the differences between patients' and practitioners' needs.

Bradshaw's taxonomy of need

* Felt need: gap between knowledge and practice
* Expressed need: new programme needs development
* Unmet need: no new programmes exist

This taxonomy can be applied to the learner and teacher in relation to modernising education. It could also be used in marketing new courses that have been developed.

Previous educational programmes relied heavily on the learner being a passive recipient of knowledge and the teacher being seen as the expert (Reece & Walker 2007). Formerly, nursing education programmes were designed to focus very much on the input of knowledge without considering the changes that take place in the individual who experiences new learning. A new graduate profession will require nurses to focus on evidence and the development of autonomous practice. Sometimes it is only long after the learner has completed a course that the real benefits of that learning can be measured. Most often, students recall learning when they apply it to a situation they currently find themselves in. For example, students in a classroom may find it hard to see the point of developing discharge planning skills. It is not until they find their new skills being called upon in practice that they realise their importance. Likewise, managing change skills may be required to develop a new service in practice settings, or leadership skills may be needed to take a new team forward.

Developing a range of new skills is essential in order to deliver the NHS agenda for 2011. Most undergraduate programmes in healthcare now have a diverse approach to delivering innovative dynamic courses.

Some examples of such innovative approaches include:

- Problem-based learning
- Reflective practice
- Virtual learning communities
- Online learning
- Clinical practice assimilations

Some of these will now be explored in more detail. The advent of problem-based learning has its origins in a number of schools of philosophical thought, such as naturalism, metaphysics, phenomenology and rationalism (Howell Major & Savin-Baden 2004).

It is a way of encouraging learners to make sense of a situation in a reasoned, guided way. In simple terms, it encourages learners to break down situations that may on the surface appear very complex. They learn to analyse what led to the situation and the factors influencing people's thoughts, feelings and behaviour.

Problem-based learning is a complex phenomenon and should not be used just as a method to deliver specific material. Problem-based learning should include all of the learning that is required and the assessment of that learning in a supported and facilitated way.

Some of the possible advantages of problem-based learning have been described by Weller (2002, p. 71):

- Increased student motivation
- Development of problem-solving skills
- Increased student responsibility
- Flexibility
- Exposure to different ideas and solutions
- Contextualisation of information
- Interactive and engaging
- Deepening of the skills of reflection and analysis

Examples of the use of problem-based learning in relation to developing and designing a course for discharge planning, will be given later in this chapter.

Online learning has become most popular, as it allows the learner to access information and courses wherever and whenever they are able. Staff working in any healthcare arena need education to be as accessible as possible. Although time is set aside to attend mandatory courses, other types of learning are usually relatively unsupported unless they form part of a more formal award such as a first degree or master's degree. Making use of online facilities opens up a wealth of opportunities for all types of students – for example, those working part-time or during the early evening as well as night shift workers.

According to Shank & Sitze (2004, p. 2):

> 'Online learning involves the use of network technologies (such as the internet and business networks) for delivering, supporting and assessing formal and informal instruction.'

They go on to say that this can be through the use of online resources and materials, electronic libraries, learning materials and courses, real-time and non-real-time discussion forums and conferencing, and knowledge-sharing forums.

The use of online learning has opened up a wealth of opportunities for the development of courses. However, a word of warning: not all material produced may be of high quality, and it may not be recognised by professional bodies for accreditation. On the other hand, employers are finding it difficult to release staff for training away from the workplace so online learning does offer a way of getting training whilst still remaining within the working environment. This ease of access could enable more staff to engage with online learning.

However, learning in isolation is not always beneficial. For instance, it does not allow students to share examples and debate issues as they would in a classroom situation. Finally, even more than ever, employers now require proof that learning is making a difference in practice. With the development of a range of new skills, e-learning may be a way of demonstrating this. It is important to take all these factors into account.

Other factors to consider when using online materials are as follows:

- Accessibility of computer equipment
- Accessibility of network
- Confidence of learner in using computer
- Copyright material
- Reviewed material
- Who is accrediting course
- Cost
- Academic currency

Most learners, especially those working in healthcare, are required to keep evidence of continuing professional development. For nurses, this is done through Preparation for Practice (PREP), as outlined by the NMC. For other allied professions, this is implemented through the Health Professions Council, which was formed in 2001 to regulate health professions. The Nursing and Midwifery Council requires practitioners to keep up-to-date evidence of study in their particular area of registration and present this periodically. Since 2005, allied health professionals have been required to keep a record of their continuing professional development, with an audit of this commencing in 2007. Updating learners' records online should help to ensure that they meet professional standards, particularly if these records are going to be used as part of a portfolio of evidence.

With the introduction of modern technologies to support teaching and learning, this is an exciting time to be developing dynamic programmes of study to meet the needs of an ever-changing NHS.

Developing a module of learning for effective discharge planning

Developing effective partnerships between education establishments and practice areas is essential when considering new courses. This can be achieved in many ways. More formally, it is done by validating and accrediting formal programmes such as initial entry nursing programmes that require 50 % of the course to be supported in practice settings (NMC 2010). Less formally, these links can be created by clinical practitioners working alongside educationalists in a research capacity or developmental role. It can be invaluable for practitioners to develop a sound relationship with university staff, so that they can guide the practitioners through the sometimes difficult process of getting courses validated and accredited.

The next part of this chapter will discuss how such a partnership can be effective in enabling new materials to be designed in an innovative and creative way. In this example, a local university worked collaboratively with a Foundation Trust Hospital to develop a course for health professionals in effective discharge planning.

Is there any need for specific discharge practice education?

In this case, the student nurses appeared to have very little knowledge of the discharge process. On taking up posts in the Trust, newly qualified nurses were only required to read the Trust's discharge planning policy. Beyond this, their education relied upon the 'goodwill' and time afforded to them by ward-based nurses who were interested in discharge planning. This shows that there is little point in formulating new government policy without also making a serious commitment to deliver the changes required in practice.

Another factor was the development of the toolkit for the multidisciplinary team in achieving timely 'simple' discharge from hospital (DH 2004). A more recent publication is the 'Ready to go?' guidance document published by the Department of Health (2010b). This stated that discharge from hospital was not simply the discharge of responsibility, but the process of transferring the care of a patient from one service to another. From a patient and carer perspective, this report identifies the following as hallmarks of good practice:

- Good communication between staff, patients and carers
- Involving patients and carers at all stages of discharge planning
- Giving good information
- Ensuring that patients and carers (where appropriate) are helped to make planning decisions and choices (DH 2010b)

Other documents have stated, when outlining the development of a nurse allied health professional initiated discharge policy, the need for education and training, with particular emphasis on:

- Core discharge skills analysis to determine areas of training required
- Competency assessment
- Competency based training and declaration of competence

When developing any new training initiatives, it is important to consider any funding implications. Developing new materials can be expensive, particularly if you intend to develop multimedia technology. A budget and schedule should always be set before starting any project, as these aspects will be crucial to its success or failure.

Developing effective relationships in any new venture is also essential: communication from all parties should be clear, prompt and transparent.

It was decided that the programme would be designed as a module of study that could be accessed by nurses and other health professionals studying at the university. The module would also be made available as a stand-alone course that could be marketed to other people outside the immediate area.

Deciding on the module content

When designing programmes of study, it is important to give some consideration to the outcomes that you wish the learner to demonstrate. The Higher Education Academy (www.heaacademy.ac.uk 2006) put forward some points for consideration when designing a training course:

- What do you want students to know?
- What do you want students to learn?
- Create a syllabus from textbooks, research papers, personal research
- Develop resources to support students' learning
- Decide how to assess the knowledge

To put the first two points another way, what do you want students to do and be able to do? Think in terms of verbs such as: listen, read, observe, discuss and argue, work independently, solve problems.

How will you know what they have learnt? What evidence do students have to provide to show that they can do something? What do students, employers, professional and statutory bodies think you should be teaching? What competencies exist in this area of practice?

Consideration should be given to all of the above when designing a programme. The overall aims of the course should put forward what you, as the teacher, will deliver to the students; and the learning outcomes should describe clearly what the students will be able to do following the session or course. The programme aim and some of the learning outcomes are shown below.

Module aim

To enable the student to understand the political, social and economic implications of effective discharge planning. In addition the student will gain an appreciation of the roles of the nurse/therapist in the discharge planning process. The module will enable practitioners to gain skills required to apply a systematic and sustainable programme of change towards introducing nurse/therapist discharge.

When formulating programme aims, it is important to remember that aims are evidence of the goals that you have set as a teacher or as a curriculum group (Reece & Walker 2007, p. 16). They set out what students will be able to demonstrate at the end of the learning experience. Module aims are fairly general and are designed to describe the overall purpose of the course.

Learning outcomes translate the module aim into something more specific and measurable in smaller components. When formulating learning outcomes, it is important to consider which particular type of learning is involved – such as psychomotor, cognitive, or affective domain. Bloom (1958) designed a taxonomy of learning that you can specifically apply to each of the domains.

Before designing your aims and outcomes, you need to set the scene by explaining why this module of study is important. This explanation should include all the relevant legislation and government policy.

Education for discharge planning

Below is an example of specific learning outcomes.

Learning outcomes specific to discharge planning module

1. Demonstrate an appreciation of the impact of government policy on discharge planning.
2. Demonstrate an understanding of the civil and legal frameworks that exist in relation to negligence and how these impact on the role of nurses and therapists who carry out the discharge of patients.
3. Explore and apply strategies of change management for the introduction of nurse/therapist-led discharge planning.
4. Critically appraise the role of the multi-professional team in ensuring effective discharge planning.

Learning and teaching strategies

It is also important to consider learning and teaching strategies when designing new innovative courses of study. Previously in this chapter we have discussed various innovations that are impacting on education. A blended style of learning has been applied to this module, and blended learning is sometimes also called 'hybrid learning'. This is a combination of delivery methods, ranging from no technology to using technology on a continuum (Shank & Sitze 2004). The methods used can also range from traditional classroom courses to self-paced learning on CD-ROM or the Internet. Introducing a range of blended learning techniques is an innovative way to develop materials.

The introduction of information technology and use of the Internet have been growing over the past ten years. Most universities now have well-developed learning management systems (LMS) and virtual learning environments (VLE). A learning management system usually includes such elements as:

- Library
- Portals
- Student record systems
- Content management systems

There has been a significant rise in the number of organisations using a virtual platform to deliver educational material, and some organisations are quicker to adopt innovations than others. Rogers (1998) suggests five categories of attitude towards innovation, which are fairly common. It may be useful to consider these, as follows:

- Innovators
- Early adopters
- Early majority
- Late majority
- Laggards

He goes on to suggest that, when early adopters make significant progress, this then becomes mainstream. It is then usually followed by the provision of extra resources and staff. It is vital that courses are designed utilising appropriate learning and teaching strategies. The following are seen as appropriate methods to include in the development of this type of module:

- Problem-based learning
- Virtual learning environment
- Online learning

At the development stage, it is important to involve relevant departments within both the university and the Hospital Trust. In the case under discussion, it was decided that part of the module would be delivered using a virtual learning environment (VLE). This would need to be designed using specific software available through the university. (It is essential that the relevant university departments are included in the original plan, as it can delay proceedings if the required software is later found not to be available.)

It was decided that a range of short case studies would be presented online and permission was sought to access health professionals who would be willing to contribute these case studies. It was thought that it would not be ethical to involve real patients in this exercise, as formal consent might be difficult to obtain.

Staff could be approached to provide short video clips. A mock interview, discussing their role, and a mock ward round/case conference could also be set up. The following table lists ideas for developing short video clips that could be used within a virtual learning environment.

Job title	Subject for video topic
Intermediate care manager	Intermediate care services Single assessment process
Discharge liaison nurse	Discharge liaison roles and responsibilities MDT meeting
Social services manager	Coordination of social services
Continuing health manager	Re-imbursement and re-charging
Lead nurses	Nurse-led discharge Estimating dates for discharge Protocol development Training needs analysis
Capacity manager Clinical site practitioners Clinical leads for discharge planning	Coordination of bed management in large NHS Trust

(Rowntree 1999, p. 9)

Education for discharge planning

Some other ideas that could also be considered for making short video clips for virtual learning environments would be:

- A ward round
- A post-take ward round
- A multidisciplinary team meeting
- A bed management meeting
- An emergency assessment area
- Interview with a patient who has been discharged (not a real patient)

Before embarking on lengthy, costly projects, it is worth having a few issues clear in your mind, as suggested by Rowntree (1999):

- Who is expecting what of you?
- What resources can you call on when developing your project?
- How will you schedule your time?

It is also worth considering whether you have chosen the right materials to elaborate your points. Rowntree (1999) suggests thinking about the following questions:

- What media are available?
- If using video, have you got editing support?

Perhaps the most useful question to ask is:

> 'What is the simplest/cheapest medium or mix of media that will satisfactorily (even if not perfectly) meet our learners' needs?'   *(Rowntree 1999, p. 65)*

When designing online materials, it is essential to start by ensuring that you have the right aim and learning outcomes. Have you considered learner support and how this will be accessed? Have you also considered existing materials that could support your new module?

As part of your plan, put some time aside to develop scripts for your video clips and work out how you will sequence your ideas. Will you need graphics experts and information technology support?

In the specific example under discussion, the module material also included problem-based learning. This was designed using case studies that highlighted both the positive and negative aspects of patient discharge. Using such case studies, learners would be expected to engage online with a support group to identify solutions and ways of improving discharge planning.

The module material would need to meet the requirements of the SENDA (2005), so it is important that equality and diversity are considered at all levels. Most universities have special departments set up to make sure these requirements are met in any new material produced. These provisions are intended to widen participation in education, and make education inclusive and not exclusive.

Assessment of learning should be clearly laid out. In this particular module, the following assessment strategy was decided upon by the university. However, the appropriate method of assessment also depends on what experience the learner is bringing to the module. For instance, a particular individual may have many years of experience, which could enhance the experience of others.

Two-part assessment: 50% each of total marks

a) Completion of a reflective analysis of the discharge or transfer of a patient from hospital to home or other care setting. (2000 words)

b) Completion of range of online tasks relevant to discharge planning. (1000 words)

The assessment strategy should test what learning has taken place and how this can be embedded in practice.

Mode of delivery

It is envisaged that the module would be delivered in several ways, including:

1. An induction day to introduce the learning material and provide student support for developing information technology skills.

2. Online learning time, in which activities would be assessed in an ongoing way. These activities would be formative and summative components of the module.

3. Tutorial support to ensure that students are progressing with online material and that they have a sound level of knowledge in order to develop a range of reflective skills.

4. An evaluation day to consolidate ongoing learning and evaluate assessment strategy.

The module would be delivered over a period of months, as part of a formal academic semester or year. Some students might not access the formal assessment but perhaps just wish to carry out the learning as an informal development exercise. Academic credits can only be awarded to students who have successfully achieved a pass grade in all aspects of the assessment strategy. Usually awarding universities have a formal process for awarding academic credits. Students who wish to have acknowledgement of credits would usually be required to register with the awarding university.

Piloting training materials

Having designed material for inclusion in a formal module or unit of learning, it is important to consider how and what training is required for staff developing materials and students who will be accessing the courses. All too often, it is left to chance that students will know how to engage with the technology. However, the reality is that many of them are not that proficient and soon become disheartened and de-motivated. Innovative styles of delivery should be well planned and produced to a very high standard. Going back to the planning stage is advisable to see if information on how to access materials is clear. It may be best to pilot your course with a few volunteers, before publishing it for the wider community. Indeed, Rowntree (1999) suggests that piloting may be the most crucial aspect of the whole project. The motto should be: Write it … try it out … improve it.

Feedback from pilot stages is essential to ensure that your final version is credible and marketable. This feedback should include critical commenting, piloting and continuous monitoring. Most online and virtual learning environments have sophisticated ways of recording how many learners have utilised the resource, and immediate feedback is usually available.

Other questions that need to be considered when designing materials for online teaching are as follows:

- What type of learner is the course aimed at?
- How can you encourage self-directed learning?
- Do staff members have access to computers via libraries and on ward areas?
- Is mandatory training for any new staff provided as part of an induction programme?
- Do you have access to the most up-to-date media system for computer use?

Evaluation of training materials

In evaluating your module you may need to consider a stakeholder analysis. A stakeholder analysis looks at all of the interested parties and how this programme has impacted upon them. A list of interested parties in a typical stakeholder analysis is shown below.

Stakeholder analysis for evaluation of module

- Any co-authors
- Colleagues or managers
- Learners
- Pilot learners and tutors
- Foundation Trust colleagues
- Consultants
- Accrediting bodies
- Others
- Patients and carers

It is important to make the technology cost-effective and for production costs to be clearly thought out. Most universities have a set price for the cost of the module delivery. This can range from as little as £100 to as much as £1000, depending on the level and mode of delivery. You also need to consider the cost of updating information, which can quickly become out of date in the health service arena.

You also need to consider the long-term delivery platform. Educational and practice areas could gain invaluable experience in delivering online courses, so putting off development of online material may not be an option at all. This type of innovation can also lead to new developments such as the use of mobile phones as a means of providing learning materials for students.

Marketing the module or course is another important factor. Events such as conferences and networking meetings can provide a platform to market new and innovative educational packages.

Evaluation of course material can take many forms. Evaluation needs to be immediate and materials should be appraised in a positive and constructive way. Some major problems may show up straight away. For instance, some students cannot even begin the course because their computers do not have the right software to open the existing materials!

Lees, Price & Andrews (2010) carried out a comprehensive evaluation of a part-time, post-registration discharge practice education module. The module was validated by a local university and successful candidates were awarded 12 credits at degree level. The evaluation included outcomes and impact of the learning and the assessment strategy. A total of 10 work-based projects were implemented in clinical practice, and the Trust discharge standard was a significant factor.

Based on their evaluation, they made the following recommendations:

- Currently discharge practice is not integrated
- In future, patients' perspectives on their discharge experience should be included
- Study days could be used to present a condensed version of the module for organisations that find it difficult to release staff from clinical areas

(Lees, Price & Andrews 2010)

Other considerations should include, as outlined by Lewis and Allan (2005):

- Overall design principles
- Methods and techniques
- Individual learning
- Development of knowledge
- Changes in professional practice
- Impact on the organisation
- Impact on the virtual learning organisation

Training time for all students and staff should be built in to the overall timetable of events; as previously mentioned, the cost of this should be included in the overall cost of delivering the module.

Conclusion

Developing learning materials for effective discharge planning is an exciting initiative. The module discussed in this chapter was produced for practitioners who had gained an initial qualification in their own area of practice, which could have been nursing, physiotherapy, occupational therapy or social work. This is to assist members of the multidisciplinary team to assess their own level of knowledge and skill in the discharge planning process. It should help to identify training needs and it could be studied alone or as part of a more formal programme of learning such as a diploma or degree or a higher award such as a master's degree or doctorate.

The components of the module and the interactive material could be adapted to cover other staff such as healthcare assistants and students from all professions. Newly qualified staff could study this module as part of a development programme or supervisory programme. Expert practitioners and consultants could use the material as a reflective aid to ensure they were delivering best practice in the area of discharge planning.

Tips for success

- Use a collaborative approach when developing new training material.
- Follow professional practice guidelines.
- Utilise expertise to develop interactive materials.
- Ensure that learners are supported.

References

Age UK (2010). Factsheet 37. Hospital discharge arrangements. Age UK.

Bloom, B.S (1958). *Taxonomy of educational objectives.* Boston, USA: Pearson Education.

Bradshaw, J. (1972) A taxonomy of social need. *New Society.* March: 640–643.

Conole, G. & Oliver, M. (2007). *Contemporary Perspectives on E-Learning Research.* Themes, Methods and Impact on Practice. Oxfordshire, UK: Routledge.

Department for Education and Skills (2003). 'The Future of Higher Education'. London: HMSO.

Department of Health (2004). 'Achieving timely "simple" discharge from hospital – A toolkit for the multi-disciplinary team'. London: HMSO.

Department of Health (2010a). 'Liberating the NHS: Developing the Healthcare Workforce'. London: HMSO.

Department of Health (2010b). 'Ready to go? Planning the discharge and transfer of patients from hospital and intermediate care'. London: HMSO.

Department of Health (2010c). 'Using the Commissioning for Quality and Innovation (CQUIN) Payment Framework: a summary guide'. London: HMSO.

Economist Intelligence Unit (2008). 'The Future of Higher Education: How technology will shape learning'. London.

Health Commission (2004). 'Patient Survey Report'. London: Health Commission.

Health Professions Council (2005). 'Continuing Professional Development Key Decisions'. London: Health Professions Council.

Higher Education Funding Council (2004). 'Learning and Teaching: Teaching Initiatives: Centres for Excellence in Teaching and Learning.' www.hefce.ac.uk/learning/tinits/cetl/

Higher Education Academy (2006). 'Some ways of designing a course page'. www.heacademy.ac.uk/1555.htm

Howell Major, C. & Savin-Baden, M. (2004). *Foundations of Problem-based Learning.* Society for Research into Higher Education and Open University Press. Berkshire, UK: Open University Press.

Jisc infonet (2006). Infokit. Analytical Tools and Templates. www.jiscinfonet.ac.uk

Lees, L., Price, D. & Andrews, A. (2010). Developing discharge practice through education module development, delivery and outcomes. *Nurse Education in Practice.* **10**, 210–215.

Lewis, D. & Allan, B. (2005). *Virtual Learning Communities: A guide for practitioners.* The Society for Research into Higher Education and Open University Press. Berkshire: Open University Press.

Nursing and Midwifery Council (2004). *The Prep Handbook.* London: NMC.

The Nursing and Midwifery Council (2010). http://standards.nmc-uk.org/PreRegNursing/Pages/Introduction.aspx

Quality Assurance Agency for Higher Education (2006). 'The Quality Assurance Agency for Higher Education: An Introduction'. www.qaa.ac.uk/aboutus/intro.asp

Reece, I. & Walker, S. (2007). *Teaching, Training and Learning: A practical guide incorporating FENTO standards.* (sixth edition). Sunderland, UK: Business Education Publishers Ltd.

Rowntree, D. (1999). *Preparing Materials for Open Learning and Distance Flexible Learning.* London: Kogan Page.

SENDA (2005). 'The Special Educational Needs and Disability Act 2001'. London: HMSO.

Shank, P. & Sitze, A. (2004). *Making Sense of Online Learning: A Guide for Beginners and the Truly Sceptical.* San Francisco: Pfeiffer.

Weller, M. (2002). *Delivering Learning on the Net: The Why, What and How of Online Education.* London: Routledge Farmer.

Weller, M. (2008). *Virtual Learning Environments: Using, Choosing and Developing Your VLE.* Oxfordshire: Routledge.

Chapter 16

Competency in discharge planning and role development
Denise Price

In the late 1990s, nursing roles proliferated, and competency frameworks were developed to ensure that individuals possessed the skills and ability needed to practise safely and effectively without the need for direct supervision (UKCC 1999). As new ways of working and national policy pushed the boundaries of professional practice further, competency frameworks continued to feature in the development of new services, even though their impact varied according to local organisational culture, and individuals' personal and professional desire to develop new roles in response to changing patient need (Price *et al.* 2007).

Are competencies still relevant?

We know, through 'Front Line Care', the Prime Minister's Commission Report on the Future of Nursing and Midwifery (DH 2010b), that competence remains central in determining what skills nurses and midwives require to practise effectively. This report clearly states the need for competencies when designing new models of service delivery. Competencies continue to support nurses working effectively in different settings, within existing and new roles and when they change jobs (Price *et al.* 2007).

There is considerable evidence available in relation to the potential effectiveness of using competency frameworks, not least their ability to provide skilled, knowledgeable and confident practitioners (DH 2010d, Price *et al.* 2007, RCN 2006). The evidence as to how the use of competencies has improved the overall shift in the skills of individuals is less obvious. However, this may be due to the fact that the assessment of competence varies across organisations, ranging from formal sign-off to individual reflection in practice.

Price *et al.* (2007) describe how developing competencies is the first step required when considering new or changed roles as part of service redesign. By beginning with competencies, you align specific knowledge and skills to patient outcomes. In this way, you allow the development of roles to support pathways of care provision thereby supporting delivery of patient outcomes, rather than the traditional development of roles based on the known and historic delivery of care (Watts *et al.* 2007, DH 2010b, NHS Institute 2009a). At an individual practitioner level, using a competence framework effectively applies knowledge, understanding, skills and values within a designated area of practice; and there is a general consensus that this is good practice (DH 2010e).

New partners and methods of planning

The decision to deliver a patient-led NHS (DH 2005) signalled a change in how and where services were developed and commissioned, with services being designed that best suited patients' needs, bringing care closer to home and being delivered with 'the right skills in the right place'. This was further supported by the 'Next Stage Review – High Quality Care For All' (DH 2008) which provided a more clinically led focus for the redesign of services, placing a greater emphasis on multi-professional roles and specialist roles, and increasing levels of care delivered in non-acute settings.

'Front Line Care' (DH 2010b) describes how nursing and midwifery delivery has changed and adapted in response to changing healthcare settings and different models of delivery, which provide greater access, improved choice and greater freedom for patients. The report clearly describes the nurse's potential contribution in utilising existing legal and professional capacities and competencies in referral and discharge. Whereas discharge was previously seen primarily as a task and function of acute settings, the delivery of care in differing environments has increased the focus on discharge in this wider context and subsequently on a much broader group of staff (Day *et al.* 2009).

Have the requirements for discharge practice competencies changed?

Competencies are statements that often describe specific tasks which practitioners are required to undertake in the workplace, as part of their individual role or function, or as part of a team. They are underpinned by knowledge, experience and skills. They often cannot be separated from an individual's professional values and beliefs. Collectively, they represent competence in its broadest sense to colleagues, service users and carers (DH 2010b, DH 2010e, Price *et al.* 2007).

The 'Revision to the Operating Framework for the NHS' (DH 2010f) proposed that hospitals should be responsible for patients for the 30 days after discharge. (For more on this, see Chapter 2.) If a patient is readmitted within 30 days, the hospital will not receive any further payment for the additional treatment required. This raises the expectation that the quality and timing of discharge will have to improve, and gives greater urgency to the task of improving discharge practice and the overall competency of individuals and teams.

As delivery of care currently involves organisations and roles in a variety of settings (including primary care, privately financed walk-in centres and community-based services), the need for competency frameworks has increased greatly, given that all these staff could otherwise potentially be working to differing standards and variable levels of competency. This is where a competency framework really adds value, by ensuring that the right skills are in place across the whole pathway of care, regardless of the provider, and keeping the focus on the final outcome for the patient.

The recent consultation White Paper 'Liberating the NHS: Commissioning for Patients' (DH 2010c) described the increased freedoms for healthcare to be provided by non-NHS organisations, potentially signalling the move to a free market. While this may benefit patients, by giving them increased choice and more personalised care, it also has the potential to develop practitioners to differing sets of standards, and competencies guard against this. It is anticipated that the revised operating framework will make the discharge process more 'joined up' and better focused on patient outcomes (DH 2010f).

Against this backdrop, it is clear that competencies remain a valuable tool to ensure consistency of practice and definition of roles and responsibilities. According to Price *et al.* (2007), the key starting point is deciding on the particular competencies required to deliver effective discharge planning. We then need to identify the most effective jobs to deliver, or be trained to deliver, to ensure consistency, which will be dependent on the complexity of the task and the requirements of the service overall (NHS Institute 2009a, Griffiths & Robinson 2010, DH 2010b).

Price *et al.* (2007) outlined how competencies (described by the RCN as being achieved at four different levels of practice: competent, experienced, advanced and consultant), could be used to map competencies for discharge planning onto the Knowledge & Skills Framework (KSF). While this approach is still relevant, it does not take into account the increasing numbers of non-NHS organisations that are now prevalent in the delivery of care, in which the KSF is not used.

We know that competencies enable us to evaluate and assess clinical practice and they play an important role in professional development (Lee-Hsieh *et al.* 2003, Price *et al.* 2007, NHS Institute 2009a). More importantly, as discharge planning encompasses many more organisations as part of effective care pathway delivery, competencies can be developed across teams and pathways of care, ensuring that the skills and expertise of each discipline are used to identify and implement the best strategies for the patient (Watts *et al.* 2007, Lees 2010). However, Watts *et al.* (2007) argued that increased benefits to patients would be seen if professionals clearly outlined their roles in relation to discharge planning. This reinforces the need to be clear about roles and responsibilities.

Huang *et al.* (2005) described how a lack of clearly defined roles and responsibilities in the multidisciplinary team can negatively affect the discharge process. With the involvement of increasing numbers of providers, this issue can have a significant impact on discharge planning and should be considered carefully when designing the care pathway (NHS Institute 2009a).

Commissioner influence

'Commissioning a Patient Led NHS' (DH 2005) placed the responsibility for commissioning health services for local populations with local Primary Care Trusts (PCTs). This strategy was aimed at reducing health inequalities and ensuring the provision of safe and effective healthcare, and it brought clinicians across organisations together to work on redesigning care pathways to improve patient experience and health outcomes.

'Front Line Care' (DH 2010b) describes how commissioning will be an increasingly important driver for quality by means of commissioning services across pathways, and ensuring that appropriate roles, skills and competencies deliver effective care. The launch of the Department of Health 10 key steps (DH 2010d) also enables commissioners, through a whole systems approach, to ensure that patient choice and independence is maximised through the development of care pathways, with improved personalised care and discharge planning. This is agreed by providers and embedded in contracts.

Achieving competencies across pathways and providers of care

Lees & Emmerson (2006) and Maher & Fenton (2010) described how the active management of discharge planning requires nurses to make decisions, balance risks and avoid delays. Huang *et al.* (2005) also described how effective discharge planning depends on successful multidisciplinary team working between health and social care professionals, and how using a whole systems approach recognises the contribution of all partners to the delivery of high-quality care. Griffiths & Robinson (2010) and the Prime Minister's Commission on the Future of Nursing (DH 2010b) recognised that developing a role and competency framework facilitates the transition of jobs between organisations, where the delivery of care is then viewed across a pathway of care, not organisation specific.

When discharging patients across a wide range of different care providers, a common set of competencies to support good discharge planning is essential, to ensure effective transfer and handover of care to different professionals (Marsh & Brady 2007, NHS Institute 2009a). While the use of competencies has never been mandated, more work-based learning, and the development of consistent pathways of care across differing providers, will enable us to ensure that consistent skills and knowledge are developed whatever the setting (Thomas & Ramcharan 2010).

Mapping competencies to specific outlines and levels

Evidence supports the concept of discharge being either complex or simple (Lees 2010, Thomas & Ramcharan 2010, DH 2004). The Department of Health (2010c) defines simple discharge as 'those patients who can be discharged to their own homes and who have simple health care needs which can be met without complex planning'. Simple discharge is undertaken by all staff responsible for the admission and transfer/ discharge of patients to an alternative setting, usually where an inpatient stay is on a day case basis or the length of stay is 3–4 days maximum. Where inpatient care is longer and the patient's needs are multifaceted, both in terms of health and social care needs, then these are often described as complex discharges, requiring a broader level of competency.

While some organisations may be less familiar with competency frameworks, their use and overall assessment in practice, many competency frameworks support the novice practitioner. Evidence suggests that, to simplify the use of competencies to support practice, competencies could be grouped into generic discharge competencies, where all staff are required to undertake a number of specific tasks, supported by a range of specific competencies aimed at roles whose primary function is discharge planning, care coordination or discharge liaison (Griffiths & Robinson 2010, Lees 2010, Thomas & Ramcharan 2010, NHS Institute 2009a, Marsh & Brady 2007). (For more on this, see Chapter 10 on discharge coordinator roles.)

Alternatively, competencies could be grouped to reflect levels of practice, as described by the RCN – in other words, competent, specialist, advanced or consultant level, with generic competencies embedded in all roles and specific competencies aimed at specialist or advanced level roles (DH 2004, Lees & Emmerson 2006, RCN 2006, Hickman *et al.* 2007, DH 2010b). The benefit of this approach is that generic competencies are transferable across health and social care, supporting staff whatever their working environment (Price *et al.* 2007)

Competencies and the assessment/appraisal process

While there is little evidence to support the use of competencies within the appraisal process, the KSF (Knowledge and Skills Framework) has been used across the NHS to assess the actual skills and development needs of individuals. Given the diversity of providers already involved in the delivery of patient care, using the KSF in isolation could place non-NHS practitioners at slight odds with NHS colleagues. Competencies can therefore be used as part of the appraisal process, to assess actual skills and knowledge and identify development needs.

Competencies can be assessed using a number of different methods, mainly based on workplace learning and assessment. Although assessment has to be undertaken by trained assessors who can demonstrate adequate experience, competencies do provide the flexibility to assess in the clinical area and help link theory to practice (Price *et al.* 2007). The key to using competency frameworks, however, is ensuring that they are consistently applied across an organisation or care pathway, and utilising commonly agreed approaches to support multi-professional education and training (Lees & Emmerson 2006, Lees *et al.* 2010, DH 2010b). In this way, competency frameworks transcend organisational differences, providing a common footprint for all training, development and service redesign, whereby the competencies required to undertake a particular role, in any setting, become a 'common language' (Price *et al.* 2007, NHS Institute 2009a).

Practical implications for effective discharge planning

Continuity of care in discharge is an important quality issue. Yet there remains considerable evidence to demonstrate that poor discharge planning leads to increased likelihood of readmission, poor adherence to therapy and treatments, reduced patient reported outcomes and poor patient experience overall (Flower 2005, Walker *et al.* 2007, Day *et al.* 2009, DH 2010d, Watts *et al.* 2007, Thomas & Ramcharan 2010). Day *et al.* (2009) outline the differences between acute and primary care providers and the emergence of discharge planning as a complex area of practice, as the dependency and co-morbidity of patients increases.

Hickman *et al.* (2007) and the NHS Institute (2009a) demonstrated that one of the interventions that was critical in providing optimal health outcomes for older people admitted to acute care was an increased emphasis on discharge planning, particularly a multidisciplinary team approach, with communication strategies that emphasise discharge planning.

In March 2010, the Department of Health launched a document entitled 'Ready to go', which provided a practical resource or guide for practitioners and organisations, to make improvements in the discharge and transfer of patients (DH 2010d). The guide outlines ten key steps to achieving safe and timely discharge, underpinned by ten key principles according to which practitioners work together and work with patients and families. While not technically a competency framework, these ten steps and key principles enable the development of competencies to reflect the practitioner level (i.e. competent, experienced or advanced level in whatever discipline, allowing a multi-professional approach, as reflected in the table on page 250).

The table broadly identifies competencies of assessment and planning, of care in collaboration with the patient and family, of communication (verbal and documentation), of partnership working both within and outside the organisation, of leadership, of action planning and of problem-solving, decision-making and team working (Flower 2005, Walker *et al.* 2007, Day *et al.* 2009, Huang *et al.* 2005, Santry 2009, DH 2010b, Lees 2010, Lees *et al.* 2010, Thomas & Ramcharan 2010).

This approach has been further supported by the launch of the 'High Impact Actions for Nursing and Midwifery' (NHS Institute for Innovation and Improvement 2009a), giving eight good practice examples that deliver quality and productivity, and reduce costs.

One such example is 'High Impact Action Ready to go – no delays' (2009a), which aims to increase the number of patients in NHS-provided care that have their discharge managed and led by a nurse or midwife where appropriate. The move towards nurse-led discharge is mainly in response to an overall increase in discharge activity, due to shorter lengths of stay, increasing patient throughput and the increasing acuteness of patients' medical conditions. As simple discharges make up 80% of all discharges, changing the way in which simple discharges occur will reduce delays in discharge, improve patient experience, and reduce the risk of healthcare-associated infections (Maher & Fenton 2010). It is estimated that a reduction in length of stay of between two and six days per patient could save NHS Trusts between £15.5 and £46.5 million annually (NAO 2000).

This finding was further supported by the 'Essential Collection', a collection of good practice case studies, based on the practical experiences of implementing the 'High Impact Actions' (NHS Institute 2010). The 'Ready to go – no delays high impact action, provides a number of case studies with excellent examples of improving discharge, and makes particular reference to the use of competency-based training to support the development of nurse-led discharge.

Planning the discharge and transfer of patients from hospital and intermediate care, adapted from 'Ready to go?'

	Set an expected date of discharge (EDD) and discuss with patient/carer	Develop a clinical management plan within 24 hrs	Coordinate the discharge/transfer process through effective leadership
Advanced practitioners (Expert)	Able to: Undertake full assessment of the patient Demonstrate excellent knowledge of the clinical condition Estimate the length of stay needed to complete treatment Review and revise EDD based on new assessments/data	Able to: Develop clinical management plan based on full assessment Implement and review plan developed by another member of MDT Make effective discharge decisions	Able to: Lead a team effectively Demonstrate collaborative working Communicate effectively with team and patients Develop/implement plan Identify and agree shared goals
Practitioners (experienced)	Able to: Undertake partial assessment of the patient Use protocols/guidelines to support planning Prompt MDT to estimate EDD Prompt review of EDD based on assessment	Able to: Implement aspects of the plan and coordinate care Assess the patient for discharge using guidelines Identify when patient's condition has deteriorated	Able to: Understand individual roles as part of MDT Communicate effectively with MDT/patients Anticipate information required from decision-making Demonstrate high level of knowledge of discharge process
Newly qualified (Competent)	Able to: Carry out basic components of assessment Follow instructions and report variances Demonstrate awareness of discharge model	Able to: Demonstrate understanding of plan Implement aspects of the plan Demonstrate understanding of effective communication	Able to: Demonstrate an awareness of MDT roles Understand the importance of effective and timely discharge

(DH 2010d) and Price et al. (2007), pp. 70–71

Roles and responsibilities – the ideal versus the reality

Although access to competency frameworks and discharge planning guidance has been extensive over the last few years, its application in practice remains variable (Watts *et al.* 2007, Day *et al.* 2009, Huang *et al.* 2005, Ward *et al.* (2010) describe how nurses have become disengaged from the management of patient admission and discharge, and feel pressurised into speeding up discharge because of the demands of bed capacity and increasing patient turnover.

Evidence indicates that inter-professional education and training is a way of improving and understanding roles and responsibilities but in practice this does not always occur (Atwal 2002, Pethybridge 2004). Bowles *et al.* (2003) and Day *et al.* (2009) all demonstrated that lack of knowledge, experience and competence were important concerns relating to discharge planning effectiveness. They advocated the inclusion of discharge training in induction and staff development programmes.

Lees *et al.* (2010) highlighted the need to link education and training to service and clinical priorities and demonstrated that, by aligning training with the needs of patients and clinical delivery at local level, clinicians and managers would be truly accountable for improvements in practitioner practice. They also demonstrated the importance of practice development in linking nursing objectives (excellent care for patients) and those of the organisation (service development and redesign) to the delivery of positive outcomes for patients (Lees *et al.* 2010, p. 211).

Impact from support-level roles

The NHS currently employs over 303,000 support-level staff for doctors and nurses, and a significant proportion of these are healthcare support workers. Numbers of non-NHS support staff, across the health and social care sector, are likely to be even greater. Clearly, the support workers who work alongside nurses providing direct clinical care have gained a more prominent role, especially since the introduction of higher-level support workers in the form of assistant practitioners (Griffiths & Robinson 2010, Sandall *et al.* 2007).

In reviewing healthcare support worker regulation, Griffiths and Robinson demonstrated that healthcare assistants not only undertook practical tasks such as bathing and feeding patients but they were also involved in a range of administrative tasks traditionally undertaken by registered nurses such as care planning, and discharge planning. This finding has been supported by other studies that have shown how roles can drift from purely supportive functions to include tasks such as discharge planning which impinge on professional practice (Bridges *et al.* 2003, Sandall *et al.* 2007). Evidence suggests that, in 2008, 72% of healthcare support workers were studying at NVQ levels (level 2 – 35%; level 3 – 62%; level 4 – 1%), with considerable variation across acute trusts (Griffiths *et al.* 2010). A survey of support workers in 2007 demonstrated that they were spending increasing proportions of time in non-supervised roles.

Defining roles and responsibilities within discharge planning is clearly imperative in order to secure sustainable improvement. While healthcare support workers play a valuable role, evidence suggests that the ratio and involvement of registered nurses directly influences patient outcomes. The role of healthcare support workers in discharge planning should be carefully and fully considered in the context of safe and effective care (NNRU 2009, Hickman *et al.* 2007).

In view of the move to an all degree-level registration for nursing, there is potential for employers to consider the use of healthcare support workers more (DH 2010b). It is therefore vital to clarify both the role and function of support workers if they are to continue to play any role in the discharge planning process. This may include collecting relevant information to support the discharge process; ensuring that key steps along the discharge planning route are completed in a timely way; and keeping the patient and family fully informed and briefed about progress, to allay concerns.

While support workers may have training in discharge planning, this does not confer the right to undertake the task. The decision to discharge remains with the supervising registered practitioner, and the needs of the patient and the organisation are paramount (DH 2010b, DH 2010e).

Conclusion

Given the increasing range of healthcare providers, the diversity of care pathways and the implications of the 'Revision to the Operating Framework for the NHS' (DH 2010f), it is imperative to consider the number and breadth of roles and the use of competency frameworks to support discharge planning in order to effect maximum improvement.

We know that the current pace and scale of change in healthcare is unprecedented, and this conclusion is reinforced by the white papers 'Liberating the NHS: Commissioning for Patients' (DH 2010c) and 'Equity and Excellence: Liberating the NHS' (DH 2010a), both of which propose a very different model of commissioning and delivery for the NHS. Evidence suggests that timely discharge supports the overall strategy of shorter stays in hospital and rehabilitation in non-acute settings. It also delivers patient-centred care and improves the patient experience (DH 2004, Flower 2005, Santry 2009, NHS Institute 2009b), thus signalling the continued importance of the role played by nurses and others in discharge planning.

Hickman *et al.* (2007) demonstrated that early comprehensive discharge planning improved outcomes for patients through improved use of medicines, greater awareness of potential complications and being less concerned about managing their own care at home. However, the key factor is, and always will be, how we apply best practice and the evidence base consistently across an ever-changing NHS landscape. Let us truly acknowledge the relevance and value of good discharge planning to patients, use the tools and examples of best practice to guide us, and embed competencies into everyday practice once and for all, to ensure delivery of consistent, high-quality care to patients.

References

Atwal, A. (2002). Nurses' perceptions of discharge planning in acute health care: a case study in one British teaching hospital. *Journal of Advanced Nursing.* **39** (5), 450–458.

Bowles, K.M., Foust, J.B. & Naylor, M.D. (2003). Hospital discharge referral decision making: a multi-disciplinary perspective. *Applied Nursing Research.* **16**, 134–143.

Bridges, J., Meyer, J., Glynn, M., Bentley, J. & Reeves, S. (2003). Inter-professional care co-ordinators: the benefits and tensions associated with a new role in UK acute health care. *International Journal of Nursing Studies.* **40** (6), 599–607.

Day, M., McCarthy, G. & Coffey, A, (2009), Discharge planning: the role of the discharge co-ordinator. *Nursing Older People.* **21** (1).

Department of Health (2004). 'Achieving timely "simple" discharge from Hospital. A toolkit for the multi-disciplinary team'. London: DH

Department of Health (2005) 'Commissioning a Patient Led NHS'. London: DH

Department of Health (2008). 'Next Stage Review – High Quality Care For All'. London: DH

Department of Health (2010a). 'Equity and Excellence: Liberating the NHS'. London: HMSO.

Department of Health (2010b). 'Front Line Care: Report by the Prime Minister's Commission on the Future of Nursing and Midwifery in England'. London: HMSO.

Department of Health (2010c). 'Liberating the NHS: Commissioning for patients'. London: HMSO.

Department of Health (2010d). 'Ready to go? Planning the discharge and the transfer of patients from hospital and intermediate care'. London: HMSO.

Department of Health (2010e). 'Responsibility and Accountability: Moving on for new ways of working to a creative, capable workforce. Best practice guidance'. London: HMSO.

Department of Health (2010f). 'Revision to the Operating Framework for the NHS in England 2010/11'. London: HMSO.

Flower, L. (2005). Evaluating the development of a nurse-led discharge scheme. *Nursing Times.* **101** (6), pp. 36–38

Griffiths, P. & Robinson, S. (2010). Moving forward with healthcare support workforce regulation. A scoping review: evidence, questions, risks and opinion. National Nursing Research Unit, London: King's College London.

Hickman, L., Newton, P., Halcomb, E.J., Chang, E. & Davidson, P. (2007). Best practice interventions to improve the management of older people in acute settings: a literature review. *Journal of Advanced Nursing.* **60** (2), pp. 113–126.

Huang, T & Liang, S. (2005). A randomized clinical trial of the effectiveness of a discharge planning intervention in hospitalised elders with hip fracture due to falling. *Journal of Clinical Nursing*. 14, 1193–1201.

Lee-Hsieh, J., Kao, C., Kuo, C. & Tseng, H. (2003). Clinical Nursing Competence of RN–to-BSN Students in a Nursing Concept Based Curriculum in Taiwan. *Journal of Nursing Education*. 42 (12), 536–546.

Lees, L. (2010). Exploring the principles of best practice discharge to ensure patient involvement. *Nursing Times*. 106 (24), 10–14.

Lees, L. & Emmerson, K. (2006). Identifying discharge practice training needs. *Nursing Standard*. 20 (29), 47–51.

Lees, L., Price, D. & Andrews, A. (2010). Developing discharge practice through education module development, delivery and outcomes. *Nurse Education in Practice*. 10 (4), 210–215.

Maher, L. & Fenton, K. (2010). Implementing the eight high impact actions to transform healthcare and boost efficiency. *Nursing Times*. 106 (3), 12–14.

Marsh, L. & Brady, J. (2007). 'Occupational therapists and nurses: Working in partnership to achieve effective discharge planning' in Lees, L. (ed) *Nurse Facilitated Hospital Discharge*. Keswick: M&K Update Ltd.

National Audit Office (2000). Hip Replacements: Getting it right first time. London: NAO.

National Nursing Research Unit (2009). RN+RN = better care. What do we know about the association between Registered Nurse staffing levels and patient outcomes? *Policy Plus*. Issue 20. London: NNRU, King's College.

NHS Institute for Innovation and Improvement (2009a). 'High Impact Actions for Nursing and Midwifery.' Coventry: NHS Institute.

NHS Institute for Innovation and Improvement (2009b). 'High Impact Actions for Nurses and Midwives, Rapid Review of Economic Data'. Coventry: NHS Institute.

NHS Institute for Innovation and Improvement (2010). 'High Impact Actions for Nursing and Midwifery. The Essential Collection'. Coventry: NHS Institute.

Pethybridge, J. (2004). How team working influences discharge planning from hospital: a study of four multidisciplinary teams in an acute hospital in England. *Journal of Interprofessional Care*. 18 (1), 29–41.

Price, D. & Garbarino, L. (2007). 'Competency and role development' in Lees, L. (ed) *Nurse Facilitated Hospital Discharge*. Keswick: M&K Update Ltd.

Royal College of Nursing (2006). 'Core Career and Competency Framework'. London: RCN.

Sandall, J., Manthorpe, J., Mansfield, A. & Spencer, L. (2007). 'Support workers in maternity services: a national scoping study of NHS Trusts providing maternity care in England in 2006'. London: King's College London.

Santry, C. (2009). Call for nurse-led patient discharge to improve care. *Nursing Times*. 105 (41).

Thomas, C. & Ramcharan, A. (2010). Why do patients with complex palliative care needs experience delayed hospital discharge? *Nursing Times*. 106 (25), 15–19.

United Kingdom Central Council (UKCC) for Nursing, Midwifery and Health Visiting (1999). 'Fitness for Practice: the UKCC Commission for Nursing and Midwifery'. London: UKCC.

Walker, C., Hogstel, M., Cox, O. & Curry, L. (2007). Hospital discharge of older adults. *American Journal of Nursing*. 107 (6), 60–70.

Ward, L., Fenton, K. & Maher, L. (2010). The high impact actions for nursing and midwifery. 8: ready to go – no delays. *Nursing Times*. 106 (34), 16–17.

Watts, R., Pierson, J. & Gardner, H. (2007). Co-ordination of the discharge planning process in critical care. *Journal of Clinical Nursing*. 16, 194–202

Chapter 17

Blended learning using computer assisted technology (CAL)

Vanessa Lockyer-Stevens

This chapter explores the use of computer-assisted learning (CAL) as part of a portfolio of learning about discharge planning (Koch *et al.* 2010). The use of CAL in planning the discharge of a wheelchair-dependent young woman following a fall is described as an example.

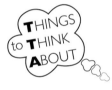 Things to Think About (TTA) icons in the design of e-learning packages are used to illustrate how web-based education technologies can complement a blended approach to flexible ways of learning.

Background

Learning is an active life-long process of critical reflection that influences and affects the way we interact with others, helping us gain an understanding of the world around us (Brown *et al.* 1983; Ramsden, 1992). Both these authors argue that understanding arises when the learner can demonstrate mastery of the field of study, rather than merely being able to manipulate facts about the subject being studied. Educationalists enjoy creating new ways of developing learning to achieve this understanding, and computer-assisted learning is one these methods.

The past two decades have witnessed an increase in the popularity and use of CAL (Koch *et al.* 2010). Most nursing and midwifery graduates use CAL platforms such as MOODLE or Blackboard, also known as virtual learning environments (VLEs), to complement face-to-face teaching as one of many types of learning used in university education. Learning in hospitals remains largely face-to-face and, with the burden of mandatory training, release from clinical areas can be difficult to achieve. In the light of all these issues, there is a pressing need to adopt more flexible ways of learning.

Education for discharge planning

Training practitioners to continue striving for excellence in delivering high-quality, evidence-based patient care is everyone's business. Finding new ways to tailor hospital-based education to particular working environments is increasingly important in today's rapidly changing healthcare settings (Koch *et al.* 2010). This is particularly crucial where the need to satisfy regulatory and mandatory requirements, whilst constantly working within the evidence-based framework, has become increasingly burdensome. Patterson Lorenzetti (2008) argues that the need to make efficiency savings whilst fulfilling consumer demand means finding a complex balance that is sometimes difficult to achieve. Recognising that we live in a world of constantly changing working practices does, however, provide compelling reasons to explore contextually sound methods of web-based learning. Rapid changes in information technology (IT), including CAL, have therefore brought learning closer to the bedside.

The Heart of England NHS Foundation Trust (HEFT) has recently purchased MOODLE to host a variety of learning opportunities that provide innovative ways of acquiring knowledge. Whilst many staff members were already familiar with more conventional means of learning and teaching, the introduction of MOODLE has proved useful because of its greater flexibility and interactivity. The discussion forum has been particularly stimulating as a means of debating and sharing ideas. Whilst the value of face-to-face teaching is generally undisputed, web-based resources provide immediate, 'any-time, anywhere' access to patient-centred learning.

A number of studies have explored users' anecdotal and experiential history of using CAL, including their perceptions of increased time, their lack of knowledge and skill in using CAL, and their intentions and actual behaviour when it comes to using CAL. As Posey & Pintz (2006) remind us, today's nurses need to work collaboratively with others to problem-solve in increasingly complex healthcare settings, and it is important for them to take a fresh look at flexible learning strategies in the interests of quality and standardisation of knowledge.

Collaborative learning engages learners as active, critically reflective thinkers. Learning is no longer confined to talk-and-chalk, as forums in particular provide growing emphasis of the incidental growth of communities of practice. Wenger *et al.* (2002) note that learning and teaching are social processes from which learning groups such as MOODLE parties, naturally form. These groups interact with existing organisations (boundary processes) and subsequently define members' sense of agency or identity (Maley *et al.* 2010). Wenger *et al.* (2002) argue that engagement, imagination and alignment are three social processes that involve the collaborative participation and flexible ways of learning required for discharge planning. Engagement, for example, recognises the learning group and its journey from observer to participant. Those with imagination construct new learning techniques, while alignment with and to others creates a platform for storytelling and shared narratives about the participants' learning. Likewise, Garrison (2003, p. 47) observes that online education nurtures independent thinkers in an interdependent collaborative community of enquiry.

CAL therefore complements existing modes of learning, and offers a number of ways in which learning about discharge planning can take place.

Computer-assisted learning (CAL) for discharge planning

CAL is a global term used to describe the role of computers in supporting a portfolio of learning activities including web-based content. Also known as online or electronic learning, it has many different uses. Interactive quizzes, podcasts, reusable learning objects or RLOBS (Blake 2009), video and audio conferencing, lecture clips, self-assessments, narrated Power Point® presentations, animations, virtual and digital animations and video clips are all educational tools supported by CAL (Koch *et al.* 2010).

Glen (2005, p. 416) describes electronic learning as a way of 'integrating information technology into the learning/teaching process, which is delivered by the Internet'. Jefferies (2006, p. 55) elaborates on this by talking about the value of discussion forums, chat rooms and email in supporting an online community of learners, which can include teachers, subject experts and other students.

Online resources such as articles, video clips and text can combine or supplement materials developed locally. Educators can develop diverse, innovative, novel and contextually sound methods, especially as they are also subject experts. Pedagogic support may be required in the development of these resources. Many developers claim 'novice' status, though this may be partly due to their perceived lack of time to prepare and develop the use of these materials (Blake 2009).

Tung & Chang (2008) ascribe this anxiety to perceptions about the relative usefulness and ease of using a computer. This, they state, can create computer anxiety and computer self-efficacy problems. Computer anxiety is defined as 'a fear of using computer technology' (Chua *et al.* 1999), and self-efficacy refers to individuals' belief (or otherwise) in their own ability to use a computer (Compeau & Higgins 1995). There was a clear correlation between computer self-efficacy and behavioural intention. Tung & Chang (2008) found that this affected whether or not users engaged with CAL. In other words, if an individual is confident in using a number of computer activities such as learning, it is easier for them to engage with and use CAL.

Moreover, consistency of design plays a part. If activities and courses are developed with similar standards of quality and simplicity, and consistent instructional and navigational design, not surprisingly this makes them easier to use and appears to increase self-efficacy.

On the other hand, e-learning can also bring about considerable change and reorganisation, and in some instances, it may be seen as a threat. Kotter & Schlesinger (2008) claim it sometimes causes a 'disturbance of the status quo, a threat to people's vested interests in their jobs, and an upset to the established way of doing things'.

Despite such anxieties, a number of studies report the positive value of CAL (Koch *et al.* 2010, Blake 2009, Pullen 2006). For some, enthusiasm for using CAL was independent of computer or internet skills (Pullen 2006). Some claim to prefer CAL to face-to-face learning. Our experience at Heart of England appears to confirm this. We have purchased MOODLE as a VLE hosting platform, and have found its architecture user-friendly.

One of the biggest advantages of CAL is for 'just-in-time learning'. Computer technology can help users find and confirm required knowledge in a way that engages them and enables them to provide a rapid response, thus improving the quality of patient care. These are all important considerations when producing engaging and purposeful e-learning resources for discharge planning.

Advantages and disadvantages of CAL or e-learning

Advantages	Disadvantages
Builds a positive attitude towards learning (pedagogic) value. Offers new ways of delivering learning and training (e.g. bespoke educational programmes).	A lack of confidence and time to develop teaching materials (Blake 2009). Not ideal for all learning.
Can accommodate flexible study patterns (Blake 2009). For example, some study better at night whilst others in the morning.	No computer facilities, network or insufficient broadband width to view or participate in. Some may feel obliged to study 'out of hours'.
Reduces need for face-to-face teaching. Can be used as part of a blended approach (Blake 2009).	May be perceived as replacing the value of face-to-face learning.
Provides a range of delivery styles. Architecture of CAL is user-friendly.	Success can't be guaranteed, as it partly depends on computer self-efficacy, i.e. individuals' belief in their own ability to use a computer (Compeau & Higgins 1995).

Advantages	Disadvantages
Good as a revision tool. For example, people can see results and follow trends in improving through repeated practice.	May prefer to read books, talk to others and read journal articles.
Mobile access to learning via on-the-move technology, e.g. ipad, iphone, blackberry.	Risk of loss of large amounts of work if a personal computer, laptop or other e-learning device is lost or stolen.
Provides an opportunity to view recorded lectures and tutorials when unable to attend actual session (Koch *et al.* 2010).	May disadvantage those for whom English is not their first language.
Online courses allow learners to cover topics most relevant to professional practice that accommodate just-in-time learning (Pullen 2006, Blake 2009).	Perception that face-to-face teaching is irreplaceable.
Offers 24-hour access to any-time, anywhere, self-paced learning as favoured by healthcare professionals (Pullen 2006, Hare *et al.* 2006). Can help improve work/life balance (Sit *et al.* 2005) by providing learning materials, at a time and place that suits individuals' needs.	May feel obliged to study 'out of hours'. Encroaches on personal time.
Convenient way for educationally and geographically diverse groups of healthcare professionals to update knowledge and view best practice.	Some may feel isolated and don't enjoy learning alone (Wedlake 2010).
Reduces travel time, costs and ward release time (Blake 2009).	Some individuals can't afford or do not want to have a computer at home.
Online forums provide extra learning; an online chat room can enable learners to learn from each other.	Some may prefer to learn alongside peers and tutors in the classroom.
Creates computer-literate, confident staff who feel comfortable with IT.	Anxiety about how to use a computer and navigate their way around computer programs such as MOODLE. This creates a general anxiety about computers (Tung & Chang 2008, Chua *et al.* 1999).
Privacy and security can be ensured by giving each individual a protected password (Hare *et al.* 2006).	

Computer-assisted learning – plan well to win hearts and minds

It is important to start by methodically gathering information about the benefits and value of e-learning, if it is to be successfully adopted by the learner. Underlying (sometimes negative) perceptions of its relevance, user-friendliness and quality require leaders to champion its development. Content, in particular, needs to be relevant to professional role and training. Here are some things to think about:

THINGS to THINK ABOUT

- Who is the target audience – nurses, healthcare assistants, medics?
- What kind of e-learning activity is best suited to the audience?
- How long will the e-learning activities take?
- Does the programme require piloting?
- Is there an assessment requirement attached to the programme? If so, are there formative (practice) exercises and/or summative (attracts a final mark) elements for completion?
- Does the learner know how to use a computer?
- Do teachers know how to develop e-learning materials?
- Is technical support available from an IT department?
- Can the available broadband width support the use of video clips and podcasts?

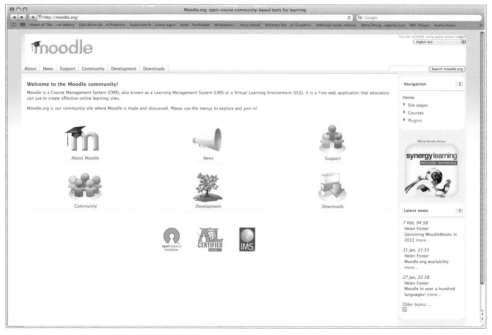

A MOODLE computer screen display.

Sample scenario: Grace

The following examples illustrate a number of e-learning activities centred on the discharge of a young woman called Grace.

Grace, a 19-year-old woman with cerebral palsy, had a fall from her wheelchair, in which she suffered a fractured tibia. She is now ready for discharge, following hospital treatment. She lives in sheltered accommodation, and has a daily carer to help with washing and dressing, as she is unsteady on her feet. Despite this, Grace is normally able to transfer from bed to wheelchair with the aid of one person. Grace has a below-the-knee Plaster of Paris, following surgery for internal fixation and plating of her fracture. Her family live some distance away.

Planning Grace's discharge generates a number of questions, some of which are listed below:

- What type of transport will be required on discharge?
- How can we assess Grace's understanding of how much care she will require following discharge?
- Who will ensure that carers are aware of Grace's discharge?
- What is the role of the district nurse in the care of Grace's fractured leg?
- How often and where should fracture clinic appointments take place?

> **Learning Activity**
> Based on the questions listed, decide what web-based resources and activities would best support learning about Grace's discharge?

Creating web-based learning activities about discharge planning

Introducing an e-learning module

Welcome to this module designed to enhance your knowledge in planning the discharge of Grace, a young adult with cerebral palsy

There are a number of interactive learning activities, each with an aim and learning outcomes. You can watch a video clip and a narrated Power Point®, and test your knowledge using a number of multiple-choice questions. You can study at your own pace, at a time and place convenient to you. You can see your results, print and add them to your learning portfolio, and share ideas with peers and teachers if you wish, in the discussion forum

Good introductions to learning are invaluable. They need to be clear and concise, engaging, easy to follow, interactive and relevant to the learner's sphere of practice (Longman & Gabriel 2004). This example takes account of the flexibility that online learning offers.

Figure 17.2 Introducing an e-learning module

Using Power Point®

Design a Power Point® presentation about, say, the role of the district nurse in helping with Grace's personal hygiene whilst she is in plaster. The presentation could include pictures of below-the-knee plaster, listing reasons for protecting it from wet damage, and explaining the role of district nurses in teaching the carer how to check for possible pressure points (including discoloration and smell).

There is some clever software that allows you to narrate each Power Point® slide. It works by using a voiceover tool to elaborate on the subject heading identified on each slide. It's a similar principle to writing in the printed notes section of a paper copy, which acts as a memory jogger (see below).

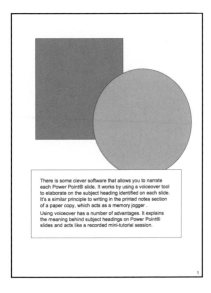

Figure 17.3
Power Point® notes page.

Using voiceover has a number of advantages. It explains the meaning behind subject headings on Power Point® slides and acts like a recorded mini-tutorial session.

Discharge planning for Grace

- **Role of Carer** (digital video clip depicting role play between discharge nurse and carer OR audio narrative about the role carers play in supporting those with a disability to maintain a normal life).

- **Role of Residential home** (audio voiceover talking about nature and purpose of residential care for the disabled).

Figure 17.4
Power Point® slide with ideas for audio or digital video clip to elaborate on key themes identified on PP slide

Blended learning using computer assisted technology (CAL)

Using multiple-choice questions (MCQs)

When developing MCQs, you need to ask a number of questions. First, prioritise learning into 'must know', 'should know' and 'nice to know' categories. Then ask yourself, will multiple-choice questions be sufficiently sensitive to confirm whether learning has taken place?

Secondly, ensure that questions are constructed in a clear and concise way. They need to be easy to follow and relevant to Grace's needs in the context of the discharge policy of the organisation.

THINGS to THINK ABOUT

Tips for writing MCQs:

- Ensure that you clearly identify one or more answers that are correct for each question.
- Write short unambiguous answers.
- Ask a colleague to proof read your work.
- Ensure that distracter questions (i.e. incorrect options) are plausible in some way. Example: Grace may not require an ambulance.
- The use of improbable answers should be avoided Example: Grace can make the journey home by bus.
- Always arrange the questions vertically not horizontally on the page.

Here's an example of an MCQ relating to transport home:

Grace requires transport home. Which one of the following is correct? Would you:
- a) Ask Grace what type of transport she thinks is needed?
- b) Assume that Grace needs an ambulance?
- c) Ask someone from Grace's residential home to collect her?
- d) None of the above?

Correct answer: (a)

Another question might focus on the issue of gaining access to accommodation.

Grace's transport home is arranged for late afternoon. What do you need to check in order to ensure that Grace can gain entry to her accommodation? Choose two of the following.
- a) Ring Grace's parents to find out what entry arrangements are in place after 5 pm.
- b) Ask Grace what arrangements are in place to gain access to her accommodation.
- c) Ask Grace if she has keys.
- d) Assume that Grace has a door key to her room.

Correct answers: (b) and (c)

Using true or false questions

Based on lecture or tutorial notes, video clips or narrated Power Point®, true or false questions (or interactive quizzes) are designed to prompt the learner to choose whether or not a statement is truthful. For example:

> All adults with cerebral palsy are cognitively impaired.
> True or false? _____
>
> Many adults with cerebral palsy do not require specially adapted homes.
> True or false? _____

Using short-answer questions

These questions are designed to elicit a 'constructed response'. In other words, they require the learner to create an answer themselves. Typically, responses ranging from one word to a few sentences are required. 'Fill in the blank' is an example of a short-answer question. Here is an example:

Internal fixation of fractures generally requires a .... anaesthetic.

Using synchronous learning (discussion boards)

Most virtual learning platforms, such as MOODLE or Blackboard, have an online discussion area, where learners share and debate knowledge and ideas about their learning. Similar to an online chat room, virtual classrooms or discussion boards are useful in facilitating learning from each other, through online group work and exchange of information.

Conclusion

This chapter has explored the merits of using CAL to facilitate learning about discharge planning. The main strength of CAL lies in its flexibility, which allows the learner to study at a time and place that best suits them (Tung & Chang 2008, Koch *et al.* 2010, Wedlake 2010). A number of studies have found computer anxiety to be prevalent among users, particularly where, for example, they fear that mistakes made online cannot be corrected, as seen in self-assessment (Posey & Pintz 2006, Blake 2009). However, Marakas *et al.* (2000) found that the more familiar learners became with IT, the greater their intention to use it. This is an important point to bear in mind when designing education resources. Lastly, web-based learning is still ideally seen as complementing face-to-face learning, not replacing it (Wedlake 2010).

The most important take-home message is therefore that those who believe online learning is useful are more likely to use it. However, course materials must also be perceived as being user-friendly (Tung & Chang 2008). Educational support for developers of web-based materials is vital to its success, as is IT support to maintain easy and consistent access to CAL.

References

Blake, H. (2009). Staff perceptions of e-learning for teaching delivery in health care. *Learning in Health and Social Care*. **8** (3), 223–234.

Brown, A.L., Bransford, J.D., Ferr Brown, A.L., Bransford, J.D., Ferrara, R.A. & Campione, J.C. (1983). Learning, remembering and understanding. In Flavell, J. & Markman, E. (eds.) *Handbook of Child Psychology* (fourth ed). *Cognitive Development*. **3**, 77–166. New York, USA: Wiley.

Chua, S.L., Chen, D. & Wong A.F.L. (1999). Computer anxiety and its correlates: a meta analysis. *Computers in Human Behavior*. **15**, 609–623.

Compeau, D.R. & Higgins, C.A. (1995). Computer self-efficacy: development of a measure and initial test. *MIS Quarterly*. **19** (2), 189–211.

Garrison, D.R. (2003). Cognitive presence for effective asynchronous online learning: the role of reflective inquiry, selfdirection and metacognition. In Bourne, J. & Moore, J.C. (eds), *Elements of Quality Online Education: Practice and Direction*. Needham, MA, USA: The Sloan Consortium.

Glen, S. (2005). E-learning in nurses' education: lessons learnt? (Editorial). *Nurse Education Today*. **25**, 415–417.

Hare, C., Davies, C. & Shepherd, M. (2006). Safer medicines administration through the use of e-learning. *Nursing Times*. **102** (16), 25-27.

Jefferies, P. (2006). Developing e-learning materials. In Glen, S. & Moule, P. (eds) *E-learning in Nursing*. Basingstoke & New York: Macmillan.

Koch, J., Andrew, S., Salamonson, Y., Everett, B. & Davidson, P.M. (2010). Nursing students' perception of a web-based intervention to support learning. *Nurse Education Today*. 30, 584–590.

Kotter, J.P. & Schlesinger, L.A. (1 July 2008). *Choosing Strategies for Change*. (HBR Classic). Harvard Business Review.

Longman, S. & Gabriel, M. (2004). Staff perceptions of E-learning: A community care access centre looks at current practices and approaches to better meet individual learners' needs and the educational and fiscal needs of the organisation. *The Canadian Nurse*. **100** (1), 23–27.

Maley, M.A., Lockyer-Stevens, V.A. & Playford, D.E. (2010). Growing rural doctors as teachers: A rural community of medical education practice. *Medical Teacher*. 983–989.

Marakas, G.M., Johnson, M.D. & Palmer, J.W. (2000). A theoretical model of differential social attributions towards computer technology: when a metaphor becomes the model. *International Journal of Human-Computer Studies*. **45**, 529–552.

Patterson Lorenzetti, J. (2008). Cost-effective marketing for online programs. *Distance Education Report*. **12** (5), 6–7.

Posey, L. & Pintz, C. (2006). Online teaching strategies to improve collaboration among nursing students. *Nurse Education Today*. **26**, 680–687.

Pullen, D. (2006). An Evaluative Case Study of Online leaning for Healthcare Professionals. *The Journal of Continuing Education in Nursing*. **37** (5), 225–232.

Ramsden, P. (1992). *Learning to Teach in Higher Education*. New York, USA: Routledge.

Sit, J.W.H., Chung, J.W.Y., Chow, M.C.M. & Wong, T.K.S. (2005). Experiences of online learning: students' perspective. *Nurse Education Today*. **25** (2), 140–147.

Tung, F. & Chang, S. (2008). Nursing students' behavioural intention to use online courses: A questionnaire survey. *International Journal of Nursing Studies*. **45**, 1299–1309.

Wedlake, S. (2010). Examining midwives' perceptions of using e-learning for continuing professional education.

Midwifery Digest. **20** (92), 143–149.

Wenger, E., McDermott, R. & Snyder, W. (2002). Communities of Practice: A guide to managing knowledge. *Organisation.* **7**, 225–246.

Section 5

Discharge practice case studies

Part A

Case studies from surgery, elective care and care pathways

Chapter 18

Nurse-facilitated discharge for adult surgical patients
Sarah Coombes

This case study outlines the approach adopted to introduce nurse-facilitated discharge in a district general hospital across its surgical and orthopaedic units. The criteria used in the orthopaedic setting are shared as an example that can be followed in other settings.

Organisational challenges

Achieving safe and timely discharge is crucial to ensuring patient flow through organisations. Nurses have always played an integral role in discharge planning and they now have a crucial role in facilitating a patient's actual discharge from hospital DH (2010). Around 80% of patients discharged from hospital can be classified as simple discharges, where a self-limiting condition has responded to surgery/treatment. Nurse-led and nurse-facilitated discharge has been high on the government's agenda for a number of years but organisations have struggled to implement and/or sustain the practice (Lees 2007).

In this case, the organisation had previously tried to implement nurse-facilitated discharge (NFD) with little success. Complicated protocols, training packages and assessment criteria had failed to engage nursing staff, making the process appear very complicated and 'not worth the risk of undertaking'. It had therefore been discarded as not worth pursuing. A new approach was tried a couple of years later. A task and finish group was resurrected, to review what had not worked previously and what was required in order to achieve this key objective. The composition of the task and finish group was of paramount importance in order to drive it forward.

Composition of task and finish group

Divisional lead nurse	Surgery and Cancer
Modern matron	General Surgery
Ward managers	Orthopaedic Elective General Surgery Wards
Practice educator	Surgery and Cancer
Risk/governance manager	Surgery and Cancer

Consultant surgeon colleagues were well briefed on the concept and fully supported the initiative, working closely with the team on developing the criteria for discharge and policy. As one consultant commented, 'this legitimises what nurses have been doing for years'.

Nurse-facilitated discharge is not complicated but we had previously made it extremely complicated, time-consuming and onerous. This time, the key was to keep it simple, maintain high-quality care, and comply with Clinical Negligence Scheme for Trusts and Trust standards.

A new approach to implementing NFD

Criteria for selecting nursing staff for NFD

Rather than make nurse-facilitated discharge the sole responsibility of Band 7 ward managers (as previously tried), we decided that registered nurses could initiate nurse-facilitated discharge as long as they had:

- The ability to assess and make critical decisions regarding discharge
- 'Prerequisite knowledge'
- A position in which they would have the need and opportunity to initiate and authorise discharge
- Access to – and the support of – the multi-professional clinical team
- The desire and opportunity to attend the in-house nurse-facilitated discharge training session

Training for NFD

'Prerequisite knowledge' was defined as having a minimum of two years' clinical experience of the specialty. Suitable nursing staff members were identified by their ward managers, following appraisal. The training programme was reduced from two days to one half-day session focusing on the perceived benefits not only for the patient, but the healthcare professional and the organisation. The components of nurse-facilitated discharge covered are outlined the table below.

Topics covered in the discharge training session

Identifying simple discharges
Using 'Criteria-led discharge'
Predicting date of discharge
Discharge against medical advice (self-discharge patients)
Professional and legal requirements

Professional and legal requirements had been identified as one of the key issues causing concern for nurses in undertaking this role previously. A clear professional and legal policy was approved by the organisation and this was covered during the training session.

Assessing competence in NFD

Following selection and appraisal from their ward manager and attendance on the half-day training session, the practitioner had to be assessed and deemed competent in the following:

- Mid Cheshire Hospitals NHS Foundation Trust Nurse Facilitated Discharge Policy for Adult Patients and its implementation
- Professional and legal responsibilities
- Documentation required
- Multidisciplinary team working
- Estimating date of discharge
- The use of clinical management plans
- Making referrals
- Identifying abnormal results and reporting
- Decision-making in NFD
- Discharge against medical advice

Competency was assessed using a variety of methods: direct questioning; observation of practice; and written evidence (supervised records of undertaking NFD and audit of completed NFD documentation).

The components of NFD were also linked to the NHS Knowledge and Skills Framework (DH 2004):

- Core 1   Communication
- Core 4   Service Improvement

Discharge practice case studies

- Core 5   Quality
- HWB 2   Assessment and Care Planning
- HWB 3   Protection of Health and Wellbeing
- HWB 6   Assessment and Treatment Planning
- HWB 7   Interventions and Treatments
- G1   Learning and Development
- IK1   Information Processing

This relates to a Band 5 Registered General Nurse job description within the organisation.

Statement of Competence

STATEMENT	Circle your response	COMMENTS	DATE & SIGN
1. I have read the MCHFT Nurse-Facilitated Discharge Policy for Adult Patients and understood the documentation relating to Nurse-Facilitated Discharge.	YES/NO		
2. I understand my responsibilities relating to the extended role of Nurse-Facilitated Discharge.	YES/NO		
3. I am confident about how to apply the Nurse-Facilitated Discharge Policy, and how to assess a patient's suitability for home according to the criteria-led discharge protocols used in my clinical specialty.	YES/NO		
4. I understand when it is appropriate to seek medical advice/opinion with regard to discharging a patient.	YES/NO		
5. I know where the NFD resource folder is on the ward and I am aware of its contents.	YES/NO		
6. I know who the Nurse-Facilitated Discharge team are, for advice and to discuss issues with.	YES/NO		
7. I have undertaken supervised discharges of patients using all the Criteria-Led Discharge Protocols for my clinical area of practice.	YES/NO		

Criteria development

As discussed previously, nurses currently guide the medical staff in the decision to discharge. With the help of clear protocols, training and assessment, clinical engagement and partnership working, NFD is achievable.

A set of guidelines was devised for a particular procedure/condition that enabled patients to be discharged without the need for further medical review (see table below for an example of the criteria used for a patient who had an elective hip replacement).

Elective Hip Replacement NFD Criteria

Patient label

CRITERIA-LED DISCHARGE

Total Hip Replacement
In order to facilitate efficient and safe early discharge, please indicate medical criteria and parameters to trigger a criteria-led discharge without further medical review. All patients will be reviewed by a Band 6 nurse or above on the day of discharge, prior to leaving the ward. Please tick, date and sign to indicate TTO prescription has been completed.

(tick) ☐   (date) _____ / _____ / _____ (sign)_____(bleep)_____

Criterion 1 Patient is experiencing minimal discomfort	Range/parameter Any pain is relieved by regular analgesia. Operation site is checked; no visible signs of infection apparent. Patient is taking diet and fluids. Patient has had bowels opened in previous 24 hours.	Achieved ☐ (Sign)

Criterion 2 Patient is mobilising safely	Range/parameter Patient has been assessed by physiotherapist/senior nurse as safe for discharge. Relevant equipment has been provided by Occupational Therapy. Stairs/step assessed and safe for discharge. Aids for mobilising supplied.	Achieved ☐ (Sign)
Criterion 3 Vital signs	Range/parameter Vital signs are within patient's own normal parameter. Temperature <37.5 over previous 24 hours. Patient is not scoring on EWS.	Achieved ☐ (Sign)
Criterion 4 Post-operative discharge arrangements	Range/parameter Wound clean and dry. Arrangements made for removal of clips. Additional dressings and clip removers supplied if required. District Nurse referral phoned through. Patient assessed by nursing staff as safe to administer Clexane Injections until 28 days post-operatively or alternative arrangements made. Blood card completed for check. Platelets on 14th day. TTO's ready for patient. Electronic Discharge letter completed. Verbal advice given to patient regarding precautions as stated in Total Hip Replacement booklet.	Achieved ☐ (Sign)

		Achieved ☐
		(Sign)
		Achieved ☐
		(Sign)

If the above criteria and parameters are met, I agree to this patient's Criteria-Led Discharge by nursing staff (completed sticker in Healthcare Records).

Nurse: _____   Signature:_____

Date:_____   Time of Discharge:_____

Comments:

Reproduced with permission from Mid Cheshire Hospitals NHS Foundation Trust.

As shown in this table, the nurses use a strict set of medically approved criteria to assess whether the patient can be discharged home. Any deviation from the criteria protocol results in the patient reverting back to a medical review and discharge.

Record-keeping

In accordance with the Nursing and Midwifery Council Code of Conduct (NMC 2008) and local policy, accurate documentation must be maintained. Nurses authorised to discharge must ensure that patients are aware of the scope and limitations of nurse-facilitated discharge. Informed consent is obtained from the patient by the Registered Nurse. Medical staff document in the healthcare records that the patient is suitable for nurse-facilitated discharge (see below). The completed criteria checklist is filed in the patient's healthcare records and the discharge checklist is completed.

Medical sticker within case notes

**NURSE-FACILITATED DISCHARGE
FOR ADULT PATIENTS**

I agree that this patient can be discharged
against a set of agreed criteria.

> **PATIENT LABEL**

Date ....

Signature ....

Print name ....

The ward record/log book is completed for each discharge, to identify any delays in nurse-facilitated discharge and to monitor the number of patients discharged via NFD. The ward record/log book information feeds into monthly team meetings and performance reviews. A bi-annual audit of NFD is undertaken. This not only focuses on the number of patients discharged but also on length of stay and readmission rates.

Professional and legal responsibilities

As mentioned earlier, this was the area that concerned nursing staff the most. Professionally, the nurse must have knowledge of personal accountability for their practice, acknowledging limitations of professional competence, and must only undertake and accept responsibility for those activities for which he/she is competent (NMC 2008). Legally, there is no reason why nurses cannot take more responsibility for the discharge process, including the decision to discharge.

Two legal standards apply, as follows:

- Constitutional standard (rule of law), which requires the nurse to act within the law

- Minimum quality standard (rule of negligence), which requires that if a nurse takes on a role or task that was previously performed by a doctor, he or she must perform that role or task to the same standard as a doctor

The Trust, as an employer, will assume vicarious liability for the actions of nurses authorised to discharge, providing that:

- They have undergone the necessary preparation
- They are deemed competent to undertake the role by their line manager
- The framework for authorised discharge has been followed
- The member of staff has been authorised by the Trust to undertake the role
- The provisions of the Trust's NFD policy have been followed by the member of staff at all times

Meeting the challenges of implementing NFD

Registered medical staff must have reviewed the patient up to 48 hours prior to discharge and this review must be documented in the healthcare records. A completed sticker MUST be placed in the patient's healthcare records. Medical staff must prescribe take-home medication in a timely manner, ideally when identifying that the patient is suitable for nurse-facilitated discharge.

One of the main challenges is to avoid nurses seeing NFD as yet another addition to their already heavy workload. Instead, they need to see it as part of their routine patient care. Successful implementation of NFD requires good leadership, tenacity in reminding consultant colleagues to complete the sticker and a determination to embed NFD in the 'culture' of the ward and the wider organisation.

Final tips

- Keep it simple
- Ensure clinician 'buy-in'
- Don't over-complicate training requirements
- Ensure strong leadership from the beginning to embed NFD

References

Department of Health (2004). 'The NHS Knowledge and Skills Framework'. London: HMSO.

Department of Health (2010). 'Ready to go? Planning the discharge and the transfer of patients from hospital and intermediate care'. London: HMSO.

Lees, L. ed. (2007). *Nurse Facilitated Discharge from Hospital*. Keswick: M&K.

Mid Cheshire Hospitals NHS Foundation Trust Joint Discharge Policy and Process (2007).

Nursing and Midwifery Council (2008). 'The NMC Code of Professional Conduct: standards for conduct, performance and ethics'. London: NMC.

Chapter 19

Integrating predicted date of discharge to reduce length of stay

Melanie Webber-Maybank and Helen Luton

The following case study will discuss using estimated/predicted dates of discharge in an elective orthopaedic ward. The benefits to patients, clinicians and health boards will be examined. Helpful tips on integrating estimated/predicted discharge dates to reduce length of stay have also been included. Throughout this case study, the word 'predicted' will be used – even though the terms 'estimated' and 'estimated length of stay' are synonymous and are used in other referenced work. This work took place in Wales (see Chapter 7 for further discussion of Welsh policy in relation to discharge planning).

Key points:

- Better planning and awareness of predicted discharge dates can shorten length of stay and improve bed management.
- Patients who spend less time in hospital are less likely to be exposed to healthcare-associated infections, and cutting length of stay reduces NHS costs.
- The ticket-home system is visible, accessible and simple, and improves communication between patients and staff and between members of the multidisciplinary team (MDT).
- Although this system was implemented on an elective orthopaedic ward, it is easily applicable and transferable to other clinical specialties.

Background

Careful planning of patients' predicted discharge date clearly has a significant part to play in improving healthcare and reducing NHS costs. Ensuring that patients and their carers are aware of their predicted discharge date (PDD) from the time of admission is recognised as good practice and improves patient experience (Lees & Holmes 2005).

Discharge practice case studies

The 'Orthopaedic Plan' (WAG 2004) states that ensuring a sustainable orthopaedic service is about making better use of resources through improved management and innovative ways of working. In the Healthcare Commission's 2004 national patient survey, patients identified delays in discharge as a key area for improvement (DH 2004).

The ideal system should involve minimal delay and patients should be fully informed about when they will be able to leave hospital (DH 2004). Managing the patient's journey is crucial to improving patient experience and making the best use of beds (DH & RCN 2003).

Patients have a right to know how long they are expected to be in hospital and what time they will be discharged so that they and their families can plan accordingly. Patients do not want to be in hospital longer than necessary, and they would rather recuperate in the more familiar and comfortable surroundings of their own home. Patients and their carers need to be involved in the discharge process from the time of admission (Lees 2010).

Context

Cardiff and Vale University Local Health Board provide health services for over 500,000 people living in Cardiff and the Vale of Glamorgan. Nursing staff on the elective orthopaedic ward at University Hospital Llandough identified a need to reduce patients' length of stay. The aim was to improve the flow of patients through the system by ensuring increased focus by multidisciplinary teams and patients on the predicted discharge date. The 'ticket-home' initiative started in August 2008. Ward West 3 is a mixed-sex ward that cares for patients undergoing major orthopaedic surgery, and it already had many systems in place to improve discharge (Webber-Maybank & Luton 2009):

- PDDs were displayed on patient status boards at nurse's station
- PDDs were displayed on the clinical workstation computer program
- Discharge board focused MDT attention on potential discharges
- There were daily MDT meetings at which every patient's discharge arrangements were discussed

Despite all these proactive systems already being in place, the nursing team felt that more could be done. The predicted date of discharge was not visible to patients or their families and they were therefore not as involved in the discharge process as they could have been.

Developing the ticket home

We started with a series of challenging creative thinking sessions by clinical leaders.

During these sessions, staff developed the ticket-home discharge tool. This is an A4 laminated card, which is placed on each patient's bedside locker, where it is easily visible to the patient and their carers and all members of the multidisciplinary team. The visual management technique was key to the tool's design, to ensure that everyone (including the patient) could see the status of the discharge plan at a glance.

According to Ad Esse Performance Improvement Consultants (2007), 'Visual management has a number of benefits which include greater involvement, motivation, control and better communication.'

The ticket home states the patient's name and consultant and there are sections for the physiotherapist and occupational therapist to fill out when the patient is discharged. It also contains information about whether the patient needs transport home, and whether their X-ray and take-home medication have been completed. The final and most important part is the section where the planned date for going home is written. The language on the ticket was kept patient-friendly so that there was no confusion over terminology. The phrase 'predicted discharge date' was not used on the ticket. Instead, we used the term 'planned date for going home', as we felt that this was more patient-friendly and easier to understand.

The new discharge tool was explained to the multidisciplinary team to ensure complete engagement from all participants. Outpatients and preadmission staff were also informed so that they could tell future patients that this system was in place.

Putting the ticket home into practice

On admission, the ticket is explained to patients and their predicted discharge date is filled in. As they meet their multidisciplinary discharge goals, further information is added until all goals are achieved. Patients are then identified as fit for discharge. In this way, patients are engaged in the discharge process from the time they are admitted to the ward. They are also informed about the process in preadmission and orthopaedic education classes.

The discharge process should be a multidisciplinary effort with consistently high standards for all patients (Athwal 2002). The ticket-home system is a tool to help ensure that these high standards are achieved. The predicted discharge date is clearly visible to patients and staff and the ticket home identifies the goals that need to be achieved before discharge is possible (such as physiotherapy and occupational therapy assessments, transport needs, prescriptions and X-rays). However, staff and patients are made aware that this is only a guide and is subject to change, as safe discharge is always paramount.

To aid nursing teams in accurately setting the predicted discharge date and to ensure standardisation, a list of appropriate lengths of stay for specific surgical procedures or clinical diagnoses was put together. This ensured equality in predicting the discharge date for patients. However, it is recognised that in other specialties this may not be as straightforward.

Safety is always paramount and patients are only discharged on or before their PDD if they are clinically fit to be sent home and all members of the multidisciplinary team have discharged them. Unplanned, rushed or poorly coordinated discharges can be unsafe (Alshire 2010). Common reasons why patients are not discharged are recorded at ward level, and recurring reasons can then be used as action points for further development.

Once the patient has met their goals and is safe to be discharged, the laminated card is wiped clean and can be used for the next patient. As the clinical area is an elective ward and the team had already set standardised lengths of stay for common procedures, the predicted date of discharge could be written on the ticket-home tool before the patient arrived on the ward. This ensured that, from the time the patient arrived with their carers and family, they were aware of their potential date for going home.

Outcomes

It was important to evaluate the ticket-home system, and data from the Trust was used to monitor its implementation.

- Before the ticket-home system was introduced, the average length of stay for total hip replacement patients was 7.4 post-operative days.
- After the ticket-home system was introduced, the average (measured over 13 months) post-operative length of stay for total hip replacement patients was 4.3 days.

This equated to a reduction of 3.1 days in average length of patient stay.

Also, before the introduction of ticket home, 33 % of total hip replacement patients achieved their predicted discharge date. After implementation of the tool, 67 % of patients hit their predicted discharge date – an improvement of 34 %.

In addition, patient flow through the discharge process was far smoother.

It was also discovered that, as a by-product of the ticket home, discharges of patients before 12 pm had increased across orthopaedics. It is well recognised that discharging patients before 12 pm results in effective and efficient bed management (DH 2004). It seems that improved communication about discharge in the team and better collaborative working enabled this to occur.

The system also led to an increase in the number of discharges over the weekend, which had previously been irregular and unplanned. Since the implementation of ticket home, weekend discharges are now part of the whole system and patient flow.

A key recommendation for achieving timely simple discharge from hospital (DH 2004) is establishing weekend discharge as standard, to reduce fluctuations in numbers of beds needed.

Data is still being collected on the impact of ticket home via Cardiff and Vale University Local Health Board Trust's central information warehouse, but ward-level data collection suggests the positive trend is continuing. Data is collected each month, and displayed for patients, carers, staff and other healthcare disciplines to read in graphs and tables to ensure that progress is shared.

Patient involvement

With the ticket-home system, patients and their carers are able to start their patient journey with the end in mind, and plan accordingly. The patient's expectations are set as soon as they come into hospital, and they are aware that discharge is part of their patient journey. The ticket home can be seen by both patients and their carers, as it is on the patient's locker where all their belongings are kept. This gives them immediate ownership of their discharge date, and they become part of their discharge process and not just a spectator. They have control of their discharge and become proactive rather than reactive (Lees 2010).

The ticket home empowers them to take part in the discharge process. As each discharge goal is achieved, the relevant section on the ticket home is completed and patients can see this process happening visually.

Here are some of the comments made by patients:

'I only need to tick those two boxes and I can go home.'

'Last time I came in I didn't know what was happening – now I do.'

'I will beat that ticket and go home earlier.'

'My daughter will take Thursday off work to collect me.'

'It gives us confidence to go home.'

It was important for the ward team to know that patients were happy with ward processes, as patient satisfaction is paramount. Patient surveys were designed and the data collated at ward level. Results indicate that 100 % of patients are happy with the discharge process and that being told their predicted date of discharge is useful to them and their families. Patients also felt that they were adequately prepared to return home and that the discharge was well organised. Discharge no longer comes as a surprise to patients and their carers/relatives. They are aware of what stage of the journey they are at, and they know that they are potentially going home the day before discharge if they achieve the final goal.

Case study

Mrs X was a 65-year-old lady who underwent a primary total hip replacement. During the preadmission process, the ticket-home concept was explained to her. This was reinforced on her planned admission to the clinical area. On her day of admission, the ticket home was completed, with a predicted date of discharge of four days after her surgery. During this time, Mrs X and her husband had the opportunity to discuss any concerns about discharge. The nursing staff also explained that the predicted date of discharge was used as a guide and that she might go home before the date if she was safe and fit to do so, or she might go home a day or two later. Staff reinforced that the ultimate goal was a safe and timely discharge from hospital. At this point, Mrs X told the staff and her fellow patients that she was going to tick all the boxes on the ticket home and beat the predicted date and aim to go home earlier.

Mrs X underwent her surgery and had no post-operative complications.

On the day following her surgery, the physiotherapist began Mrs X's rehabilitation. She made good progress and underwent her occupational therapy assessment on day two.

All members of the multidisciplinary team worked with Mrs X to achieve her predicted discharge date of four days following surgery. On day two, the orthopaedic surgeon said Mrs X was medically fit for discharge after reviewing her X-ray and blood results. The discharge medication was arranged and that section of the ticket home completed.

Mrs X now only had to get two more boxes ticked on the ticket home to be safely discharged. As she could see her progress, she was even more determined to go home on day three, and discussed this with the nursing staff during bedside handover.

On day three, the occupational therapist delivered equipment and completed her section of the ticket home. Mrs X was now on crutches and only had a stair assessment to complete; this was completed satisfactorily during that morning.

Mrs X's husband arrived on the ward to collect his wife at 11 am. Mrs X and her husband were thrilled that she had achieved all her goals and had beaten her predicted date of discharge. They commented on how they felt that they were key members of the team, and could visually see her progress on the ticket home.

Conclusion

Setting and achieving predicted discharge dates gives patients goals to work towards, and a sense of achievement when they reach them. Not all patients will meet their predicted discharge date (due to surgical complications or complex social care arrangements) but, even for those who miss the target, it ensures that there is a focus on discharge arrangements and it accelerates the discharge date.

Some clinical areas are more suited to the ticket-home system than others, and elective care is an ideal clinical environment. Other areas, such as emergency care and medicine, will need to follow different principles to ensure that the ticket meets their needs but the system is easily modifiable. Some specialties, due to their caseload and patient mix, will be able to achieve a higher compliance with predicted discharge dates and some fewer, but a tool that helps to improve discharge efficiency – to whatever degree – will benefit both clinicians and patients.

Through strong clinical leadership and teamwork on the orthopaedic ward at University Hospital Llandough, there has been a recognisable culture change and patient discharge is now the focus of attention for all healthcare professionals, patients and relatives. The simplicity of the tool has contributed to its success. The time taken from the creation of the idea to implementation of the tool was just 48 hours. The team came up with the idea on Friday and the ticket home was in place on the Monday. Quite simply, the team 'just did it', and assessed and evaluated the tool while implementing it. The cost of developing the tool came to £10, which was for the laminating pouches. The rewards that have been reaped have been immeasurable – reduced length of stay, increased patient satisfaction and enhanced staff satisfaction, to name a few. The challenges to the process have been relatively few, but it is recognised that each clinical area has its own challenges and some will have greater hurdles to overcome to reduce length of stay.

Since the initial implementation, no modifications have been made. The visibility, accessibility and simplicity of the ticket-home system ensured that the cultural change quickly became embedded in the clinical area.

References

Ad Esse Performance Improvement Consultants (2007). http://www.ad-esse.com/media/11662/visual_man.pdf

Aleshire, B. (2010). 'How to plan for a safe discharge'. (online source). http://ezinearticles.com/?expert=Brent_Aleshire

Athwal, A. (2002). Do multidisciplinary integrated care pathways improve interprofessional collaboration? *Scandinavian Journal of Caring Sciences*. **16** (4), 335–435.

Department of Health (2004). 'Achieving timely "simple" discharge from hospital: A toolkit for the multidisciplinary team'. London: HMSO.

Department of Health & Royal College of Nursing (2003). 'Freedom to practise: dispelling the myths'. London: HMSO.

Lees, L. (2010). Exploring the principles of best practice discharge to ensure patient involvement. *Nursing Times.* **106** (25), 10–14.

Lees, L. & Holmes, K. (2005). Estimating a date of discharge at ward level: a pilot study. *Nursing Standard* **19** (17), 40–43. www.nursing-standard.co.uk

National Leadership and Innovation Agency for Healthcare (2008). *Passing the Baton – A Practical Guide to Effective Discharge Planning.* NLIAH.

Tierney, A. & Closs, J. (1993). An evaluation of hospital discharge. *Nursing Times.* **89**, 11–12.

Webber-Maybank, M. & Luton, H. (2009). Making effective use of predicted discharge dates to reduce the length of stay in hospital. *Nursing Times.* **105**, 15.

Welsh Assembly Government (2004). 'An Orthopaedic Plan – Getting Wales Moving'. Cardiff: WAG.

Chapter 20

A 'bed-less service': Cataract surgery

John Deutsch and Nursing Team (Bree Coleman, Viv Hoare, Julie Young and Claire Craige)

Cataract surgery has made a gargantuan leap in the last 15 years, having changed from a procedure requiring a four-day inpatient stay to an outpatient procedure with an integrated care pathway. This has required a major change in practice and the development of new roles. The concept of a care pathway has helped coordinate primary and secondary care, as well as a large multidisciplinary team. This service now has no beds, and discharge planning (beginning at preadmission screening) takes this into account within the care pathway.

This chapter describes the development of a patient-centred approach delivered through a care pathway, concluding with a case study and learning points regarding discharge planning.

The historical background

In 1991, the provider–purchaser split and GP fund-holding were introduced in the UK. Like many other elective services in the UK, secondary eye care services were caught in a system where elective demand far outstripped clinical need. Waiting lists were up to two years long. Secondary care services were under pressure, short of clinical resources, quite rightly prioritising emergency over elective care.

Hereford was a 23-bedded single-specialty hospital in a semi-rural setting. In common with many other eye departments in the UK, it was a financially efficient centre, with low staffing numbers, running an excellent service for those who made it through the doors. Only ten years earlier, eye services ran outpatient clinics in open halls, and consultations were held at high desks (rather like old-fashioned railway station ticket offices). This system delivered a cheap and effective service but often at some cost to privacy and quality.

Gradually, the need for more services (partly as a result of the development of better equipment and surgical processes) was recognised. Provider-purchaser split, GP fund-holding and payment by results, together provided the mechanism by which secondary care was able to increase provision in shortage specialties by appointing more staff and allocating more resources for services that were in demand. This was particularly true of cataract treatment, and there has since been similar service expansion in the treatment of glaucoma, diabetic eye disease and age-related macular degeneration, amongst other conditions.

Over a decade, in England and Wales, rates of cataract surgery doubled, from around 150,000 in 1998 to 300,000 in 2008 (RCO). The increase in surgical turnover put pressure on existing beds. In 1983, cataract surgical patients were usually operated on under general anaesthesia and remained as inpatients for about four days (with associated risks of urinary retention, deep vein thrombosis and infection). Very few units had recognised the possibility of day-case surgery with its attendant efficiency and patient benefits. (Ingram *et al.* 1983).

Local context

A standard ophthalmic surgical list in Hereford had three or four cataract patients and there were five lists per week. By 1995, most patients were given local anaesthesia and kept in for one night. There were seven lists per week, with four to five patients per list. Our unit now runs a total of between 11 and 14 lists per week, with between five and eight patients per list, over three sites (Brecon, Llandrindod and Hereford), with an inpatient stay rate of under ten patient bed days per year over the whole eye service (almost entirely non-cataract-related). Similar transformations have been seen nationally.

Further pressures to reduce length of stay resulted from the dissolution of specialist eye hospitals, including our own, and the competing pressures on beds in a multi-specialty environment.

Process-driven change

The first cataract care pathway, 1994

The increased demands on the Eye Department services, although serviced by an increase in staff and facility, also demanded a rationalisation of the process. With this came the introduction of protocols and care pathways. The cataract care pathway started with a very simple format, consisting of two sides of paper. The process was divided into: pre-operative assessment; biometry (measurement of the eye); day of surgery, including the surgical and anaesthetic record (if required); the post-operative arrangements; and review visit.

Early evolution of the cataract care pathway

As the service developed, nationally driven measures impacted on our care delivery. These included more extensive pre-operative assessment requirements, site of surgery forms, venous thromboembolism risk assessments (yes, for cataract!). In addition, the Royal College of Ophthalmologists introduced guidelines for best practice in cataract surgery – four revisions to date (RCO).

Extension of the care pathway to include primary care services

Action on Cataracts (DH 2000) set further parameters for change. The pathway now includes the optometric assessment and referral pathway and an optometric follow-up pathway.

The future

Plans for the future include same-day pre-operative assessment. There are logistical barriers to this in a small unit with a large number of mixed patient clinics. Specialist clinics can ring-fence staff and this can create inefficiencies in space/staff utilisation. The challenge here is to develop a cataract clinic that offers the patient a one-stop service, without compromising on clinical quality or safety and still maintaining an efficient work flow. It is also important to allow some time between the patient agreeing a surgical plan and its execution (a cooling-off period).

Case study

A 91-year-old lady, Mrs X, lives alone and is referred for cataract extraction. She has rheumatoid hands and home carers call in twice a day to assist her with hygiene and meal preparation. She is independent in her activities of daily living but lives in an isolated rural Welsh cottage without easy access to public transport.

She is placed on the waiting list and subsequently reviewed in the ophthalmology pre-operative assessment clinic. This clinic is run by specialist ophthalmic staff. The assessment process involves a discussion regarding provision of post-operative care, and how to engage her and her carers in the post-operative period of two to four weeks, during which she will require eye drops four times daily. If Mrs X cannot have reliable post-operative medication then surgery may not be actionable. The choice always remains with Mrs X.

This focuses the attention of Mrs X and her carers and relatives to engage as a partnership. All those involved invest in the process, and the patient and carers are motivated to fulfil the goal of improving Mrs X's vision and thereby improve her quality of life and independence.

Mrs X's carers could not agree to administer the eye drops, as this would have necessitated an increase in the care package. Instead, her neighbours agreed to assist as much as they could manage. Mrs X is given a bottle of artificial tear drops to try at home. She gains confidence in instilling her own eye drops and proceeds with the plan.

The day of surgery proceeds routinely. Mrs X is reviewed and discharged within half an hour of her surgery and is collected from hospital by taxi. The surgeon is otherwise occupied in theatre, and in normal circumstances the discharge process is entirely nurse led.

Her surgery and post-operative recovery is uneventful. The post-operative review is with her own optician four weeks later. The optician completes a report of the visual outcome and patient satisfaction with the service. This audit form is returned by post to the Eye Unit. The patient is discharged from the pathway and the audit data is collated by the surgical service for later review.

Learning points

Change can be threatening and may be perceived as stepping on many professional toes. The evolution of our cataract service has followed national trends and has been in response to national directives and local need for change. There have been many benefits, quite apart from reducing costs, most particularly to the patients.

Managing the expectations of the professional and patient

Initially, on implementation of the change, many patients still received inpatient care. Over a period of time, the expectations of the patients and the team changed. Change took time to embed.

A detailed information leaflet was developed and is now given to the patient at time of listing. At pre-operative assessment, detailed social factors are considered. Why does this patient need to stay in hospital? Are there any advantages or disadvantages to the inpatient stay in any particular case? The issue is not age or rurality. The fact that a 90-year-old patient is living alone, in a very rural setting 30 miles from the hospital, has to be planned for but does not mitigate against day-case surgery. They may well be quite competent at instilling their own drops post-operatively, or they may have carers who can supervise treatment, in the same way as meeting their other needs. Indeed the patient is much more likely to get the correct dose and frequency of treatment at home, rather than on a busy ward where drops are seen as 'secondary' to acute care and 'can wait'. The patient is empowered and motivated to participate in their own care rather than be a passive recipient, whatever their age.

We now all assume that the patient is going home. The question of inpatient stay almost never arises and has increased our day-case rate to over 99%. It may well be that cataract surgery is perceived quite differently now. It has become a 'simple procedure', rather than a complicated operation. The technical aspects and team may have become a lot more sophisticated but the delivery, and the view from the patient's perspective, is characterised by simplicity, speed and efficiency.

The patient journey

The time and trouble taken by the typical cataract surgery patient, from diagnosis to the final post-operative visit, has been vastly reduced. In 1984, the patient was subjected to a total wait of up to two years, five days' inpatient stay and the consequences thereof (including risks of deep vein thrombosis and urinary retention), as well as many medical and nursing interventions in the course of the treatment, including at least five hospital visits and two visits to the optometrist.

Now, the journey is complete within 18 weeks (national target) and a four-week follow-up period. The interventions include one or two pre-operative visits to the hospital in uncomplicated cases, no hospital follow-up visits (in 95% of cases, local audit data), two optometric visits, an audited process with recorded outcomes, no inpatient stay, a three-hour day of surgery hospital stay, and a change of spectacles as required at the end of the process.

Integrated service – the need for a care pathway to connect the team

The care pathway evolved to connect primary and secondary care, and a multidisciplinary hospital team. The care pathway defines each practitioner's responsibility and the next step. It has been kept simple, and has been further simplified at each revision as far as possible, in order to maintain practitioner engagement and cooperation. Form-filling is onerous at the best of times and can lead to complacency and completion by rote. Each item on the form has a purpose. The form has remained at four sides of A4 and is filed in the patient record.

The optometric outcome sheet is one side of A4 and doubles as the variance (exceptions) record and audit sheet with final visual outcome. Orthoptic, nursing, healthcare assistants, medical and optometric staff use the same form and pathway in an integrated process, removing duplicated forms and processes. For example, vision testing, drug history, social history and other observations would previously have been repeatedly recorded. An electronic patient record is eagerly awaited but needs to be integrated across the primary and secondary interface. In addition, the English and Welsh systems are to date incompatible.

The multi-professional input into the care pathway has given us a much fuller picture of the patient and their needs, with each aspect complementing the other parts of the record. Care needs to be taken in developing and revising parts of the pathway so that duplication continues to be avoided. Some previously 'doctor-led tasks' have been appropriately delegated to other members of the team, who require training and competency assessments to assure standards. In fact, this has often led to better data collection and recording than previously. 'Professional ambitions' and 'perceived must dos' have to be carefully managed and abbreviated. A long, onerous pathway is an ineffective one.

Conclusion

Care had to be taken to integrate all service elements. This service took 15 years to evolve to its present state and has spawned a low vision pathway, glaucoma pathway and macula pathway. We have yearly 'stakeholder' events for the whole team in primary and secondary care, to inform and develop new and old pathways. This particular pathway continues to develop. Recent considerations have been to integrate 'correct surgical site and side checks' and 'deep vein thrombosis checks'. However, national directives with limited relevance can lengthen and complicate the pathway process. It should be remembered that generic edicts can derail many efficient local processes.

A commonsense approach needs to be applied. At each revision point, the two key questions need to be considered:

• How does the patient benefit from this change?
• And can we make it simpler still?

References

Department of Health (2000). 'Action on cataracts: good practice guidance'. London. HMSO.

Ingram R.M., Banerjee D., Traynar M.J. & Thompson, R.K. (May 1983). Day-case cataract surgery. *British Journal of Ophthalmology.* **67** (5), 278–281.

Royal College of Ophthalmologists
http://www.rcophth.ac.uk/page.asp?section=100&sectionTitle=Information+and+Advice+for+the+General+Public

Chapter 21

Using integrated care pathways to support the discharge of dying patients to their preferred place of care

Claire Whittle and Jill Main

This chapter outlines the care of Mary, an elderly lady who wants to be discharged home as her health deteriorates, highlighting the ways in which long-term conditions impact on people's health and well-being. The chapter explores the importance of recognising the dying phase and how high-quality, safe care can be provided through the use of an integrated care pathway. It also emphasises the need for early discharge planning to support end-of-life patient choice.

Key tips for timely discharge:

- Ensure that there is clear communication with the patient and their family regarding discharge planning and care options
- Start discharge planning as part of the admission process
- Review discharge planning throughout the inpatient stay
- Consider in advance the services and equipment required for safe discharge, and organise their provision as early as possible
- Ensure rapid discharge protocols are in place, including a clear communication strategy for transfer of information to the patient's GP and other care agencies
- Recognise the dying phase and respect patient choice regarding discharge and care at end of life

Mary's story, part 1

Mary is a 75-year-old lady who was diagnosed with hypertension 15 years ago. Two years ago, she had a myocardial infarction. She has been suffering from increasing breathlessness and has been admitted to hospital on a number of occasions as her symptoms have worsened. During one of these visits, she was given the diagnosis of heart failure. Mary lives at home with her 78-year-old husband Jack. They have two daughters, Amy and Sarah (both married with children), who live locally.

Over the last year, Mary has become increasingly depressed, as she feels her quality of life is becoming poor. She used to take care of her grand-daughter regularly for her daughter Amy but her breathlessness means that she can no longer do this. She is also becoming socially isolated because her mobility is now affected by her increasing breathlessness, and she has lost confidence in her ability to go out on her own. Stewart and McMurray (2002) observed that people with heart failure, most of whom are elderly, often have an extremely poor quality of life.

The three trajectories of illness

Heart failure can be considered to be one of the organ system failures described by Lynn *et al.* (2004) in relation to the three trajectories of illness. Murray *et al.* (2005) outline how the illness trajectories described by Lynn (2004) provide a broad timeframe that can help clinicians plan and deliver care that integrates active and palliative management. They also suggest that an understanding of these trajectories ensures that end-of-life care is considered at an earlier stage.

Trajectory 1 describes the typical cancer journey, with a steady progression and usually a clear terminal phase.

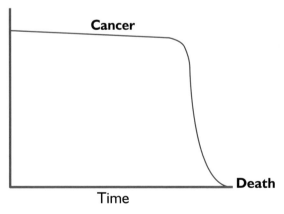

Figure 21.1 Trajectory 1

Trajectory 2 (figure 21.2) describes how those with organ system failure progress towards the end of life. Here, there is a gradual decline, punctuated by episodes of acute deterioration and some recovery, and ending with a more sudden and seemingly unexpected death.

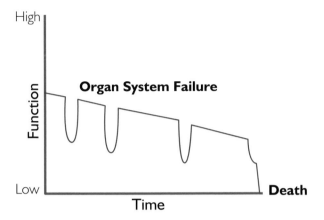

Figure 21.2 Trajectory 2

The third trajectory (figure 21.3) is described by Murray *et al.* (2005) as 'prolonged dwindling'. Figure 21.3 plots an individual with a low baseline of cognitive or physical functioning, who may die following what might appear to be a minor event. These patients typically have very few reserves left and so a relatively minor event can prove fatal.

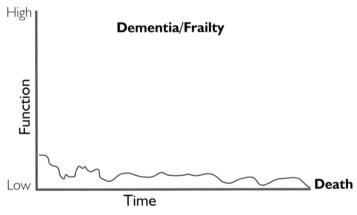

Figure 21.3 Trajectory 3

Illness trajectories reproduced with kind permission from Joanne Lynn and David M. Adamson, 'Living Well at the End of Life: Adapting Health Care to Serious Chronic Illness in Old Age', Santa Monica, California: RAND Corporation, WP – 137, 2003. Online at http://www.rand.org/pubs/white_papers/WP137/

Discharge practice case studies

Patients with long-term conditions are more likely to fit into the second and third trajectories, typically with a pattern of short-term admission to a hospital for care during an acute exacerbation of their illness. This is particularly pertinent to Mary.

Mary's story, part 2

Mary was once again admitted to hospital after falling at home. This was her third admission in the past 12 months and she was taken to an elderly care ward. The consultant geriatrician felt that Mary's heart failure had progressed significantly and he considered that she was now in the final stage of her life. He felt she would probably not survive this latest exacerbation, and so she should now be considered for palliative care. This is often a very difficult decision to make, and others have commented on the problems of making such a decision due to the unpredictable nature of the heart failure illness trajectory (Stewart & McMurray 2002, While & Kiek 2009).

Palliative care is the active holistic care of patients with an advanced progressive illness. Effective management of pain and other symptoms, and the provision of psychological, social and spiritual support, are paramount. The goal of palliative care is to achieve the best possible quality of life for patients and their families (NICE 2004). Therefore the medical team commenced the end-of-life integrated care pathway (ICP), to support Mary's care and management during the palliative phase of her illness.

The medical team discussed with Mary and her family her care and management plan using the end-of-life care pathway as a framework. The decision not to attempt resuscitation was included in the pathway documentation, and this information was passed to all appropriate members of staff.

Talking about death and dying can be very awkward for both patients and healthcare professionals. The hospital consultant spoke to Mary and her family in an open and honest way about her prognosis, using advanced communication skills and following the breaking bad news policy. She expressed a wish to die at home, as this was her preferred place of care at the end of her life.

Preferred Priorities for Care (PPC)

The Preferred Priorities for Care or PPC (DH 2007), previously known as Preferred Place of Care, is a document that individuals hold themselves and take with them to different places where they receive care. It allows them to record their thoughts and feelings about their care and choices, including if possible where they would want to end their life. This information can therefore be made available so that anyone involved in their care is aware of what matters to them and can assist them with seamless care. As care needs change, the PPC can be updated to reflect this. It is never too early to start a PPC plan, particularly for people with long-term conditions who may live with their deteriorating condition for many years. Identifying each person's preferred place of care was also highlighted as important by Lord Darzi, who reported that the 'sick and elderly should have the right to choose to die at home' (DH 2007).

Mary's story, part 3

As Mary had made her wishes clear, the need for rapid discharge was acknowledged by the multidisciplinary team, and the rapid discharge process was commenced. She was referred to the occupational therapist, who assessed the need for, and ordered, a commode and a pressure-relieving mattress. For those patients discharged under the rapid discharge process, to enable them to die at home in the place of their choice, equipment provision is fast-tracked so that it can be delivered the same day. It is important that the family and carers are made aware of how to use equipment, and the clinical teams (liaison nurses/key worker) need to ensure that carers are taught appropriately. This was particularly important, as Mary had a urinary catheter.

The ward nurses taught Mary's daughters how to empty the drainage bag. Her daughters were apprehensive regarding Mary's discharge home but they were prepared to help with their mother's care as much as possible, as this was what she wanted. Mary was also referred to the heart failure specialist nurse, who visited her on the ward to offer advice and support, assessing her symptoms prior to discharge and advising staff accordingly.

The medical team in the hospital informed the GP of the discharge, ensuring that the GP was aware that Mary was being discharged to die at home. The details of Mary's condition and the management plan were confirmed via fax, stating that Mary had been commenced on the end-of-life care pathway. The medical team also ensured that medications were ordered in a timely manner, to be ready whenever the discharge go-ahead was given. These medications would then be available in Mary's own home, whenever she needed them, to ensure that she was comfortable and pain-free. Medications were ordered for pain, agitation, restlessness and nausea and vomiting. A member of the medical team sat with Mary's daughters and went through the discharge medications. They asked many questions and were reassured that the district nursing team would be visiting regularly to ensure that Mary remained comfortable.

Prior to discharge, Mary was referred to the social care team and the district nursing team for assessment at home, with a view to more support being provided. Mary was allocated a key worker who was a member of the district nursing team. Those caring for Mary wanted to avoid readmission due to inadequate communication or the patient not being adequately supported at home.

The key worker ensured that Mary was registered by her GP on the Gold Standards Framework (2008) register. The ward team coordinated with the key worker regarding the time of discharge and the time of the district nurse's first visit. A discharge letter for the district nurses, with details of care, was completed and sent home with Mary, together with the end-of-life care pathway. An ambulance was booked and Mary travelled on a stretcher, accompanied by her daughter in the ambulance. The ambulance crew were aware of the DNAR decision written in the pathway document. Using a pathway ensured that a coordinated approach to Mary's care was achieved, as described by Panella & Vanhaecht (2010): 'Care pathways are a necessary tool to generate efficiency, achieving the best clinical and care outcomes utilising appropriate resources'.

Mary's condition continued to deteriorate. With support from the district nursing team and the community palliative care heart failure nurse, Mary died peacefully at home 48 hours later. Her final few days were managed using the integrated care pathway (ICP) to arrange her end-of-life care.

The ICP supported staff and enabled them to give high-quality care by ensuring that all Mary's physical, psychological and social needs were addressed, as well as supporting her family. Her medication was reviewed on a regular basis, her symptoms were assessed and, very importantly, her wishes about where she wished to be cared for, and where she wanted to die, were reviewed. Mary did die at home, as she wished. However, some patients may initially express a wish to remain at home, but later find themselves overwhelmed by their symptoms and needing the security of the 24-hour care that is available in a hospital or hospice. The care pathway also contained prompts to ensure that the out-of-hours service staff were aware that she was a palliative care patient at the end of life, to prevent unnecessary or avoidable hospital admission. All patients with chronic, progressive, and eventually fatal illness, need the kind of high-quality, well-organised end-of-life care (Main *et al.* 2006) that Mary received. Her death was managed well in her own home, as she wished, and her end-of-life symptoms were well controlled.

Conclusion

The benefits of using integrated care pathways to manage all aspects of care have been well documented over many years (Panella & Vanhaecht 2010). They provide a structured approach by focusing on a particular condition or group of patients, streamlining care and providing a template or prompt to ensure best practice and standardised high-quality care.

Integrated care pathways form part of a continuous quality improvement cycle and their effectiveness should be regularly reviewed. This review should include evaluation of the achievement of both process and outcome standards. This includes the monitoring of safe and effective discharge so that any necessary amendments can be made to the rapid discharge section of the end-of-life pathway.

When considering seamless discharge, pathways should be developed by primary and secondary care staff working together. As described by Ovretveit (2010), when teams develop a pathway together, this should be viewed as part of an overall strategy to develop inter-professional cooperation. In Mary's case, primary and secondary care staff worked well together to facilitate her rapid discharge home, according to her wishes, by utilising the care pathway approach.

References

Department of Health (2007). 'Our NHS Our Future: NHS next stage review – interim report'. London: HMSO.

Lynn, J. (2004). *The Solid Facts: Palliative Care*. Geneva: Europe WHO.

Main, J., Whittle, C., Treml, J., Woolley, J. & Main, A. (2006). The development of an Integrated Care Pathway for all patients with advanced life limiting illness – the Supportive Care Pathway. *Journal of Nursing Management*. **14** (7), 521–528.

Murray, S., Kendall, M., Boyd, K. & Sheikh, A. (2005). Illness trajectories and palliative care. *British Medical Journal*. **330**, 1007–1011.

National Gold Standards Framework Centre (2008). The Gold Standards Framework Prognostic Indicator Guidance. http://www.goldstandardsframework.nhs.uk/Resources/Gold%20Standards%20Framework/PIG_Paper_Final_revised_v5_Sept08.pdf (accessed 30/09/2010).

National Institute for Health and Clinical Excellence (2004). 'Improving supportive and palliative care for adults with cancer'. London: NICE.

Office for National Statistics (2004). 'Focus on Older People'. http://www.statistics.gov.uk/downloads/theme_compendia/foop05/Olderpeople2005.pdf

Ovretveit, J. (2010). The future for care pathways. *International Journal of Care Pathways*. **14**, 76–78.

Panella, M. & Vanhaecht, K. (2010). Care pathways and organisational systems: the basis for a successful connection. *International Journal of Care Pathways*. **15**, 45–46.

Panella, M., Marchisio, S., Demarchi, M.L., Manzoli, L. & Di Stanislao, F. (2009). Reduced in-hospital mortality for heart failure with clinical pathways: the results of a cluster randomised controlled trial. *Quality and Safety in Health Care*. **18**, 369–373.

Discharge practice case studies

Stewart, S. & McMurray, J. (2002). Palliative care for heart failure. *British Medical Journal.* **325** (7370), 915–916.

Vanhaecht, K., Panella, M., Van Zelm, R. & Sermeus, W. (2010). An overview on the history and concept of care pathways as complex interventions. *International Journal of Care Pathways.* **14**, 117–123.

While, A. & Kiek, F. (2009). Chronic heart failure: promoting quality of life. *British Journal of Community Nursing.* **14** (2), 54–59.

Chapter 22

Benefits of nurse-facilitated discharge for paediatric day-case surgery
Corrina Hulkes

This chapter describes the process of nurse-facilitated discharge (NFD) in a paediatric ward, which was successfully introduced to improve the quality of discharge.

The process of admission to and discharge from hospital can be distressing for patients and their families. Across the paediatric wards within the children's services department of a large teaching hospital in the eastern region, patients and parents were facing delays of up to eight hours – just to see a doctor to confirm they could go home. The nursing team felt their young patients were getting a raw deal – waiting around for a routine discharge, which the nurses could easily do. The long delays meant that children became fractious and parents frustrated, when they had already seen the surgeon in recovery and been assured that the operation had gone well. Most were happy to go home and wait until the follow-up appointment to see their surgeon again.

Background

The 'National Service Framework for Children, Young People and Maternity Services' says that discharge planning should be considered throughout a patient's hospital admission, in the expectation that discharges should be smooth, timely and developed in partnership with the child and their parents (DH 2007). This requires a change of culture and involves the whole multidisciplinary team. Considering the high percentage of patient care that is delivered by nursing staff, it is clear that nurses can have a huge impact on preventing discharge delays.

The paediatric wards had up to 80 different visiting specialties and a large proportion of patients would have to wait until the end of the day, when the surgeon or a member of their team was free from theatre to visit the ward. As well as staff spending time reassuring families, nurses were also regularly chasing busy doctors to request the discharge of a patient.

Making the change towards nurse-facilitated discharge

Having identified issues around delayed discharge by carrying out two audits, a project steering group was set up to identify ways to prevent delays, improve the patient experience and enhance clinical efficiency and productivity. Nurses led the programme from the outset. They identified the issues, gathered strong evidence, found solutions, consulted and developed a programme and changed previously accepted ways of working.

The project steering group consisted of:

- A modern matron for general paediatrics
- Senior sisters representing an inpatient ward and a day-case unit
- A project nurse
- A practice development nurse
- An admissions coordinator

Nurses are able to gather information from their patients effectively, due to the close working relationships they develop with them. Nurses are also aware of the services the patients are likely to need upon discharge because they observe the patients' needs and the services they already access. However, the discharge planning process should not be undertaken solely by the nursing teams but in conjunction with, and with support from, the multidisciplinary team. A nurse-facilitated approach to discharge planning allows nurses to take responsibility for the proactive management of the discharge of the patients in their care (Lees 2007).

Baseline data

It was identified that there were a significant number of delayed discharges, which were causing a bottleneck with regard to admissions, and also causing frustration for the nursing staff. Therefore, in order to gather objective data, an audit of the discharge process was undertaken to identify where the main issues occurred. It was hoped that this would highlight areas for change and service development.

The aim of the audit was to identify the delay between children being fit for discharge and the actual time of their discharge or transfer. Details of the reasons for these delays beyond four hours were collected. We also wanted to find out if the expected date of discharge (EDD) was being completed in the nursing notes on admission, and how many children were admitted the night before treatment or surgery in order to secure their bed.

Weekday discharges from two inpatient wards, for the month of October 2007, were included in the data collection. Children discharged at weekends were not included in the data, due to the data collector not being available.

This was a baseline audit; it was therefore decided to focus on those patients who left the ward more than four hours after they were deemed fit for discharge by the nursing staff.

Details of 175 discharges were recorded, and 68 (39%) were delayed by four hours or more.

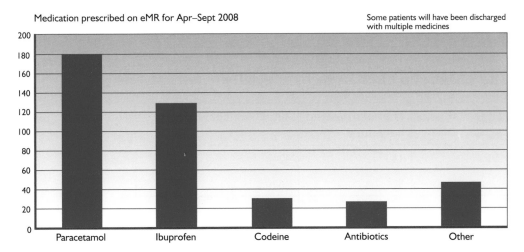

Figure 22.1 Medication prescribed on eMR for April–September 2008

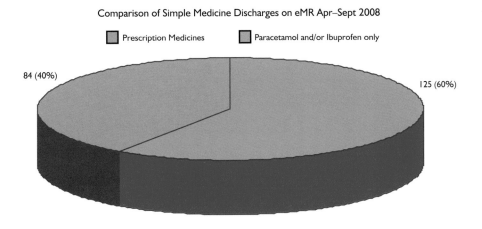

Figure 22.2 Comparison of Simple Medicine Discharges on eMR for April–September 2008

Discharge practice case studies

Table 22.1 Delayed discharges

Delay	Number of patients	
(hours)	Number	% of total discharges
4+	68	39%
6+	37	21%
8+	19	11%
10+	5	3%
24+	2	1%

Table 22.2 Delayed discharges by specialty

Specialty	Number delayed 4+ hours	Total Number	%
Paediatrics	15	42	36%
ENT	5	26	19%
Orthopaedics	13	24	54%
Paediatric Surgery	6	22	27%
Plastic Surgery	11	21	52%
Neurosurgery	4	7	57%
General Surgery	3	6	50%
*Paediatric Oncology	1	6	17%
Paediatric Urology	3	5	60%
Ophthalmology	2	4	50%
Oral Surgery	2	4	50%
Paediatric Neurology	1	3	33%
Urology	1	3	33%
Neurology	0	1	0%
Unknown	1	1	100%

*This does not represent all discharges for this speciality.

The reasons for the delays were varied; by far the most common reason was that the child was waiting for medical review – this was the case for 99 children (57% of those delayed). The only significant other reason was delay in going to theatre, which led to a delay in the time they were expected to be discharged but not necessarily a delay once they were actually physically fit to go.

It is clear that delays in medical review were the most common (57% of those delayed). One might have expected that such delays would be most common for specialities where medical staff were not based on the ward but this was not the case.

Undertaking nurse-facilitated discharge within this environment allowed the nursing team the flexibility to offer care on an individual basis, with the intention of providing children with a quicker and more efficient discharge process that was more responsive to the child's and family's needs and made the best use of the nurse's skills. It was hoped that, once established, this practice could be implemented on all the children's wards within the department.

Development of principles

The steering group met at monthly intervals to organise a plan of development and implementation. The new developments, along with the audits that had been carried out, were presented at consultant meetings, to ensure that information regarding nurse-facilitated discharge was disseminated throughout the department and in order to gain support for this new process.

To begin with, the discharge procedures and policies already in place within children's services were reviewed and amended in order to incorporate nurse-facilitated discharge into the discharge planning process. A new procedure for nurse-facilitated discharge was developed, to outline the scope of the practice, detailing the nursing staff boundaries and guidelines that enabled them to undertake this extended practice safely.

The key principles underpinning the role of nurse-facilitated discharge were agreed upon and outlined, to ensure that all nurses undertaking this extended skill were aware of the principles by which the idea was developed.

Key principles of nurse-facilitated discharge:

- Patient safety is paramount
- Benefits to patients and the NHS
- Coordination and cooperation
- Communication between all involved in the discharge process
- Voluntary partnership
- To support and not to replace multidisciplinary care
- Educational preparation

Source: Cambridge University Hospitals (2008)

Training

Training was considered a key factor for successful implementation and ongoing practice. The training was delivered by the practice development team and was offered to nurses with at least two years' experience in their chosen speciality. A training package was developed in line with the Trust's competency framework, to enable the participating nurses to explore the issues of risk management and accountability, as well as identifying the practical changes associated with their additional role.

Throughout the process, the nurses were made aware that this was an extended skill and was not a compulsory element of their posts; they had the opportunity to opt out at any point if they felt it necessary to do so. This was seen as a vital tool in managing change within the ward environment; if the nurses had enough information and felt included in the processes then they were empowered to undertake the role and implement and sustain the new practice.

Documentation

New documentation was developed in line with the Trust's procedures, to give the nurses guidance on the discharge criteria for children. The documentation consisted of a checklist by which nurses could identify when the child had achieved all the expected criteria and was therefore deemed suitable for discharge. The criteria consisted of questions surrounding the child's recovery from the procedure, for instance whether their observations were within acceptable limits and whether they were tolerating diet and fluid, as well as questions regarding training and information given to parents or carers and follow-up care. If any criteria were not met, then the child had to be reviewed by a member of the consulting team prior to discharge.

The pilot

It was intended that the pilot would take place over a six-month period and the process would be reviewed by audit at three-monthly intervals. The audit would identify which specialities had been discharged by the nurse-facilitated discharge process, and would also identify the reasons why some cases had not followed the nurse-facilitated discharge process. To carry out this review, the audit would use the discharge letters of the children who had attended the day-case unit.

All the nurses working on the day-case unit were accepting of the new practice and undertook the necessary training to allow them to practise this role autonomously. They were introduced to the new documentation and asked to provide immediate feedback, communicating any problems with the process to a member of the steering group, so that problems arising could be dealt with efficiently.

Report on nurse-facilitated discharge audit, April to September 2008

Total number of discharges:	588
Nurse-facilitated discharges:	410
Non-nurse-facilitated discharges:	178

When the 178 non-nurse-facilitated discharges were analysed, the number of discharges that could have been nurse-facilitated amounted to 152.

The first audit (undertaken after three months of the pilot) identified that there was a large variation in the ratio of nurse-facilitated and non-nurse-facilitated discharges for the different procedures and specialities. Having identified these, the steering group was able to focus on specific areas and identify reasons why these patient groups were not undergoing nurse-facilitated discharge.

Discussions with the consultants in the relevant teams revealed that this was commonly due to lack of knowledge regarding the new practice, which allowed children to be discharged without a review from the consulting team so long as they had fulfilled all criteria for discharge. Throughout the subsequent three months of the pilot, further education and discussion was undertaken with consulting teams to highlight the benefits of nurse-facilitated discharge and to discuss any concerns the teams had.

Outcomes

- At the end of the six-month pilot, 95% of children were being discharged by nurses from the day-case unit.
- Nursing staff felt empowered and motivated and the patient journey became smoother and more efficient.
- Families appreciated not having to wait for doctor review after they had finished in theatre. They valued the time and advice given by nurses and this was demonstrated through completion of comment cards.
- Doctors were now more accepting of nurse-facilitated discharge, and more confident of this process.
- Reduced length of stay of patients resulted in increased activity, as there was better usage of beds.
- The unit was able to utilise beds for morning sessions and separate afternoon sessions.
- There was no increase in readmission rates.

Obstacles to the introduction of NFD

Slow acceptance from consultants

As previously discussed, at the halfway point in the six-month pilot, it was identified that, despite initial talks with consultants about NFD, a large number of teams still felt that a child required a medical review prior to discharge. But, with further discussion, and an acceptance of writing in the child's notes and that specific parameters should be written in the medical records, along with the statement that '(Child's name) is suitable for nurse-facilitated discharge', we saw an increase in the second three months of the pilot.

Tablets to take out (TTOs)

The majority of the discharge letters undertaken by doctors were due to medications being required and the fact that the nurses on the ward were not nurse prescribers.

Simple medication discharges were those that contained non-prescription, over-the-counter medicines, ibuprofen and paracetamol. This therefore informed our decision to introduce Patient Group Directives (PGDs) on to eMR letters. However, following discussions with pharmacy, an alternative method of dispensing the drugs was introduced. We also promoted the idea that parents should ensure that they had simple analgesia at home prior to a child's elective surgery. Parents were informed of this through an information leaflet, sent out to them with their appointment letter. This also had the added benefit of cutting our medication costs.

Electronic discharge summary

There were increasing numbers of eMR letters being written in theatre, which were then printed and sent along with the patients down to the ward area. This was encouraging, as it showed that the doctors were aware of the importance of discharge letters and were able to write them during theatre to ensure that all the information was accurate.

There were a few instances when patients did not have any eMR letters completed prior to discharge. This was sometimes because eMR was unavailable at the time of writing and then had not been followed up. The other reason could have been that there was no one available to do the eMR letter, especially if the senior nurses on the ward were not on shift at the time of discharge. (The protocol only allows Band 6 and 7 nurses to undertake nurse-facilitated discharge.) Therefore it was identified that the training should also be rolled out to experienced Band 5 nurses.

Nursing perception of time pressure

At the start of the project, and during the introduction phase, the nurses were concerned that undertaking this additional task would be very time-consuming. However, in comparison to the amount of time that they had previously been spending chasing doctors, and in view of the increased job satisfaction they gained, they found that the time involved was relatively short, and the benefits made it worthwhile.

Sustainability

Following the successful introduction and evaluation of NFD, the next step was to roll it out to the other paediatric ward areas. Yearly updates on discharge planning in the ward environment are in place to keep the nurses' skills and knowledge as up to date as possible, based on ongoing package development by the Paediatric Practice Development Team. Annual reviews of the processes will be undertaken by the steering group to ensure that the process is meeting the aims and objectives outlined within the policy, as well as meeting the needs of the service users. Feedback from service users in the form of comment cards (a service offered within the Trust) will also be monitored, to highlight any praise or complaints regarding the process. In conjunction with this, the bed management process will be monitored for signs of improvement or regression.

Conclusion

The key points are:

- A senior sister or other designated senior nurse (i.e. practice development nurse) on each ward can certify NFD competency for the senior staff nurses on the ward (two years' post-qualification experience).
- The senior sister on each ward is responsible for keeping a list of all competent nurses.
- Each nurse will have to be assessed, completing five nurse-facilitated discharges in order to be certified as competent. Once a nurse is declared competent, the competency assessment checklist should be kept in that nurse's personal development file.
- All children should be reviewed daily with the medical staff, and children considered suitable for nurse-facilitated discharge identified. Parameters should be written in the medical records, along with the statement that '(Child's Name) is suitable for nurse-facilitated discharge'.
- The nurse should then assess any potential barriers to discharge, such as social circumstances, and ensure that these are resolved prior to the child's discharge.
- Before discharge, the nurse should review the parameters. For instance, if the discharge is pending a blood result, they should ensure that the results are available and have been assessed prior to discharge.
- If there is any deterioration in the child's condition or the parameters are not met, medical staff should be informed immediately.

References

Cambridge University Hospitals NHS Foundation Trust (2008). Nurse Facilitated Discharge Policy. On Trust Intranet.

Department of Health (2000). 'The NHS Plan: A plan for improvement, a plan for reform'. London: HMSO.

Department of Health (2003). 'Discharge from hospital: pathway, process and practice'. London: HMSO.

Department of Health (2004). 'Achieving "simple" timely discharge from hospital: a multidisciplinary toolkit'. London: HMSO.

Department of Health (2007). 'National Service Framework for Children, Young People and Maternity Service'. London: HMSO.

Lees, L. (2007). *Nurse Facilitated Hospital Discharge*. Keswick: M&K Publishing.

Part B

Cases from medicine, care of older people, and unscheduled care

Chapter 23

The role of the Rapid Emergency Assessment and Communication Team (REACT)

Jo Brady and Liz Lees

This chapter describes a Rapid Emergency Assessment and Communication Team (REACT) based at the Heart of England NHS Foundation Trust in Birmingham. The chapter offers a context and rationale for the establishment of the team. It also explores three case studies in order to demonstrate how such a team, working in an acute environment, can benefit patients who are being discharged.

Context

The Rapid Emergency Assessment and Communication Team (REACT) is an admission prevention team, which was established in January 2010, following a service redesign. Currently the team responds to referrals on the Heartlands Hospital site, which is one of three sites comprising the Foundation Trust.

REACT interfaces with key areas in a non-elective patient pathway, predominantly the Acute Medical Unit (AMU), Clinical Decisions Unit (CDU), Emergency Department, patients referred from Fracture Clinic and occasionally, Physiotherapy Outpatients Department.

Referrals are accepted for patients who have not been admitted and are deemed medically fit (or are awaiting confirmation of this, following a consultant review) and who have social/ physical or functional needs identified by nursing or medical staff, who make the referrals. Referrals are relatively informal and usually involve a discussion of the patients' case on the 'shop floor'. A full social and functional history, together with a joint occupational and physiotherapy assessment is conducted. On assessment, the needs of the patient are identified and services/equipment are signposted accordingly.

Background

Many patients present to ED with complex medical/social needs, over and above their clinical cause for attendance. Elderly people are likely to be affected more by acute injury or a period of ill health (Hendriksen & Harrison 2001). Incomplete assessment of social and functional needs, particularly of older people within ED, may play a part in re-attendance (Hendriksen & Harrison 2001). Historically, emergency departments focus on treating the patient's acute illness or injury, and the related functional consequences of the illness or injury are not always acknowledged as a priority (Hendriksen & Harrison 2001). For example, elderly patients in the ED are not necessarily routinely asked if they are able to manage their basic activities of living (Nankhonya 1994, cited in Smith & Rees 2001). There are assessment frameworks, however, which do explore social and domestic issues and can be used as part of an initial nursing assessment (Lees 2005).

Hann (1997) suggests that an occupational therapist is uniquely placed as part of a multidisciplinary team to provide assessment and identify the functional needs of the patient when they present at the ED. A study by Hardy (2001) found that a fast-track occupational and physiotherapy team on the Emergency Department floor can help to successfully identify patients who are suitable for discharge home to the care of a community-based team. This can save an average of 4.6 bed days per patient. The Health and Social Care Agent Team is in agreement. It produced a good practice guide in January 2004, on 'avoiding and diverting admissions to hospital', in which it highlighted the need for therapy and social work teams in the ED (DH 2004).

Development of the team

Hence, with this evidence in mind, we approached senior management with the concept of developing a therapy team working at the 'front door' (ED) in a bid to prevent unnecessary social admissions to the acute hospital setting.

The aims of the REACT service are to:

- Enable rapid functional and social assessment, leading to discharge of appropriate patients
- Reduce the number of patients admitted for functional and social reasons
- Help achieve a four-hour target in ED by moving patients through the system more efficiently and towards discharge where safe and appropriate
- Reduce pressure on base ward beds by keeping people safely out of hospital where possible
- Provide a coordinated, timely and seamless approach, whereby the patient can connect to services as required

- Minimise duplication through integration of therapy at the outset
- Create a patient-centred service that is responsive to patients' needs
- Provide care that keeps patients at home or out of acute setting
- Reduce healthcare costs – assessment visit versus inpatient stay
- Direct patients towards other services and other sources of information
- Build relationships/confidence in medical teams to enable them to decide not to admit patients
- Develop trust in assessments between acute and primary care settings

In order to realise these aims, a service review was conducted, details of which are listed below.

Service review

Existing service	Existing service provision
Short Stay Medical Unit 1 x OT B7 & 1 x B3 OT Tech Acute Medical Ward 1 x OT B6 & 1 x B3 OT Tech Flex Capacity Ward 1 x OT B5 0.5 & B3 0.5 General Medical Ward 1 x OT B5 0.5 & B3 0.5 General Medical Ward 1 x OT B6 & 1 x B3 OT Tech	Monday to Friday: 8 am–4.15 pm

Following a series of meetings and discussions with the OTs, the service redesign below was adopted. In addition, staff training was arranged around a competency framework, with all OT staff gaining baseline physiotherapy assessment skills and physiotherapists gaining OT skills. This approach enables the first-contact clinician to conduct baseline assessments and commence discharge planning, which prevents duplication and improves the patients' experience.

Service redesign

Service redesign	Service provision
1 x Band 7 OT 3 x Band 6 OT 1 x Band 6 Physio 2 x Band 4 Multi-skilled Tech 1 x Band 2 Multi-skilled Ass 1 x Band 5 W/E OT Covers: ED, CDU, AMU1, AMU2, Short Stay Med Ward, General Medical Ward, Flex Capacity	Offering a seven-day, extended-hours service: Monday–Friday: 8 am–6.15 pm Saturday: 10 am–2 pm Sunday: 11 am–3 pm

The role of REACT

The multi-professional team plays an active role in triaging new referrals and assessing and treating patients' symptoms and functional problems. REACT enables the wider multidisciplinary team to gain a broader understanding of each patient's circumstances, providing support for effective decision-making and signposting of services for patients. The service ensures that patients receive timely, coordinated care and support that is planned around their needs and choices, including care closer to home. The team provides an integrated service, ensuring that good communication and planning occur during the patients' transition between the ED, the AMU team and primary care services. Three case studies follow, to demonstrate the input of the REACT service in expediting discharge from acute settings.

Case study 1

22.37 pm	A 74-year-old male attended the ED with fall/knee pain
09.45 am	Referral received from Clinical Decisions Unit Nursing staff for REACT assessment
10 am	Information gathered from medical notes; nursing and medical team ready to commence initial interview with patient
10.10 am	Initial interview completed, with patient's consent; identified the following: • Lives with wife in ground-floor level access flat • Has care package of three calls per day • Previously independently mobile with delta frame • Has 'foot drop'; recently supplied with foot splints – in situ Problems identified: • No suitable footwear available for mobility assessment • Patient stated that delta frame at home was broken
10.20 am	Delta frame provided from REACT stock for mobility assessment
10.30 am	REACT referral to Orthotics for suitable specialist footwear – referral fast-tracked and collected
10.45 am	Mobility assessment conducted; new delta frame and footwear supplied to patient to prevent further falls at home
10.55 am	Identified care agency number for patient's care package via Google, as information not available from patient's notes
11 am	Contacted hospital-based Social Work Department and identified allocated Community Social Worker
11.20 am	Telephone call to Care Agency to inform them that the patient was to return home today; care package recommenced for pm calls

11.30 am	Handed over to nursing staff and patient assessed, then discharged from REACT, as safe to go home
11.40 am	Doctors wrote discharge letter; discharge medication given to patient
11.55 am	Patient discharged home, left hospital – bed now available.

This case demonstrates that knowing where to access resources and conducting a functional assessment in the acute setting can enable the discharge process to be expedited, to the benefit of the patient. In addition, good communication with the agencies providing care may assist the smooth transition to home and thereby prevent readmission to hospital acute services.

Case study 2

09.45 am	A 43-year-old female attended the Acute Medical Unit via GP referral with decreased mobility and lethargy; she had a history of multiple sclerosis
11.45 am	Referral received for REACT assessment
12.00 pm	Information gathered from medical notes; handover from medical and nursing staff, ready to commence initial interview for nursing assessment with patient
12.15 pm	Initial interview completed, with patient's consent; identified the following: • Lives with husband and two children in privately owned house • No formal care or support in place; husband and family provide support as needed • Previously managed personal hygiene independently; husband assists with showering • Mother helps with housework, shopping and childcare as required • Sleeps upstairs, toilet upstairs Problems identified: • No stair rails in situ • Increased fatigue during activities of daily living • Decreased mobility • Steep step up to front and back door
12.30 pm	Mobility and stair assessment conducted – wheeled zimmer frame issued; recommended stair rail be fitted at home – patient agreed
12.55 pm	Contacted specialist OT technician requesting site visit (to patient's house) to measure for rails
1 pm	Discussed energy conservation techniques, adaptive equipment and support available in the community

1.30 pm	Telephone call received from OT technician, measurements gained, permission received from patient to fit all necessary rails around home; deliver and fit identified equipment
1.50pm	Referral made to MS Specialist Nurse in Community, MS Society information leaflet provided; patient declined referral to Social Services – telephone number provided for future reference
2 pm	Referral made to Wheelchair Services for assessment
2.20 pm	Handed over to nurse and doctor – assessment completed, outlined actions, nil barriers to discharge; discharge letter and medications completed
3.15 pm	Patient discharged home, left hospital – bed now available
3.30 pm	Telephone call received from OT technician: stair rails, grab rails to front and rear door, shower cubicle and beside toilet fitted; commode and perching stool delivered Patient discharged from REACT

This case demonstrates the REACT team making key early interventions before the situation at home reached a point at which the patient perhaps would not have coped in the future. This type of access to an assessment in the community would have been initiated via a GP visit, and referral for OT. However, in the meantime, she might have been readmitted to acute services. The equipment supplied was very timely. Referral to other services meant that she was linked to support if and when required.

Case study 3

03.11 am	An 86-year-old female attended the ED via ambulance, following a fall from bed; she had a history of hypertension, she was partially sighted with arthritic hands, and lived alone in a privately owned house
12.30 pm	Referral received for REACT assessment
12.50 pm	Information gathered from medical notes, handover from medical and nursing staff, ready to commence initial interview with patient
1.15 pm	Initial Interview completed, with patient's consent; daughter in law present; identified the following: • No formal care in place; family provide support with housework and shopping • Manages personal hygiene independently • Mobile, with a wheeled zimmer frame • Due to previous fall on stairs, patient sleeps downstairs; toilet downstairs. • Patient reports increasing difficulty preparing meals; son has recently contacted Social Services to arrange Meals on Wheels

	Problems Identified: • Meal preparation • Decreased confidence with mobility
1.40 pm	Transfer and mobility assessment conducted; patient independent and safe with wheeled zimmer frame
1.55 pm	Discussed pendant alarm (information given) and intermediate care (IMC) referral to support with meal preparation and confidence building; patient agreed to referral
2.05 pm	Referral made and accepted by IMC for supported discharge to prevent admission
2.15 pm	Telephone conversation with patient's son, advised of actions taken, happy with plan Advised patient's son to move bed against wall Son to meet patient at her home on discharge
2.20pm	Handed over to nurse and doctor – assessment completed, outlined actions, nil barriers to discharge Discharge letter and medications completed; requested nursing staff contact IMC once patient has left hospital; discharged from REACT
3 pm	Patient discharged home, left hospital – bed now available

This case illustrates that, although new equipment was not required and arrangements for meals had been previously instigated by the son (awaited a service), intermediate care services were able to support the patient's discharge through home visits to improve her confidence – often a key factor in cases where a fall has occurred. Knowledge of intermediate care, and what it is set up to do, is essential in order to work in a collaborative manner with the patient at the centre of the process.

Evaluating REACT

Regular audits are conducted to monitor effectiveness. The table below shows REACT admission prevention data and comparative data from a four-week period in January 2010 and January 2011.

Four-week evaluation of REACT, January 2010 and January 2011

	January 2010	January 2011
Number of referrals received	70	166
Number of admissions prevented	40	122 (+ 16 rapid assessment and discharge)
Number of admissions following REACT assessment	30	14

	January 2010	January 2011
Number of bed days saved	304	884.5
Savings	£33,440	£229,970
Estimated saving over one-year period	£421,520	£2,759,640

Conclusion

On 12 July 2010, the White Paper 'Equity and excellence: Liberating the NHS' set out the government's vision for the future of the NHS. The White Paper outlined the government's commitment to ensuring that Quality, Innovation, Productivity and Prevention (QIPP) supports the NHS to make efficiency savings, which can then be re-invested in the service to continually improve quality of care.

By implementing the QIPP ethos, REACT's success continues to grow. The model is being adopted across all Trust sites within HEFT and the team is currently discussing with senior management a number of new projects that will improve services for our patients.

References

Burns E. (2001). Older people in accident and emergency departments. *Age and Ageing.* **30**, 3–6.

Carill, G., Hawkins, G. & Hawkins, G. (2002). Preventing unnecessary hospital admissions: an occupational therapy and social work service in an Accident and Emergency Department. *British Journal of Occupational Therapy.* **65** (10), 440–445.

Crane, K. & Sparks, L. (1999). An admission avoidance team: its role in the Accident and Emergency department. *Accident and Emergency Nursing.* **7**, 91–95.

Department of Health (2004). 'Avoiding and diverting admissions to hospital: a good practice guide'. Health and Social Care Change Agent Team. London: HMSO.

Hann, C. (1997). Use of occupational therapists in A & E. *Emergency Nurse.* **5** (6), 26–30.

Hardy, C., Whitwell, D., Sarsfield, B. & Maimaris, C. (2001). Admission avoidance and early discharge of acute hospital admissions: an accident and emergency based scheme. *Emergency Medicine Journal.* **18**, 435–441.

Hendriksen, H. & Harrison, R. (2001). Occupational Therapy in Accident and Emergency departments: a randomised controlled trial. *Journal of Advanced Nursing.* **36** (6), 727–732.

Lees, L. (2005). 'A framework to promote the holistic assessment of older people in emergency care'. *Journal of Older People's Nursing.* **16** (10), 16–21. www.nursingolderpeople.co.uk

Smith, T. & Rees, V. (2004). An audit of referrals to Occupational Therapy for older adults attending an Accident and Emergency department. *British Journal of Occupational Therapy.* **67** (4), 153–158.

Chapter 24

Evidence that nurse-facilitated discharge works in practice in acute medicine

Dr Kiaran Flanagan and Ann-Marie Cannaby

Nurse-facilitated discharge has become an integral part of elective surgical practice, outpatient clinics, post-acute care and community setting healthcare. However, its potential has yet to be fully realised in an acute medical environment. The medical complexity of patients' conditions in this area of clinical practice has traditionally meant that care has been led by doctors.

Acute medicine was recognised as a sub-specialty of medicine by the Specialist Training Authority in 2003, and subsequently as a full specialty of acute internal medicine by Parliament in August 2009. This has enabled significant innovation and improvement in the quality and safety of service delivery in the initial phases of acute unplanned medical care. It is a genuinely multi-professional specialty, which has created many opportunities for expanded nursing practice, as shown by the increasing numbers of nurse practitioners in this area.

As the specialty of acute medicine has matured, it has been recognised that many acute unplanned medical admissions present with specific diagnoses, and only require a short length of stay, often with simple discharge needs. This cohort of patients can be considered appropriate for nurse-led care and nurse-facilitated discharge.

This chapter describes how nurse-facilitated discharge has been successfully practised in an acute medical setting at University Hospitals of Coventry & Warwickshire (UHCW). The chapter focuses on the following issues:

- Understanding the need
- Getting started
- Tools required
- Understanding success
- Challenges in implementation
- Lessons learned and sustainability: Where are we now?

Understanding the need

National context

The discharge process has come under intense scrutiny as result of increasing demand for capacity, a reduction in bed numbers and requirements to achieve national access targets. A reduction in the working hours of doctors, as a result of the implementation of the European Working Time Directive, has placed further constraints on effective working.

The 'NHS Plan' (DH 2000) stated that: 'It's about working smarter to make the maximum use of the talents of the entire NHS workforce.'

Nursing staff make up the largest proportion of the NHS workforce. Nurses work with patients 24 hours a day and can therefore identify changes in the patient's condition and can also identify when a patient is ready to leave hospital. Engaging nurses in discharge extends the capacity to discharge patients to seven days a week, 24 hours a day.

Nurse-facilitated discharge has been identified by the Department of Health (DH) as the key to shaping the future of nursing. In addition, the Chief Nursing Officer's ten key roles for nurses (2000) prompted the Department of Health (DH, 2003) to recommend that senior nurses should be empowered to facilitate the discharge of patients. More recent publications (NHS Institute 2009, Lees 2010, Lees & Field, 2011) have continued to reinforce the many ways in which nurses' involvement in discharge planning can improve patient experience and outcomes.

'Freedom to Practice' (DH & RCN 2003) included mechanisms to facilitate nurse leadership in the discharge process and gave nurses tangible support in taking on a leadership role in discharging patients.

The introduction of 'Achieving timely "simple" discharge from hospital' (DH 2004a) re-asserted and embraced the nurse's role in discharge. This 'toolkit' emphasises that changing the way in which discharge occurs can have a major impact on patient flow and effective use of bed capacity.

Finally, '10 High Impact Changes for Service Improvement and Delivery' (NHS Modernisation Agency 2004) further reinforced the case for nurse-led discharge, stating that it could potentially reduce variation in discharge and free up GP or consultant time to concentrate on medically focused work. To date, most work in this area has been in community settings and clinical areas dealing with planned, low-risk patient care (such as day-case surgery) or in a condition-specific context such as pathways to manage DVT, COPD or cellulitis. Implementing nurse-led and nurse-facilitated discharge within medicine, with its unplanned flow and complex patient population, has unique challenges and has yet to be fully implemented outside the rehabilitation setting.

Local context

University Hospitals of Coventry & Warwickshire NHS Trust is a busy tertiary centre. It serves a local population of 1 million, with approximately 20,000 unplanned admissions to acute and emergency medicine in 2009/10. The Trust operates two sites: University Hospital and Rugby St Cross Hospital. The University Hospital site receives the majority of acute medical admissions through an integrated system within the emergency department.

As in other Trusts, there has been a significant increase over recent years in the volume and complexity of patients presenting as emergencies with acute medical conditions. Pressure has increased on a fixed bed base and on clinical staff. Faced with the implementation of the European Working Time Directive and the need to meet access targets, new ways of working have had to be found.

In 2004 the acute medicine specialty was introduced to UHCW and a ward was assigned as a short-stay acute medical ward, with a view to developing a nurse-led discharge service. At the same time, a multidisciplinary Rapid Emergency Assessment and Care Team (REACT) was introduced to help implement nurse-facilitated discharge from acute areas, by providing rapid integrated assessment of holistic needs.

Applying the skills of the REACT team, supported by a framework of nurse-led discharge, to a specific population of patients with unselected acute medical conditions revealed that there was significant potential to reduce lengths of stay, minimise minor medical interventions, reduce the number of doctor hours required and improve quality of care, whilst maintaining safe practice. In 2005, a pilot project was undertaken to explore this potential.

Getting started

The core team

The first step involved identifying a project leader and a core team of enthusiastic nursing staff to champion the work and focus training. The nurses who volunteered for the core team were representative of all Bandings and experience, as long as competence was demonstrated (DH 2004b). It was considered that, if nurse-facilitated discharge was limited to nurses on higher grades, implementation would be restricted to a small number of practitioners and would have less impact.

Together, the members of the core team set the project objectives, identified training needs, agreed the target cohort of patients and set out the tools that would be required. A project brief was written, based on these discussions, and submitted to the divisional team. Key stakeholders were identified and these included medics, practice facilitators, the REACT team and managers. Engagement was sought through a series of meetings and informal discussions.

The patient pathway

The patient pathway was designed by the core team, in collaboration with key stakeholders. The objectives were:

- Rapid identification of appropriate patients
- Clear transfer of care between medical and nursing staff
- Appropriate placement of patients on the nurse-led ward
- Defined ongoing care protocol and discharge criteria
- Contingency arrangements if a patient's condition deteriorated or changed significantly
- Integration of multidisciplinary team (REACT) working

In order to rapidly identify patients, a core team member would 'outreach' to the allied acute medicine ward to highlight potential patients to the responsible physician. To ensure that appropriately trained nursing staff were always available to accept patients, the core nursing team arranged shifts so there was always one of them working on the ward. Given the risk of inappropriate patients being transferred to the ward, it was decided that, although the medical input to the ward would be reduced, it would not be removed, especially during the initial phase of the project. This supported the nursing staff but also enhanced and recognised the skills of the whole multidisciplinary team in planning discharge for patients, thus reinforcing the multi-professional perspective.

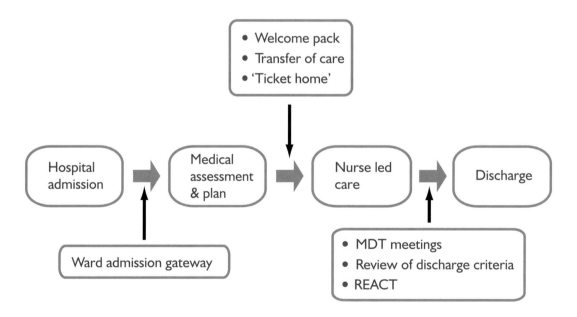

Figure 24.1 The patient pathway

Tools required

Admission gateway

In order to ensure that patients most able to benefit from nurse-facilitated discharge were appropriately placed on the nurse-led ward, an admission gateway was developed. This not only included the admission criteria but also defined the role of the outreach nurse, the time of day by which discharges should be achieved and the beds allocated (to avoid inappropriate out-of-hours transfers at times of high pressure on beds), and a contingency plan to manage inappropriately admitted patients. The following ward admission criteria were agreed:

- Anticipated length of patient stay less than seven days
- Clear medical diagnosis and discharge plan for patient
- Patient not requiring ongoing medical specialty input
- Patient not requiring permanent change to normal living arrangements

Transfer of care document

Acute clinical problems	Chronic diagnoses
Urinary tract infection Dehydration Impaired renal function	Diabetes Hypertension
Discharge criteria	Call doctor if…
If you and the patient are happy to proceed* Apyrexial 24 hours on oral antibiotics Eating and drinking normally Improving renal function (Creat < 150) Good urine output Mobilising safely, appropriate to discharge environment	Any concerns* Spikes temperature > 38 Any new symptoms Deterioration in symptoms Reduced urine output Worsening renal function

*These criteria were pre-set on all transfer of care documents.

The transfer of care document was at the core of the nurse-facilitated discharge capability. It was recognised that a formal procedure should take place to clarify lines of responsibility and ensure that patient care was transferred with the mutual agreement of nursing and medical teams. The transfer of care document also provided a summary of the active medical problems, chronic diagnoses, discharge, and hand-back/review criteria.

In view of the fact that acute medical patients are most commonly characterised by complex co-morbidity, with individual discharge needs, it was felt that a pre-written condition-specific pathway was not appropriate in acute medicine. It was also decided that multiple single-condition pathways would be confusing (especially if the patient had more than one active diagnosis). The core team therefore agreed that the care pathway and discharge criteria would be patient specific. Each transfer of care document would be written for that particular patient by the medical team, and the criteria would be agreed by the receiving nurse. The patient would be assessed daily by the nurse, according to these criteria, to allow discharge (Lees & Field 2011). The care had to be within the competency of the nurses to assess. Therefore criteria that included clinical examination findings (such as chest clear) were excluded. Biochemical markers of clinical progress could be included.

Patient information

Patient information on discharge is important, and interventions that educate patients about their discharge have been shown to be most beneficial in terms of outcomes. Different projects may require different methods of education. Nurse-led/nurse-facilitated care is a departure from the traditional model of doctor-led inpatient care. As a result, there were concerns (largely from nurses themselves) that patients would not accept this new model of care and would not understand why a doctor was not seeing them every day whilst they were in hospital.

To address this issue, a welcome pack was introduced, to describe the care on the ward and provide information for patients. Over the last few years, and in other projects within the hospital, some patient pathways have included specific information that has been mapped prior to admission, during admission and at discharge. This information is now standardised for both the patients and the healthcare professionals, to ensure that consistent information is given and to enable nurses to discharge patients. This information is used extensively by the nurses.

> *"Welcome to our ward. We hope to make your stay here as comfortable as possible. Your care here will be led by the nursing staff, supported as needed by our consultant team. Please let us know any concerns or questions you may have. Ask any of our staff, we are keen to help. We will keep you informed of all aspects of your care. On arrival you will be given a date of discharge and we can help you with any arrangements you need.*
>
> *We are an 18 bedded nurse led-ward, which cares for patients who have been reviewed by a medical consultant and have a clear plan of care to facilitate discharge. This is documented for the nursing team to follow and gives the experienced nursing team the ability to provide patient-centred care, in order to safely discharge patients from hospital."*

Figure 24.2 An excerpt from the ward information leaflet

Estimated date of discharge (EDD)

Although estimated or planned date of discharge is now recognised as being integral to effective discharge planning, and is widely implemented, this was not the case when our project first started in 2005. Estimated dates of discharge were introduced for each patient and proactively managed by the nursing team. The dates were communicated to each team member on the ward board. The patients and their carers were also involved, to enable matched expectations of care and to avoid late delays to discharge. The planned date of discharge was displayed on the board next to each patient's bed, in addition to being filled in on the ward information leaflet issued.

Since the implementation of the project, the use of estimated discharge dates and the planning of the patients' care for discharge have been further embedded across the Trust. These aspects have been formalised, using a computer system that enables all professional groups to see the patient's progress on their journey towards discharge. This has proved vital to daily discussions on the ward with the multidisciplinary team. Nurses lead this process for both simple and complex discharges (Lees & Holmes 2005, Lees 2010).

Integrated notes

One of the key changes made in day-to-day working was in the way clinical care was documented. Prior to project implementation, medical and nursing notes were kept separately. It was agreed by the core team that this negatively affected continuity of care and inhibited effective communication between the medical and nursing teams. All the multidisciplinary team members involved in the patient's care agreed to document sequentially, in the same place in the patient notes. The REACT team (and on occasion the nursing team) had supplementary records that were kept separately.

Visual management systems: Ward board and notes folders

A ward board was introduced to improve efficiency of ward practice. The information displayed included patient's name, date of admission, nurse- or doctor-led status and estimated date of discharge. 'Board rounds' were held twice daily with the multidisciplinary team. The responsible team (nurse/medical) was reviewed, in addition to the EDD, patient progress and next key steps towards discharge. This improved team communication and permitted proactive case management, helping to reduce lengths of stay, as observed (Lees 2010, NHS Institute 2010).

For ease of ward round management, patients' clinical case notes were kept in different-coloured folders, according to whether they were nurse- or doctor-led. An unintended but positive effect of this was to motivate the teams to have all the notes 'purple' (nurse-led colour). This ensured that each patient's suitability for nurse-led care was actively reviewed and changed as appropriate. Similarly, it became possible to tell at a glance how successfully the project was progressing. On week 1, the notes trolley was mostly black and by week 9 it was mostly purple.

Education and training package

A bespoke competency and training package was developed to support the project. There was little literature in existence for the required competencies to deliver a patient-specific, nurse-led care pathway in acute medicine. National competencies recommended as core framework were available in the 'Timely "simple" discharge from hospital' toolkit (DH 2004a).

Based on the 'toolkit', a competency framework that was specific to acute medicine was developed in collaboration with the Trust practice facilitators and with external expert advice. Domains included communication, record-keeping, multidisciplinary team working and leadership, IT skills, discharge letters, ward rounds, transfer-of-care procedure and clinical skills in patient assessment against specified discharge criteria.

The competency package was supported by a series of interactive and didactic teaching sessions, covering key areas and clinical conditions. These were supported by the relevant clinical nurse specialists (including diabetes, COPD and tissue viability).

Since the start of the project, nurse-led/nurse-facilitated discharge has grown across the Trust. The expansion of advanced practice roles has also encouraged many nurses to gain the skills and competencies needed to discharge patients.

Understanding success

At the outset of the project, key objectives were set by the core team. The domains of model feasibility (source of patients, % appropriate patients, diagnostic profile, hand-back rate) and patient flow (length of stay and discharges), safety (mortality and readmissions), were included.

During the nine-week pilot phase, 248 patients were admitted to the nurse-led ward. Of these, 185 were discharged from there, with 50 ward transfers and 3 deaths. Of the 185 discharges, 126 were nursing-led (68%). Only 55% of cases were appropriate for nurse-led care at the time of admission to the ward.

In total, 93% of admissions were received from acute medical areas (emergency department, MAU, acute medicine medical ward, and observation ward). In all, 69% of cases had less than 24 hours' care in another clinical setting.

A broad range of diagnoses were managed, including cellulitis, lower respiratory tract infections, urinary tract infections, gastroenteritis, TIA, asthma, Parkinson's disease, pulmonary embolism, seizure and constipation.

A total of 40 cases (29%) required further medical input after transfer of care was completed. Interventions ranged from advice only or one-off clinical consultation to transfer of care back under a doctor.

A length of stay of less than seven days was achieved in 83 % of cases. The mean length of ward stay was 4.5 days. Readmission rate was 11.4 % and this compared favourably to the readmission rate of the medical discharges from the same ward.

Challenges to implementation

As with all significant 'change in practice' projects, the biggest challenges were staff time constraints and operational pressures. The project benefited from having time released for a senior doctor to provide full-time support. Nursing staff time was given by the enthusiastic core team, over and above their contracted hours of working. Hospital capacity pressures limited the team's power to 'ring-fence' beds for appropriate patients. However, this was somewhat mitigated by proactive relationships with the source wards, which allowed patients to be 'pulled' into the nurse-led ward. Coupled with earlier-in-the-day discharges, the nurse-led bed base was often accounted for before the out-of-hours' period when most inappropriate admissions had historically occurred. The long day shift pattern worked by the core team extended the 'effective time' during which the ward was protected from external pressures.

Culture change was also a significant challenge. In this case, the medical staff fully engaged with the project but there was reluctance on the part of some nurses. Based on anecdotal evidence, the main underlying issue appeared to be 'change fatigue', with a degree of cynicism. A lack of confidence to undertake extended practice and concern about the anticipated net increase in workload without an increase in staffing also contributed. The impact on healthcare support workers was also poorly considered early in the project. As the extended roles of the registered nursing staff increased, a significant burden was placed on non-registered staff to back-fill work. Despite this, the staff affected were fully engaged and supportive.

Handy hints for implementing nurse-facilitated discharge in acute medicine

'Do's	'Don't's
Engage a core team of enthusiastic medical and nursing staff	Rush
Identify a named nurse leader for the project	Set expectations that are too high
Set key criteria for appropriate patients and enforce them	Institute the project without organisational support
Accept the need for ongoing medical support	Underestimate the impact on healthcare support workers – they will have to take on more work too

'Do's	'Don't's
Have an early understanding of the project scope and the competencies required to deliver	Leave out junior doctors
Gain the support of allied healthcare professionals	Leave out patient satisfaction as a performance indicator
Have contingency plans in place to manage patients who are not appropriate for nurse-facilitated discharge, who should not be on the ward	Forget to collect outcome data Identify success criteria and review progress

Lessons learned and sustainability: Where are we now?

The project described in this chapter was piloted in 2005. There have been significant organisational changes at UHCW since then, including a move to a new PFI building in 2006. The effect of this major change had an unanticipated negative impact on nurse-led discharge by geographically dislocating the ward from the other acute medical wards. This reduced communication, limited the ability to pull patients in, and culturally shifted the ward from acute to rehabilitation practice. Lengths of stay increased, following a fall in the number of appropriate patients admitted to the new ward. Staff turnover resulted in the core team being disbanded and sustainability was therefore not achieved.

This was compounded by the original core team's failure to fully realise the need for organisational readiness and senior nurse leader engagement. However, more recently organisational readiness to embed this capability has improved, as teams are now settled in to their surroundings following the PFI move, and roles and relationships have been established. It has become increasingly possible to embed nurse-facilitated discharge within the organisation and it is now common practice in many specialties.

The hospital has also reconfigured the acute medicine service. Following an expansion in consultant staff, the project was re-initiated in 2008/9. A senior nurse champion was recruited in a secondment post and took the lead in re-invigorating the work. Lengths of stay in the new home of nurse-led discharge have been reduced from 12 to 9 days, discharges within 7 days of ward admission have improved from 45% to 75%, monthly discharges have increased from 120 to 160 (comparable to the pilot), week-day discharge variation has been minimised, and staff sickness levels have been reduced from 11% to 4%.

The ward has now been merged to create a new 34-bed acute medicine short-stay ward. Integration of the short-stay ethos with the nurse-facilitated discharge model has opened up new opportunities for extended nursing roles and innovative practice. So, across the Trust and for the specific project, the future looks bright!

References

Department of Health (1999). Green Paper. 'Making a Difference: Strengthening the nursing, midwifery and health visiting contribution to health and healthcare'. London: HMSO.

Department of Health (2000). White Paper. 'NHS Plan: A Plan for Investment, A Plan for Reform'. London: HMSO.

Department of Health (2004a). 'Achieving a timely "simple" discharge from hospital: A toolkit for the multidisciplinary team'. London: HMSO.

Department of Health (2004b). 'The NHS Knowledge and Skills Framework and the Development Process'. London: HMSO.

Department of Health and Royal College of Nursing. (2003). 'Freedom to Practise: Dispelling the Myths'. London: Department of Health/Royal College of Nursing.

Flanagan, K. and Edmunds, M. (2005). Innovative practice: Implementing nurse led discharge in an acute/general medical ward. *Acute Medicine*. **6** (1), 2932.

Lees, L. (June 2010). Exploring the principles of best practice discharge to ensure patient involvement. *Nursing Times*. **106** (25), 10–14.

Lees, L. and Field, A. (2011). Implementing Nurse Led Discharge. *Nursing Times*. **107** (39), 18–20.

Lees, L. and Holmes, C. (Jan 5–11, 2005). Estimating date of discharge at ward level: a pilot study. *Nursing Standard*. **19** (17), 40–43.

NHS Institute for Innovation and Improvement. (2009). 'High Impact Actions for Nursing and Midwifery'. Warwick University.

NHS Institute for Innovation and Improvement. (2010). 'High Impact Actions for Nursing and Midwifery: The Essential Collection'. Warwick University.

NHS Modernisation Agency (2004). '10 High Impact Changes for Service Improvement and Delivery: a guide for NHS leaders'. London: HMSO.

Parker, G., Peet, S., McPherson, A., Cannaby, A., Abrams, K., Barker, R., Wilson, A., Lindesay, J., Parker, G. and Jones, D. (2002). A systematic review of discharge arrangements for older people. *Health Technology Assessment NHS R&D HTA programme*. **6** (4).

Chapter 25

Discharging patients from clinical decision units

Ola Erinfolomi

The recent emergence of specialist short-stay units has highlighted key areas for developing discharge strategies. These units include Medical Assessment Units, Rapid Diagnosis and Treatment Centres, and Clinical Decisions Units. Such units aim to have clearly structured management plans for patients, with well-defined, criteria-based end-points that encourage early decisions regarding admission or discharge. This chapter describes discharge practices in a Clinical Decisions Unit at the Heart of England NHS Trust. Two case studies are used from practice and an analysis of practice is offered.

Background

In the Heart of England NHS Foundation Trust, Clinical Decisions Units (CDUs) have been developed as an adjunct to the two Emergency Departments, to accommodate patients with a range of conditions, who are managed according to specified, evidence-based protocols (see list below). A maximum planned length of stay of 24 hours allows for a short period of treatment and observation and rapid access to diagnostic investigations. Each condition has a timed review point, at which a decision can be made about the patient's state of health and their physical, mental and social readiness for discharge. Decision-making is supported by flowcharts and pathways incorporated into the protocols. These protocols increase the consistency of patient management and reduce the risk of unsafe discharge. It is worth noting that units that offer best practice empower their nurses to discharge patients, based on pre-determined pathway criteria; such discharges are not dependent on further consultant ward rounds (or other medical reviews).

Conditions managed on CDUs by proforma (protocols)

- Asthma
- Anaphylaxis
- Cellulitis
- Chest pain (suspected cardiac)
- Deep vein thrombosis
- Deliberate self-harm
- Elderly care – safe discharge
- Low back pain (atraumatic)
- Minor head injury
- Procedural sedation
- Renal colic
- Seizure (first seizure)
- Suspected pulmonary embolism
- Transient ischaemic attack
- Urinary retention

Available from: http://emergencymedheartofengland.org/ClinicalPathways.aspx

Different types of CDU services

There are several different models for CDU-provided services, namely:

- Doctor-led and doctor-facilitated; the 'traditional' model, with discharge decisions made ad hoc, based on consultants' ward rounds and/or middle grade doctors' decisions
- Doctor-led, nurse-facilitated; admissions vetted by a senior doctor, subsequent patient care, including discharge, based on relevant pathways and unit-based nurses empowered to complete patient clinical journey with or without further medical input
- Wholly nurse-led; all decisions regarding admissions, management and discharge made by the nursing team
- Doctor-led and nurse-led, based on the admission diagnoses; nurses lead in managing certain conditions from arrival to discharge

Rationale and decision to discharge

The last three models in the above list provide the best opportunities for nurse-facilitated discharge. Irrespective of which model is utilised, the key to facilitated discharge from a CDU is having a clear and robust admission policy. The rationale for discharge is established before the patient arrives in the unit, based on a pre-determined pathway.

For this to succeed, the following criteria for admission to the CDU should be observed (Cooke *et al.* 2003, American College of Emergency Physicians 2008):

- The patient should be clinically stable.
- The patient should have a clearly defined, single illness/complaint, i.e. there should be a focused goal for the period of observation/treatment. This could be for diagnostic evaluation, e.g. low-risk acute coronary syndrome; a short period of observation (ideally less than 12 hours), e.g. moderate anaphylaxis; short-term therapy for an emergency condition, e.g. moderate asthma; or psycho-social needs, e.g. elderly patients.
- Patients should only be admitted if it is anticipated that a decision will be feasible within 12 to 24 hours.

Conversely, certain conditions are unacceptable for the Clinical Decision Unit. Patients should not be admitted if they are severely ill or injured. For example, a patient with unstable vital signs, myocardial infarction or comatose condition has very little chance of being discharged home after a short period of observation.

The discharge process is facilitated by protocols with defined criteria for discharge that can be utilised by medics or nurses. For the purposes of this case study, their use, development and indications for discharge will be specifically explored.

Using protocols

Protocols, pathways, guidelines, flowcharts and management plans are sometimes used interchangeably to describe strategies for patient care. However, protocols are used specifically for situations in which there are agreed structures, processes and outcomes for a closely defined problem. Indeed the Greek word *protokollon* translates as 'a note of agreement'. In healthcare, a useable definition of 'protocols' is offered by Field & Lohr (1992) as 'systematically developed statements to assist practitioner and patient decisions about appropriate healthcare for specific circumstances'.

The use of protocols for patient management has been the subject of some criticism. Clearly, not all patients have straightforward presentations and conditions that lend themselves to the limitations of one pathway or protocol. Detractors make the point that protocols can never provide answers for all eventualities and for all the decisions that practitioners have to make in what Schon (1991) describes as 'the swampy lowlands of practice'. This is true, and it reinforces the need to recognise that protocols cannot and should not replace good clinical judgement in patient care.

Discharge practice case studies

What protocols *can* offer is a safe and consistent standard of management for patients who meet certain defined inclusion criteria related to a given condition. Patients who do not meet the inclusion criteria, or who have more complex conditions and needs, are probably not suitable for an environment such as a CDU. Protocols also offer the opportunity to ensure that practice has a strong evidence base or, where strong evidence for a condition or treatment is lacking, then currently accepted best practice is utilised. For example, the evidence base for frequency of observations for patients with headache is extremely limited. However, the onset of new symptoms in acute onset headache is similar to that of head injury. National Institute for Clinical Excellence (NICE 2003) guidance on frequency of observations in head injury can thus be applied as current suggested best practice.

In order for protocols to be acceptable to practitioners and patients, they should have the key attributes of good clinical guidance outlined by Rycroft-Malone (2002, Chapter 9), of:

- Validity
- Cost-effectiveness
- Reproducibility
- Reliability
- Representativeness
- Utilisation review
- Clinical applicability
- Clinical flexibility
- Clarity
- Meticulousness
- Scheduled review

In the Heart of England NHS Foundation Trust, a consensus approach is taken to the process of protocol development. A group is recruited that includes members from all the professional groups involved with implementing the protocols – primarily representatives from Emergency Department doctors and nurses, Pharmacy, Radiology, Laboratories, and relevant medical specialties. Additional representatives are co-opted as required. The group is tasked with reviewing current evidence and best practice related to diagnostic interventions, risk stratification, and treatment and observation strategies for each condition or patient group. Each protocol must demonstrate cost-effective management, and meticulous application of evidence and best practice. Where rapid or accelerated access to radiology or laboratory services are key to protocol delivery and patient management, an operational agreement is reached to guarantee timely access to the relevant services.

Recommendations are made to the group, and a draft protocol is submitted for review. The protocol will include identification of relevant patients via inclusion and exclusion criteria; a structured management plan with suggested timescales for investigation and review; a flowchart for risk stratification; and criteria for admission or discharge. The draft protocol is piloted in practice for a short period to test validity, reliability, clarity and clinical applicability, and any issues or problems are resolved. The final protocol is agreed and disseminated. There are planned reviews of all protocols annually, or sooner if new evidence emerges.

Criteria for discharge are produced that are specific to each condition and take account of physiological improvement, mental wellbeing and social circumstances permitting discharge.

Doctor-led, nurse-facilitated services

When the CDU was being planned, there was a realisation that the diagnostic complexity of some of the patients' conditions required consistent input from medicine, and were beyond the management experience of most CDU nurses at the time. The service was thus developed as a multidisciplinary unit. The decision to admit is vetted by a nominated registrar for that shift, but the decision to discharge and subsequent arrangements can be made by either medical or nursing staff.

Case study 1: Asthma

Patients with asthma are managed on the general Emergency Department shopfloor, according to BTS/SIGN Asthma Guidelines (2008). They are then recruited to the CDU and managed on an asthma protocol if they meet the inclusion criteria of peak expiratory flow rate (PEFR) $\geq$ 50–75% of predicted best and no longer requiring regular nebulisers.

Treatment on CDU, including criteria for failed CDU admission (necessitating referral to Respiratory team), decision to discharge and subsequent arrangements are usually made by the nursing staff, but can be made by either medical or nursing staff. Where there is diagnostic complexity or uncertainty, such as an ambiguous or deteriorating patient picture, then a medical review is sought.

The treatment on CDU includes, as required, bronchodilator inhalers/nebulisers and steroids, and hourly observations of pulse, respirations, oxygen saturation and PEFR. In addition, the factors underlying the current asthma attack are explored. Patient review is at six hours and criteria for discharge are tested: of the patient being symptomatically improved with PEFR > 75% and stable for two hours. Inhaler technique is checked and an adequate supply of inhaled B2 agonist and oral steroids is ensured.

Contacts for emotional and psychological support are provided if necessary, and social circumstances are discussed with the patient to ensure safety and suitability. The importance of compliance with treatment is emphasised, and the patient is given clear written and verbal advice to return if their condition worsens. A GP letter is sent with the patient and posted, to promote continuity of care.

The provision of medications to take home or discharge prescriptions can be facilitated through appropriate patient group directions and through the development of independent nurse prescribers. Further examples of discharge criteria can be found at:

http://emergencymedheartofengland.org/ClinicalPathways.aspx

Case study 2: Elderly patients (safe discharge)

Prior to setting up a CDU, the department had an 'observation unit' that was used to admit patients awaiting specialty beds and those with no clear diagnoses. Once the CDU was set up, there were clear admission policies and procedures in place; a simplified chart is shown in Figure 25.1 (Tony Cross CDU Flow Chart) below, and a copy of the policy and procedure can be found at **http://emergencymedheartofengland.org/TonyCrossCDU.aspx**

Around 4,500 patients are admitted to the unit each year, of which about 1,100 are elderly patients admitted to facilitate safe discharge back home. With the establishment of the CDU, such patients are worked up on the shopfloor by an appropriately qualified clinician (Medical, Advanced Practitioner or Enhanced Nurse/Clinical Practitioner) before admission to the unit. They ensure that the patient is clinically stable, not safe to discharge home from the shopfloor, and has a reasonable/realistic chance of being discharged home by the next morning (that is, within 24 hours).

Once on the CDU, the nursing staff check investigative results and discuss with the medical team as appropriate. Provided that patients are medically 'fit enough' for discharge, the nursing staff initiate referral to the Rapid Emergency Assessment and Communication Team (REACT) and complete the discharge process. Prior to setting up the unit, there were no clear inclusion/exclusion criteria for admission and such patients were admitted randomly under Emergency Medicine, Acute Medicine or Elderly Care. The nursing team influence on initiating and expediting safe discharge was therefore very limited.

Is the patient fit to go home?

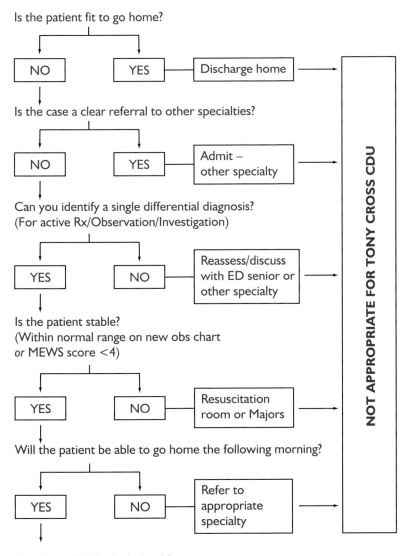

Consider CDU admission**

** Use CDU pathway as appropriate/Tony Cross CDU is an adult-only unit

Figure 25.1 Tony Cross CDU flowchart

Facilitating discharge

The first steps were to prepare a proposal for the Trust Board for support and information, to elicit support from ED staff of all cadres, from other specialties such as Elderly Care, Acute Medicine, Social Services within the Trust, Community Services and the Primary Care Trust.

We had three main options for the nursing model, namely:

- 'Specialist' nurses based solely in CDU
- Advanced practitioners (ready-trained)
- Or suitably trained general nurses rotating through the ED

We opted for the third option. We did not choose the first option because our own experience, and experience from other nearby units, had shown that 'specialist' nurses tend to leave for community posts once they have been suitably trained (and we did not want a separate workforce within the same ED). We did not choose the second option because it was prohibitively expensive, and there were no suitably qualified staff available on the market.

Though the local Higher Education Institutions (HEIs) offered a range of specialist and advanced practice modules, none would have delivered the very specific training required to manage this group of patients. Furthermore, since we had decided to have our staff rotate through the department, an education programme was developed in-house that focused on new skills and knowledge acquisition in key areas. All new staff were rotated through the main areas of the ED, namely 'Minors' stream, 'Majors and Resuscitation' stream, CDU and Paediatrics. Existing staff were required to maintain and update their skill-set in these areas on an ongoing basis.

In order to develop skill and achieve competence, the matrix on page 343 opposite was devised; staff members had to spend a three-month period in each of the following areas of the ED to support this.

These competencies were prepared based on the agreed standards of practice, plus additional competencies related to the new skills of history-taking and clinical examination, and making safe decisions regarding patient dispersal to admission or discharge. Existing standards and competencies were drawn on for validity and reliability, particularly the Faculty of Emergency Nursing Competencies for Practice (2003) and the Skills for Health Unit Competencies for Emergency Care (2005). Supervision in practice was provided by the lead nurse in each area, and day-to-day clinical supervision was provided by consultants, middle grade medical staff, advanced practitioners and established enhanced nurse practitioners.

	Clinical Decision Unit (CDU)	Minors (See & Treat / Primary Care)	Majors & Resuscitation Room	Children's Emergency Department (CED)
ANTT	✓	✓	✓	✓
MEWS	✓		✓	
PEWS				✓
Pain Assessment & Management	✓	✓	✓	✓
Initial Prep & Assessment of Patients		✓	✓	✓
Intravenous Therapy	✓		✓	
Venepuncture & Cannulation	✓		✓	
Blood Transfusion	✓		✓	
Female Catheterisation	✓		✓	
Male Catheterisation	✓		✓	
ILS	✓		✓	
PLS				✓
First Aid Interventions		✓		✓
Basic Wound Care		✓		✓
Wound Closure (Steristrip & Skin adhesive)		✓		✓
Wound Closure (Staples & Suturing)		✓		
Basic Minor Skills		✓		✓
Eye Assessment Basic Care		✓		
CDU Pathways	✓			
(History, Examination, Investigation & Management)				

The nurses continue to be regularly appraised; and for CDU, the lead nurse and lead consultant continuously appraise and support those posted to the unit, with a view to attaining and maintaining competence in managing CDU patients, based on agreed pathways. This process is extended to established nurses on an ongoing basis.

The success of our chosen model can be demonstrated in our bed occupancy rate of 1.5 patients per bed per day, due to expedited discharge based on each patient's pathway, rather than consultants' ward rounds or 'awaiting' doctors' review. Overall, the nurse-facilitated discharge model has provided benefits for patients, for nurses and for the emergency service.

Conclusion

Whilst the discharge process itself and the people making those decisions (medical and/or nursing staff) are important in facilitating discharge from a CDU, the critical factors need to be in place before the discharge decision. These factors include a robust admission policy and procedures, strong medical and nursing leadership, rapid access to diagnostic facilities, a good working relationship with other specialties, and clear pathways (including trigger points for failed CDU admission or discharge criteria). It is also important to facilitate professional development for nursing staff working on the unit. This is essential in order to ensure adherence to the pathways, thus facilitating a seamless management process, including prompt but safe discharges. There is continuous audit of the efficacy of utilisation and quality assurance of the CDU, and the unit has been cited as an example of good practice in implementing ambulatory care (NHS Institute for Innovation and Improvement 2010).

References

American College of Emergency Physicians (2008). 'Emergency Department Observation Services'. http://www.acep.org/Content.aspx?id=29204&terms=Observation

British Thoracic Society (BTS)/Scottish Intercollegiate (SIGN) Guidelines Network (2008). *British Guideline on the Management of Asthma; A National Clinical Guideline.* http://www.britthoracic.org.uk/ClinicalInformation/Asthma/AsthmaGuidelines/tabid/83/Default.aspx

Cooke, M.W., Higgins, J. & Kidd, P. (2003). Use of emergency observation and assessment wards: a systematic literature review. *Emergency Medicine Journal.* **20**, 138–142.

Directorate of Emergency Medicine, Heart of England NHS Foundation Trust (2011). 'Clinical Pathways'. http://emergencymedheartofengland.org/ClinicalPathways.aspx

Directorate of Emergency Medicine, Heart of England NHS Foundation Trust (2011). Tony Cross CDU Policy and Procedure. http://emergencymedheartofengland.org/TonyCrossCDU.aspx

Faculty of Emergency Nursing (2003). 'Competencies for Practice'. London: Royal College of Nursing.

Field, M.J. & Lohr, K.N. (1992). *Guidelines for clinical practice: from development to use.* Washington DC, USA: National Academy Press.

National Institute for Clinical Excellence (2003). 'Head injury: Triage, assessment, investigation and early management of head injury in infants, children and adults'. London: NICE.

NHS Institute for Innovation and Improvement (2010). 'How to Implement Ambulatory Emergency Care'. Coventry: NHS.

Rycroft-Malone, J. (2002). 'Clinical Guidelines' in Thompson, C. & Dowding, D. (2002). *Clinical Decision Making and Judgement in Nursing*. Edinburgh: Churchill Livingstone.

Schon, D. (1991). *The Reflective Practitioner.* (2nd ed). New York: Basic Books.

Skills for Health (2005). 'Competencies for Emergency, Urgent and Unscheduled Care'. http://www.skillsforhealth.org.uk

Chapter 26

Considerations when patients are transferred from hospital to intermediate care
Neil Fergusson

When any patient comes to hospital, we attempt to assess them and deal with them appropriately, keeping them in hospital only for the time needed for their care. In the case of the frail older person this can be difficult, and a number of additional services have been developed to assist in this process. By using examples from real practice I will attempt to cover:

1. Intermediate care

2. Improved early assessment

3. Planning care across the hospital/community boundary

Case studies will also be used to bring all the above items together. Worked examples often provide a fuller explanation.

Intermediate care

Most current community services come under the heading of 'intermediate care' (BGS 2008). It involves the expansion of community health services whilst delivering care closer to home. Whilst most services share common themes, they are never identical (Age Concern 2009). It is therefore possible to think of all services that facilitate the improved care and speedier discharge of patients under this heading (DH 2009). As well as considering how to best utilise these services, we will look at how they can be used incorrectly and could potentially hinder good patient care.

As no two intermediate care services are the same, it is useful to ask the following questions about each one:

- Does it provide service based on the hospital the patient is in, or the community health trust provider area they are from?

- Does it provide inpatient care, outpatient care, or both?

- What can it not cope with (does the patient need to be mobile with one person or do they need to have predictable care needs)?
- Can it look after demented patients and, if so, to what level?
- How quickly can the service be accessed or how can the process be speeded up?
- Are additional treatments available (such as IV antibiotics) and what is the protocol?
- Is treatment time limited and, if so, what is the time limit?

If services are community health area based, you need to be certain which area your patient comes under. Nothing is more certain to generate a complaint than to offer a service and then withdraw it on the basis of where the patient lives. At present, while services are being redesigned, and commissioning and provider services are being clearly separated, this issue is particularly pertinent (DH 2011).

Any area that plans to use these services needs to ensure that they have a full list of what is offered and how to access it. Knowing how to access services is a critical issue and not one to be overlooked. Most services have exclusion criteria. It is vital that these are known, and that evidence that they are not met is provided. Trust in assessment is essential when utilising any intermediate care service. These exclusion criteria are normally put in place in the interests of patient safety. If this information is not available, it will take longer for the necessary service to be provided and will slow down further referrals.

Rehabilitation

Most intermediate care services provide some rehabilitation involving specialist therapy and nursing teams (BGS 2008). Always consider how this will benefit the patient before suggesting it is engaged (DH 2011). In any patient interaction, it causes huge pain and disappointment to offer the hope of help, only to withdraw it. Patients and relatives often take this to mean that the patient is seen as not worth caring for. When patients are engaged in their care and choices 'they are more likely to adhere to the chosen courses of treatment' (Parsons *et al.* 2010). Any detailed look through a Trust complaints log will provide ample evidence of this.

Rehabilitation is a complex process of learning and education, which may occur over a period of weeks or months. It is sometimes approached as a 'magical black box', without first considering the following questions:

- What is the specific goal of rehabilitation?
- How possible/realistic is this goal?
- What landmarks need to be achieved (e.g. in order to walk, you must first be able to stand)?

- How can medical input assist or hinder this process?
- Where can rehabilitation be safely provided?

It is vital that everyone involved is aware of the answers to these questions before any rehabilitation is planned (Parsons *et al.* 2010).

Case study 1: Lack of a clear rehabilitation plan

BV, a 68-year-old man, was referred to be considered for rehabilitation. He was admitted with septic shock, and within 24 hours a diagnosis of mediastinitis (infection of the central part of the thorax), due to oesophageal rupture, was made. It was noted that the patient was dependent on alcohol and vomited frequently. After six hours of surgery, he was transferred to the Intensive Care Unit, where his eight-week stay was complicated by pneumonia and a bleeding stomach ulcer requiring surgery. It was noted that he had an arterial ulcer on his left leg. On transfer to the HDU, this became infected and then gangrenous, necessitating above-the-knee amputation and a further four weeks on ITU. Referral notes mentioned that he was independent prior to admission and requested consideration for rehabilitation.

This patient is a good example of a lack of thought in considering rehabilitation. An initial goal of returning to mobility, based on previous function, was never considered in the context of what had happened. He was becoming despondent, due to perceived lack of progress, and discharge seemed quite a distant prospect. Following assessment by a full team of therapists, it was suggested that a wheelchair-based existence with the independent ability to get in and out of the chair was possible. This goal was accepted by the patient and he was shortly transferred to a community rehabilitation unit for ten days and then home, where therapy input continued for two months.

Improved early assessment

It is increasingly being recognised that the largest challenge facing providers of acute care is the growing number of frail older people with medical problems (DH 2011). The systems traditionally in place to provide emergency/unplanned care struggle to cope with this group of patients, especially as the multiple illnesses encountered tend to present at hospital as a very few problems (e.g. falls, inability to mobilise, confusion, etc.). Elderly care departments provide care for some of these patients. The teams based within this speciality have accumulated a lot of expertise, but this is sadly not available to all patients.

One potential solution is to move the expert teams closer to the patients (BGS 2008). There have been attempts in the past to provide a level of specialist input at the front door (emergency department) of the hospital. This has tended to take the form of advice, or skills in providing discharge. Sadly, these models tend to be based around admission prevention and have been referred to in previous chapters such as Chapter 23. This can certainly be achieved, but they tend to view any admission as a failure. Appropriate discharge begins with admission, and the way admission is conducted can vastly improve the quality of discharge (Lees 2010). A well-considered diagnosis and treatment plan enables the patient to recover faster and allows admission to proceed more swiftly. A good understanding of expected outcomes enables the team to be ready with a comprehensive plan. It is not surprising that in complex conditions (such as stroke) specialist units have a demonstrable advantage.

The provision of a consultant physician specialising in elderly care within the Emergency Department, working with a full therapy team, fulfils these criteria. The team members' knowledge includes familiarity with all intermediate care services, and specialist medical input complements this knowledge.

Case study 2: Problem and solution

JY, a 90-year-old woman, attends the ED when found wandering in the street by her neighbours. She is hypothermic and in her nightwear. She has been suffering from cognitive decline for the past six months. It was noted by her family that she was losing weight, and they found she was no longer able to coordinate getting the bus to the local shops. Between family and neighbours, her shopping has been done, and they checked that she was OK on a daily basis. However, she has started telephoning relatives at unusual hours.

Observations are normal, and initial examination finds no abnormality, but she is kept overnight for intermediate care assessment during working hours.

Intermediate care services are unable to help. The patient does not require rehabilitation, and carer provision in the community will not be able to address the issue of night-time wandering. Assessment by the elderly care team leads to a diagnosis of delirium due to profound constipation, a side-effect of her medication. She is admitted to hospital and improves quickly. A diagnosis of vascular dementia is also made, and she is able to return home in seven days with no increase in care, with appropriate follow-up.

This case illustrates several points. The provision of intermediate care services, often with the stated goal of avoiding admission, can sometimes lead to them being used as a screening service (BGS 2008). This results in necessary admissions occurring only after a 'failed' assessment, which wastes time for both patient and service. With specialist medical and therapy input, the causes of her problems were apparent and quickly resolved, leading to a planned and structured discharge.

Case study 3: Structured care

CQ, a 75-year-old man presented with a fall and skin loss over his right hand. He was known to use CAPD, a form of dialysis that the patient can carry out at home. He had felt dizzy before he fell. Normal examination and observations revealed no cause for this. He felt unsafe to return home late at night, and was therefore admitted to the overnight stay ward.

The patient had suffered from dizziness for some time, with multiple falls in the past. This had not been explained, and he was reluctant to leave hospital. Specialist medical assessment established that he suffered from vertigo. A short course of medication was provided to ease this. Assessment of his mobility revealed a tendency to lean backwards, due to a fear of falling. The team were able to treat his problem acutely with medication, but also to provide other solutions. His vertigo and abnormal gait were both addressed by therapy provided in his own home. He thus avoided coming into hospital and has not been admitted since.

Planning care

Preventing admissions and promoting discharges require working across the somewhat false boundary between primary and secondary care. Discharge can usually be achieved when the patient no longer requires care and/or treatments that can only be provided for inpatients (see Chapter 23). Community services are often designed with this in mind. Elderly Care teams know when and how these community services can be used, and this knowledge can be very useful when planning treatment.

Case study 4: Across the boundary

JB, an 82-year-old lady, presents at hospital with a painful right leg. It has become increasingly sore and swollen over the past four days and she is now unable to walk. Her mobility is greatly limited due to arthritis and she has mild dementia. She has a large, caring family.

A diagnosis of cellulitis (a type of skin infection) is made, and treatment commenced with antibiotics. At admission, it is noted that she cannot communicate in English and becomes distressed when away from her family. Treatment with antibiotic injections begins in hospital, to ensure the therapy is appropriate. Referral is made to the community IV therapy team on the day of admission, with the plan of treatment continuing in the community if she is improving at 48 hours. This goes ahead, and she recovers fully at home.

The main point illustrated by this case is the importance of planning. The referral had to be made early, to allow for availability at the required time. Clinical knowledge was required to predict when it would be safe to continue therapy without inpatient monitoring. The whole team had to be aware of the needs of an unwell and frail individual, as well as the care resources of the family. The structure of the admission allowed for an early and safe discharge (Lees 2010).

The most commonly perceived boundary between primary and secondary care is the unplanned hospital admission (DH 2004). The frail older person is often first seen in primary care, with secondary care becoming involved when the patient can no longer be maintained in the community. Experienced staff in primary care can often predict when this will be the case. Intermediate care services can and are used to prevent admission. Secondary care can make this process more effective, but is often unable to respond to complex needs in a timely fashion. Any service that seeks to address this situation must therefore be able to respond swiftly and be easy to access.

A rapid access service is a common model in the NHS, especially when dealing with suspected cancer. This type of service can be structured to respond to the needs of older people, along the same lines as the service to improve early assessment discussed earlier. It needs to be able to formulate management plans encompassing medical and therapy interventions. The same knowledge of community services is required, to ensure maximum benefit for the patient (Parsons *et al.* 2010).

Case study 5: Easy presentation, complex problem

Mr AL is 75 years old. He initially went to his GP four weeks ago, complaining of lethargy and poor appetite with concomitant weight loss. His blood tests showed slight anaemia and mildly abnormal kidney function, with nothing of note on examination. He takes medication for high blood pressure and cholesterol.

He deteriorated over the next ten days, becoming weaker and unsteady on his feet, with one fall. His GP requested rapid assessment as she felt he would require admission if he needed to wait.

He was seen within 48 hours. He was thin with wasted muscles and struggled to stand, due to a weak trunk. He was unable to feel his feet. He complained of constant nausea and was tender in the upper abdomen. He seemed low in mood, which he felt was due to his physical decline.

Therapists immediately began to work on his walking and standing, involving their colleagues from intermediate care to continue this in the community. Medically, he was found to have low vitamin B12, which was replaced with injections by his local practice nurse. In view of his proximal muscle weakness and decline, an underlying cancer was suspected. This was found in his stomach, following an urgent endoscopy. Improvement from the replacement B12 helped intensive work from the therapy team, and medication controlled his nausea, enabling him to eat.

Four months later, he had improved greatly. His mood had lifted and he was able to undergo surgery – the first time he required admission. It is not yet clear whether this has been curative but the patient is feeling much happier.

Conclusion

Intermediate care services have a large part to play in improving discharge and preventing admission (DH 2004). However, they need to be used properly, with knowledge and thought. Specialist input early on in the deterioration of frail older people allows both hospital and community services to function well and to be accessed appropriately. The cases used to illustrate points in this chapter obviously do not cover every eventuality, but they have been chosen to stress common themes.

A good knowledge of the available services in your area and how to access them will allow you to put some of these steps into practice.

References

Age Concern (2009). 'Intermediate Care'. Fact Sheet 76. Age Concern UK.

British Geriatrics Society (2008). 'Guidance to commissioners and providers of health and social care'. www.bgs.org.uk (online access only).

Department of Health (2004). 'Avoiding and diverting admissions to hospital – A good practice guide'. London: HMSO.

Department of Health (2009). 'National Service Framework for Older People'. Standard 3, adapted from 2001 in 2009. London: HMSO.

Department of Health (2011). 'Transforming community services: demonstrating and measuring achievement: community indicators for quality improvement'. London: HMSO.

Discharge practice case studies

Lees, L. (2010). 'Exploring the principles of best practice discharge to ensure patient involvement'. *Nursing Times*. **106** (25), 10–14.

Parsons, S., Winterbottom, A., Cross, P. & Redding, D. (2010). *The quality of patient engagement and involvement in primary care*. London: The King's Fund.

Chapter 27

Estimated discharge dates: Putting theory into practice

Benjamin J. Porter

In 2009, the Care Quality Commission National Patient Survey showed that only 55 % of patients felt that they were fully involved in their discharge from hospital (CQI 2009). The same survey identified that, on the day of discharge, 40 % of patients experienced a delay in going home. In 70 % of these cases, this was due to medications not being available or because they were waiting for ambulance transport. Of the delayed patients, 54 % waited over two hours.

It is clear from these figures that much needs to be done to improve the discharge process. This will involve engaging not only the medical and nursing staff on the wards, but also the allied health professionals, social care team, hospital managers and – above all – the patients themselves as well as their carers. Discharge from hospital should not come as a surprise to patients or the staff looking after them.

In order to improve the experience for patients and staff, discharge should be seen as a process rather than a single point in time when the patient leaves the hospital (Lees 2010). This process should begin at the point of admission. After all, the main objective of a hospital admission is to significantly improve or stabilise the patient's health so that they no longer require the services offered by an acute inpatient bed.

Background

In the present economic climate, government healthcare funds are being stretched even further than before. The availability of new and costly treatments and the rising elderly population are placing a heavier burden on our social and healthcare budgets. Between 1970 and 2000, the number of NHS acute hospital beds was reduced by 30 %, despite rising caseloads (Pollock & Dunnigan 2000). Inpatient stays in secondary care are expensive, and significant efforts are being made to reduce unnecessary patient admissions and cut down on admission lengths, by improving efficiency, to save money. This means that, when a patient no longer requires the services of an acute inpatient bed, they should be discharged to an appropriate alternative place of care, whether this be in their own home or in step-down care.

Effective bed management is therefore imperative. Targets, such as the four-hour maximum wait in Emergency Departments (EDs), have improved the admissions process, but this has caused a significant mismatch between supply and demand when it comes to beds. The bottleneck has been moved toward the end of the system. Patients are processed in the ED faster and are therefore ready for admission to an inpatient bed earlier in the day, but discharges have not been speeded up to match this demand (Locker 2005, Mason *et al.* 2010). It is this mismatch between admission and discharge rates at given times of the day and week that leads to the greatest pressure on acute hospital beds.

Clearly, length of time spent in the ED does not necessarily correlate with quality of care. Instead of being admitted, some patients would benefit from spending a longer period of time in the ED and being discharged directly, following prompt investigation (Lansley 2010). This was acknowledged by the government in the 2010 White Paper 'Equity and Excellence: Liberating the NHS' (DH 2010a), and this in turn has resulted in the development of clinical indicators rather than time targets (DH 2010b).

The discharge process is therefore focused both on the individual patient and their experience of the system, but also on the system as a whole (Lees 2010). The acute hospital and the health economy as a whole have a responsibility to maintain efficient service provision by making staff and resources available. Patients and staff (both clinical and managerial) need to be fully engaged in discharge planning and the discharge process. Key to the success of this will be an understanding of the way any current discharge system works and the use of advanced planning (Lees 2010).

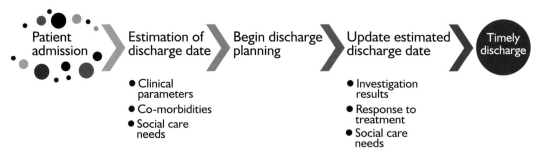

Figure 27.1 The discharge process

Using an estimated date of discharge (EDD), which is predicted on admission and updated according to the medical and social needs of the patient throughout their stay, not only allows staff to plan ahead but can also empower the patient by giving them a goal to aim for and help them prepare themselves for discharge.

This chapter will look at some of the background to estimating discharge dates and the available evidence for their use. It will also explore a case study from Birmingham Heartlands Hospital Acute Medicine Unit. The key points to remember are that:

- Discharge should be seen as a process that begins at the point of admission, rather than the single point in time when the patient leaves the hospital
- Estimated discharge dates provide patients, their carers, and health and social care staff with advance information about their discharge and post-discharge care, including follow-up
- An estimated discharge date should be identified on the day of admission. This should be documented in the patient's notes and communicated to the patient and the multidisciplinary team
- The estimated discharge date is fluid and should be updated when necessary, to reflect the patient's changing medical or social needs

The admission–discharge mismatch

In order to understand the discharge process, it is important to define the difference between number and rate, which can be defined as frequency relative to time.

National statistics show that the number of admissions has steadily increased over the past 20 years. However, the rate of admission is fairly predictable year on year, day by day, hour by hour (HES 2011). Rates are higher on a Monday and lower on a Sunday; they peak in the afternoon each day and fall dramatically overnight.

Unfortunately the same cannot be said for patterns of discharge. Hospitals usually experience far more variation in patterns of patient discharge than in patterns of admission. There is little correlation between discharge rates each day.

The overall admission and discharge numbers are, of course, fairly similar over the course of a week. If this were not the case, hospitals would soon be unable to accept any new patients. It is the mismatch between admission and discharge rates that accounts for much of the pressure faced by acute hospitals to find beds when patients are admitted. This can be seen as a relative mismatch in admissions versus discharges.

It has been demonstrated that the length of stay (LOS) will vary according to admission day. For example, patients admitted on Friday, Saturday or Sunday stay on average 0.3 days longer than those admitted on Monday to Thursday (Earnest *et al.* 2006). The main reason for this variability is the way in which processes such as ward rounds, inpatient tests and pharmacy services are managed. These differences can result in highly variable LOS, even among patients admitted with similar conditions (NHS Institute for Innovation and Improvement 2008). Generally, discharges peak on Mondays and Fridays, with a trough over the weekend.

Occasionally hospitals may experience an absolute mismatch in admissions versus discharges, for example over bank holidays. The staffing levels in hospitals are similar to weekends on a bank holiday and departments such as pharmacy and social care are often closed as well. This means that the discharge rate falls. As the admission rate remains fairly constant, there can be significant pressure on the hospital to generate extra capacity. When an absolute mismatch occurs, it can often take the hospital several weeks or months to return to its steady state. This situation is commonly seen around the Christmas period, when there are several public holidays in quick succession (Henshaw *et al.* 2000).

A study looking at the implementation of a Saturday physiotherapy service demonstrated that length of stay was reduced on average by 3.2 days if physiotherapy services were available on a Saturday. It is changes like this that will lead to improved system efficiency and timely discharge. Healthcare is in demand 24 hours a day, but many of our healthcare services only run in working hours – unless it is an emergency. Having resources such as pharmacy, physiotherapy and social services available over weekends would go a long way towards improving efficiency.

Predicting length of stay

National statistics are available, giving the mean and median length of stay for a given condition, and these can be broken down by individual hospital Trust. Clearly, not all patients will conform to these averages. In some cases the distribution is wide, but, for a proportion, length of stay is predictable. Those patients who fall outside the averages are likely to be those with medical co-morbidities or complex social problems. The Department of Health has shown that around 80% of hospital discharges can be classified as 'simple' and the remaining 20% as 'complex' (DH 2004, Lees & Holmes 2005). The criteria for these two categories are shown in the table on page 359.

The patients who fall into the complex discharge category frequently end up having their discharge delayed due to outstanding social care needs. Patients can often reach a stage where they become 'medically fit for discharge' (in other words, they no longer require the medical services of an acute hospital bed). However, due to outstanding issues with care in the community or the need to increase existing care packages, they end up waiting in hospital (Gigantesco *et al.* 2009).

One study, published in 2009, looked at 158 patients over the age of 65 on a care of the elderly ward (Jasinarachchi *et al.* 2009). It found that 36.7% had a delay in their transfer of care, with the delays most commonly affecting those who were older, had poor pre-morbid mobility or who were confused at the time of admission. They also noted that 18 patients died during their inpatient stay and five of these while the patient was 'medically fit' and awaiting discharge. Perhaps the most startling finding was that delayed discharges accounted for 682 extra bed days – an average of 4.8 days per patient.

Defining simple and complex discharges

Simple	Complex
Simple discharges relate to patients: • Who will usually be discharged to their own home or place of residence • Who have simple ongoing care needs • Who do not require complex planning and delivery. **In addition, they:** • Are identified on assessment with LOS predicted • No longer require acute care • Can be discharged directly from the ED, ward area or assessment unit.	**Complex discharges relate to patients:** • Who will be discharged home or to a carer's home, or to intermediate care, or to a nursing or residential care home • Who have complex ongoing health and social care needs that require detailed assessment, planning, and delivery by the multiprofessional team and multi-agency working • Whose length of stay in hospital is more difficult to predict.

Adapted from: DH 2004, Lees & Holmes 2005

It therefore seems reasonable to assume that a majority of patients could have a fairly accurate estimate of date of discharge generated on their day of admission; and around 80% are likely to be discharged without the need for complex discharge arrangements or social care needs. If an estimated discharge date can be formulated, then preparations for the patient's discharge can be started earlier, and variability in pharmacy services, ward round times and inpatient tests are likely to have less impact on the discharge process.

This is admittedly a very simplified way of looking at a very complex issue. Patients experience different severities of the same illness, and each patient will have their own health beliefs and attitudes that impact on their recovery and motivation towards discharge (Ogden 2000). It is conceivable that involving the patient in the discharge plans early on in their admission will improve this.

The situation where a ward round occurs and the doctor makes an 'out-of-the-blue' decision to discharge should not be a common occurrence. The patient and staff should already be aware of the estimated length of stay, and plans for the discharge should be well underway before the final decision to discharge is made. If this situation were always achieved, many more discharges could be initiated by multidisciplinary team members, such as nurses, rather than having to wait for a doctor's ward round. Using discharge checklists and/or setting clinical parameters can help achieve this (Lees 2004, Lees & Field 2011, Chetty *et al.* 2006, Ducharme *et al.* 2009).

The importance of estimated discharge dates

There is little published robust data about the use of estimated discharge dates but there is plenty of anecdotal evidence in the literature to support their use (Lees 2008, Lees & Holmes 2005, Manzano-Santaella 2009). It seems clear that setting an estimated date of discharge based on the patient's clinical and social needs will help focus the patient and multidisciplinary team (MDT) towards achieving an effective and timely discharge.

The MDT should consist of doctors, nurses and allied healthcare professionals (such as physiotherapists, occupational therapists, pharmacy staff and social workers). The more complex the discharge, the more team members are likely to be involved. The larger the number of team members, the harder it is likely to be to coordinate the discharge. Use of an estimated discharge date would provide some focus for discussion and some direction for the team.

The use of an MDT to aid the discharge process is well supported in the literature. One particular US study showed that the implementation of an MDT reduced LOS, from 61 to 15 days, for patients undergoing surgery for ventricular assist device implantation (Murray *et al.* 2009).

The use of an estimated discharge date can also help the MDT plan for the patient's discharge well in advance. It is clearly no use contacting the social worker on the day the patient is no longer in need of medical input, only to find that discharge is going to be delayed by two weeks while the social worker sets up an increased package of care.

Documentation of the estimated discharge date is also important. It has been shown that using a proforma for post-take ward rounds improves the quality of communication, and this in turn has a positive impact on patient care (Thompson *et al.* 2004, Davenport *et al.* 1995, Wallace *et al.* 1994). It is therefore recommended that any admission proforma or clerking document includes an area for documenting estimated discharge dates. This not only acts as a reminder for the clerking or post-take doctor, but also provides a standardised location for other healthcare staff to find the patient's estimated discharge date. Another option would be to use patient information boards, which are often found in ward areas and are updated frequently (Manzano-Santaella 2009, Lees & Delpino 2007), or to use an electronic system (Maloney *et al.* 2007).

Putting it into practice: **A case study**

Background

The Acute Medicine Unit (AMU) at Birmingham Heartlands Hospital (BHH) utilises a proforma clerking document. This document is used by both nursing and medical staff from the point of admission to the unit. Admissions come as referrals from General Practice, the Emergency Department or occasionally from the Outpatient Clinic.

For a university teaching hospital the size of Birmingham Heartlands, it has been estimated that around 100 beds are required each day for new emergency medical admissions. AMUs are better geared towards high turnover of patients than their medical ward counterparts. This is largely because of the higher doctor-to-patient staffing level and the fact that there is a daily consultant-led ward round in an AMU. In the BHH AMU, there is also a dedicated discharge team made up of pharmacy, physiotherapy and occupational therapy staff that is available during working hours from Monday to Saturday.

All patients are triaged on admission by the nursing staff and a full set of observations as well as an ABCDE assessment is carried out (Lees & Hughes 2009). The clerking document allows for this to be documented. The remainder of the document is used by the clerking doctor and reviewing senior to document the reason for admission, the patient's medical and social history, and a short summary of the likely differential diagnosis and immediate management plan. The final page is used by the reviewing senior doctor (usually a consultant) to review the history, amend the diagnosis as necessary and document an ongoing management plan, before the patient is transferred to a base hospital ward. As part of this senior review, there is space to write an estimated discharge date.

Methodology

In order to assess the quality of documentation and usefulness of this estimated discharge date, a short prospective audit was carried out over a five-week period. The data was collected during the rolling consultant post-take ward round that occurs between 8 am and 7 pm each day. This was a standards-based audit, with the standard being set as: '100% of patients should have an estimated discharge date documented in their notes within 24 hours of admission'.

The audit allowed for both explicit and implicit estimated discharge dates. In other words, the documentation of 'Home Tomorrow' in the medical plan was given as an implicit estimated discharge date, as well as explicit documentation of a given calendar date in the correct area of the clerking proforma.

Discharge practice case studies

Results

In total, 75 audit proformas were returned, which included one duplicate proforma and 18 incomplete proformas. Of these 18, all were fully completed retrospectively thanks to the fact that all Acute Medicine Unit documentation is scanned and electronically stored prior to the patient leaving the unit. This left a total of 74 patient episodes available for analysis.

The results showed that only 66.6% (n = 48) of patients had an estimated discharge date documented in their medical records.

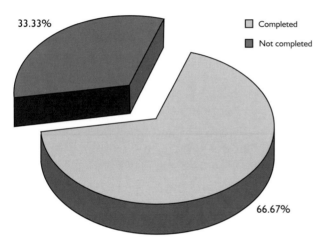

Figure 27.2 Total percentage of EDDs completed

There was significant variability in this completion figure between the six acute medicine consultants, ranging from 83.3% to 50.0%.

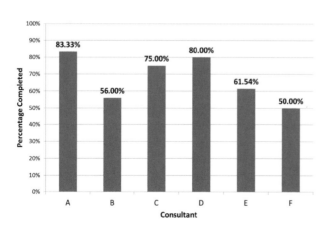

Figure 27.3 Percentage of EDDs completed by each consultant

Of the 48 patients that had an EDD documented, 52.1 % of these were accurate, with 29 % underestimating the length of stay (range 1–31 days) and 19 % overestimating the length of stay (range 1–7 days). This figure improved to 64.6 % with a variability of 1 day +/- the EDD or 81.3 % with a variability of 3 days +/- the EDD.

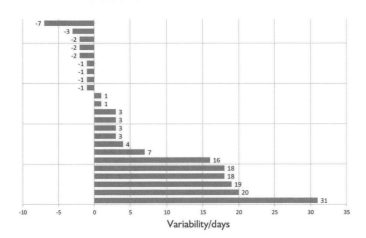

Figure 27.4 EDD variability compared to actual discharge

For those patients who had an EDD completed in the notes, the mean length of stay was 4.89 days. For those without an EDD documented in the notes, the mean length of stay was 8.65 days.

Discussion

The audit results have given the department a better understanding of the discharge process and have highlighted several issues. Most importantly, there is some difficulty in getting all staff members to engage with the use of the proforma. There are two reasons for this.

Firstly, the EDD section of the AMU clerking document is on the post-take ward round page. This page should be used by the first senior doctor who reviews the patient following admission. Unfortunately, this is sometimes overlooked and hospital paper is used to document the ward round instead. This is more often the case if the patient has been transferred off the AMU prior to senior review.

Secondly, the training sessions regarding EDDs were given to the AMU staff, and not the general medical juniors on the on-call rota who staff the unit, especially out of hours. Clearly, it will take many weeks before everyone has done an on-call shift and has been introduced to the concept of EDDs by the AMU team.

Individual doctors have differing views as to which sections of the document are pertinent to each patient. In the audit, only 66.6 % of the EDDs were completed.

Discharge practice case studies

This was partly due to the reasons highlighted above, but was also probably due to differing levels of confidence among doctors in predicting an estimated discharge date accurately.

Reliability

One of the key findings from the audit is that prediction beyond seven days into the patient stay in hospital is unreliable and that it may be best to predict EDDs based on key lengths of stay: i.e. < 24hours; 24–48 hours; 2–4 days; 5–7 days; > 7 days. One of the benefits of this type of system is that it allows patients to be better stratified into groups that are appropriate to base wards with that length of stay. For example, someone with an EDD > 7 days should not be moved to a short-stay unit, but instead might be better managed on a general medical ward or a care of the elderly ward. This system would allows acute medicine units to create capacity on a daily basis by only retaining patients who are suitable for discharge within 48 hours. In other words, an EDD < 48 hours would be required for admission to the AMU.

Grouping EDDs into key timeframes also improves their accuracy. As might be expected, allowing a larger margin of error makes for a more accurate prediction. As EDDs need to be fluid and can change depending on the patient's response to treatment or investigation results, so the EDD can be adjusted and gradually pinpointed to a specific day. For patients who are likely to have a stay of longer than seven days, an exact discharge date does not need to be decided initially, but can be honed down as the patient's clinical condition progresses.

Variability

As we have seen, the audit data demonstrated significant variability between individual consultant ward rounds, with some consultants more likely to complete the EDD than others. This is most likely due to differing training and different ward round styles, but it is an area that needs addressing. Those who take a more proactive approach and discuss discharge planning with the patient are perhaps more likely to remember to document an EDD. It is hoped that, over time, as the system becomes embedded, these variations will level out and the overall completion rate will improve. Introducing the use of EDDs requires senior leadership, and this needs to come from the whole senior management team (consultants and sisters) rather than just a dedicated few.

Feedback

The current EDD system does not allow for any feedback to individuals (apart from the results of this audit) as to their performance. Individual doctors need to be kept informed about their completion rate and the accuracy of their EDDs. The system is currently in its infancy, and feedback is vital if it is to gather momentum and have a significant impact on the discharge process.

Perhaps the most important lesson from this audit is the role of education in facilitating the engagement of both senior and junior doctors, as well as nursing and allied healthcare staff. The potential benefits and pitfalls of using an EDD need to be made clear to staff and its role in the discharge process made explicit. This in turn will help compliance and reduce complacency as the project moves forward. Staff need to be aware that it is only an estimated date and not an absolute. There is no punishment for getting it wrong, but there are large potential benefits from getting it right. Medicine does not have linear care pathways and many patients have complex medical and social needs that will affect their length of stay. EDDs are a communication tool to try to smooth out the complexity and provide a focus for the individual patient and the multitude of staff involved in their care.

Conclusion

In view of the absence of robust data in the literature, the documentation and use of estimated discharge dates will probably be a relatively new concept for most organisations. Only a handful of establishments currently use EDDs successfully, but the idea is gaining momentum.

Patients need and want to be involved in their own care, and this includes planning their discharge from hospital. Treating discharge as a process, beginning at the point of admission, rather than a single point in time, will help both staff and patients to plan ahead. The rates of admission and discharge to a hospital need to be analysed, and hospital systems need to be designed and implemented around this process, in order to reduce delays and improve patient satisfaction and organisational efficiency.

An estimated discharge date helps the patient and staff to plan the discharge process more effectively (Lees 2008). It provides a focus for both clinical and social teams, and gives the patient and their carers a prediction for their length of hospital stay.

Implementation of an estimated discharge date system will depend heavily on the engagement of senior clinical and managerial staff and will have a strong emphasis on education and training. The benefits and disadvantages of predicting length of stay need to be made clear, and staff must be kept informed of their accuracy and compliance through regular audit and review.

The use of a proforma to record estimated discharge dates is recommended, and most units should already have an admission document in use that can be adapted.

In summary, the use of estimated discharge dates is an evolving practice for which there is currently sparse literature-based evidence. There is no doubt, from national survey results, that the discharge process needs to be significantly improved across the UK, as patients do not feel sufficiently involved in the planning at present. Estimated discharge dates provide a means of supporting the discharge process, and early audit evidence from Birmingham Heartlands Hospital is promising. Further research is needed into this exciting and challenging area, and it remains to be seen if estimated discharge dates can really make a difference to hospital efficiency and patient satisfaction.

Acknowledgements

The author would like to thank Dr Phillip Dyer, Clinical Lead for the Acute Medical Unit and Consultant in Acute Medicine, Diabetes and Endocrinology, and Dr Sumeet Chadha, Consultant in Acute Medicine, both at Birmingham Heartlands Hospital, for their help and support in setting up the estimated discharge date audit and their invaluable advice and recommendations during its analysis and evaluation.

References

Care Quality Commission. Inpatient Survey 2009: historical comparisons tables [Internet]. [cited 8 February 2011] http://www.cqc.org.uk/_db/_documents/20100505_IP09_Historical_comparisons_tables_v3.doc

Chetty, M., MacKenzie, M., Douglas, G. & Currie, G.P. (2006). Immediate and early discharge for patients with exacerbations of chronic obstructive pulmonary disease: is there a role in 'real life'? *International Journal of Chronic Obstructive Pulmonary Disease*. **1** (4), 401–407.

Davenport, R.J., Dennis, M.S. & Warlow, C.P. (1995). Improving the recording of the clinical assessment of stroke patients using a clerking pro forma. *Age and Ageing*. **24** (1), 43–48.

Department of Health (2004). 'Achieving timely "simple" discharge from hospital: A toolkit for the multidisciplinary team'. London: HMSO.

Department of Health (2010a). White Paper. 'Equity and excellence: Liberating the NHS'. London: HMSO.

Department of Health (2010b). 'A&E clinical quality indicators: Implementation guidance and data definitions'. London: HMSO.

Ducharme, J., Alder, R.J., Pelletier, C., Murray, D. & Tepper, J. (September 2009). The impact on patient flow after the integration of nurse practitioners and physician assistants in 6 Ontario emergency departments. *Canadian Journal of Emergency Medicine*. **11** (5), 455–461.

Earnest, A., Chen, M.I.C. & Seow, E. (2006). Exploring if day and time of admission is associated with average length of stay among inpatients from a tertiary hospital in Singapore: an analytic study based on routine admission data. *BMC Health Services Research*. **6**, 6.

Gigantesco, A., de Girolamo, G., Santone, G., Miglio, R. & Picardi, A. (2009). Long-stay in short-stay inpatient facilities: risk factors and barriers to discharge. *BMC Public Health*. **9**, 306.

Hospital Episode Statistics. (accessed 8 February 2011) http://www.hesonline.nhs.uk

Henshaw, D., Pollock, L., Rai, G. & Gluck, T. (August 2000). A study of admissions and inpatients over the Christmas period using the appropriateness evaluation protocol (AEP). *Archives of Gerontology and Geriatrics*. 1; **31** (1), 77–83.

Jasinarachchi, K.H., Ibrahim, I.R., Keegan, B.C., Mathialagan, R., McGourty, J.C. & Phillips J.R.N. (2009). Delayed transfer of care from NHS secondary care to primary care in England: its determinants, effect on hospital bed days, prevalence of acute medical conditions and deaths during delay, in older adults aged 65 years and over. *BMC Geriatrics*. **9**, 4.

Lansley, Andrew CBE, Secretary of State. Abolition of the four hour waiting standard in Accident and Emergency [Internet]. 2010 Jun 21 (accessed 8 February 2011). http://www.dh.gov.uk/en/Publicationsandstatistics/Lettersandcirculars/Dearcolleagueletters/DH_116918

Lees, L. (2004). Making nurse-led discharge work to improve patient care. *Nursing Times*. **100** (37), 30–32.

Lees, L. (2008). Estimating patient discharge dates. *Nursing Management (Harrow)*. **15** (3), 30–35.

Lees, L. (2010). Exploring the principles of best practice discharge to ensure patient involvement. *Nursing Times*. **106** (25), 10–14.

Lees, L. & Delpino, R. (2007). Facilitating timely discharge from hospital: Combining patient name boards and discharge planning information. *Nursing Times*. **103** (29), 30–31.

Lees, L. & Field, A. (2011). Implementing nurse led discharge. *Nursing Times*. **107** (39), 18–20.

Lees, L. & Holmes, C. (2005). Estimating date of discharge at ward level: a pilot study. *Nursing Standard*. **19** (17), 40–43.

Lees, L. & Hughes, T. (2009). Implementing a patient assessment framework in acute care. *Nursing Standard*. **24** (3), 35–43.

Locker, T.E. (2005). Analysis of the distribution of time that patients spend in emergency departments. *British Medical Journal*. **330** (7501): 1188–1189.

Maloney, C.G., Wolfe, D., Gesteland, P.H., Hales, J.W. & Nkoy, F.L. (2007). A tool for improving patient discharge process and hospital communication practices: the 'Patient Tracker'. *AMIA Annual Symposium Proceedings*. 493–497.

Manzano-Santaella, A. (March 2009). Predicting length of hospitalisation and social factors. *Age and Ageing*. **38** (2), 247; author reply 247–248.

Mason, S., Nicholl, J. & Locker, T. (2010). Four hour emergency target. Targets still lead care in emergency departments. *British Medical Journal*. **341**, 3579.

Murray, M.A., Osaki, S., Edwards, N.M., Johnson, M.R., Bobadilla, J.L. & Gordon, E.A. (2009). Multidisciplinary approach decreases length of stay and reduces cost for ventricular assist device therapy. *Interactive CardioVascular and Thoracic Surgery*. 8 (1), 84–88.

NHS Institute for Innovation and Improvement. (2008). Length of Stay – Reducing Length of Stay [Internet]. Quality and Service Improvement Tools. (accessed 8 February 2011). http://www.institute.nhs.uk/quality_and_service_improvement_tools/quality_and_service_improvement_tools/length_of_stay.html

Ogden, J. (2000). *Health Psychology: A Textbook*. (2nd ed.). Buckingham; Philadelphia: Open University Press.

Pollock, A.M. & Dunnigan, M.G. (2000). Beds in the NHS. *British Medical Journal*. **320** (7233), 461–462.

Thompson, A.G., Jacob, K., Fulton, J. & McGavin, C.R. (November 2004). Do post-take ward round proformas improve communication and influence quality of patient care? *Postgraduate Medical Journal*. **80** (949), 675–676.

Wallace, S.A., Gullan, R.W., Byrne, P.O., Bennett, J. & Perez-Avila, C.A. (1994). Use of a pro forma for head injuries in the accident and emergency department – the way forward. *Emergency Medicine Journal*. **11** (1), 33–42.

Chapter 28

Advanced nurse practitioners (ANPs) in acute medicine and their role in discharge practice

Steven Close and Fiona Dey

This chapter addresses the role of the advanced nurse practitioner (ANP) in the context of an acute medical setting (RCPL 2007). In particular, the authors analyse two cases in which the role of the ANP has directly contributed to the earlier discharge of patients and assisted in patient flow.

Background

In the current climate of financial restraint, most healthcare organisations regularly face the challenges of a changing workforce. In the NHS acute hospital sector, we also have to deal with the ever-evolving, complex interaction of public expectations, out-of-hours' provision and changing demographics, which may lead to presentations to secondary unscheduled care institutions. With the shrinking and remodelling of medical workforces, the need to ensure high quality, seamless patient-centred care remains paramount, and the challenge is how best to achieve this.

Locally, for many years, we have struggled to keep up to speed with these changes, resulting in many unnecessary, lengthy, error-strewn patient journeys. Recent redesign of patient flow within medicine, restructuring of our acute medical service, and the desire to achieve the level of care required for a proposed integrated Emergency Care Centre, led us to explore the exciting prospect of developing new roles within acute medicine to provide such care.

The vision – the ANP role

Advanced nurse practitioner roles are well established both nationally and locally. In our local organisation we have ANPs based in GPs' surgeries within the community. These practitioners are managing their own caseloads and contributing to healthcare provision in the primary sector. There are also established specialist nurse practitioner roles in both primary and secondary care – such as oncology, tissue viability, care of the elderly, diabetes, epilepsy, Parkinson's disease, alcohol liaison and many more. These specialist practitioners also manage their own patient caseloads.

Acute medicine provides a challenge, in that the skills required are very general rather than specific; and the patient groups admitted to the Acute Medical Assessment Unit (AMAU) are diverse. The role of the ANP within the AMAU setting was considered, and it was felt that ANPs could help provide both consistency and the required level of care. They could also help develop and sustain new opportunities and different ways of working.

The recognised skills of ANPs include independent prescribing (which requires autonomy), and physical assessment. They also need to be able to use their clinical skills to differentiate the medical problems of individual patients. Communication skills and the ability to work within the multidisciplinary team across sectors were also seen as vital in order to achieve our goals.

While developing our acute medical service, an opportunity arose when we were setting up a 72-hour Medical Short-Stay Unit. This unit was intended to support the care and flow of patients who are often simple admission and discharge cases that, without adequate focused management, can end up as 'medical boarders' in outlying wards. Furthermore, these are patients who, due to capacity issues (availability of beds), cannot be sent to a general medical ward. Instead, their care is provided by medical physicians on a designated ward (such as surgical or gynaecological) that is not normally used for the care of acutely ill medical patients. Here, we felt, was an ideal opportunity to introduce an ANP's role in providing a nurse-led service for such patients. The ANPs will ensure that patients are followed up and discharged where possible within a defined time period, thus preventing a potentially protracted length of stay on a general medical ward.

Developments in the ANP role within acute medicine

Two individuals, both of whom were already working as autonomous practitioners to agreed protocols on the Hospital at Night Team, were appointed. These practitioners had completed a Healthcare Practitioner degree recognised by the Royal College of Nursing (RCN). They had proven competencies in taking a comprehensive patient history, carrying out physical examinations, making a provisional diagnosis and commencing planned care. They had experience of working with specialists and making referrals where appropriate (NMC 2005).

This experience was utilised to initiate the setting up of the Medical Short Stay Unit (MSSU), a 72-hour maximum length of stay, step-down area from the Acute Medical Unit. The ANPs, supported by an acute medicine consultant, reviewed non-complex patients, requested and expedited investigations, organised specialty review, completed discharge letters, and participated in criteria-led discharge. They also played a key role in liaising with nurse managers to highlight and provide solutions to blockages in the discharge process.

Over the last two years, we have managed an average of 140–180 patients per month, with an average length of stay of 3–3.5 days and only two complaints. One of the complaints received was that the patient thought the advanced nurse practitioner was 'too busy doing the doctor's work', rather than ensuring that the nursing issues were being attended to.

This led us to consider how we inform our patients about our role, and how we are perceived by our patients. There was much debate regarding what we should wear. A brief audit was undertaken, regarding the delivery of medical care on the SSMU by the advanced nurse practitioners. Patient satisfaction was taken into account, and consultant, specialist and ward-based nursing staff were asked to give feedback with their findings about the role and the functioning of the unit. The feedback was positive.

Challenges of setting up the ANP role

When establishing the ANP role in acute medicine, we aimed to:

- Have a positive impact on patient safety and the quality of the patient journey
- Integrate new roles into already established practices
- Identify where the new role would fit
- Identify the services required by each group of patients
- Support new initiatives such as electronic discharge summaries
- Improve time management
- Integrate the ANP with the medical workforce
- Stay focused on the ANP role
- Ensure that whatever systems we put in place were robust and could be used by everyone

The ANP role in practice

Two cases that have been dealt with by the ANP and the team are analysed below, to demonstrate the types of patients that can be discharged by an advanced nurse practitioner.

Case study 1

A 57-year-old male van driver presented with sudden-onset pleuritic chest pain on a Thursday afternoon. He was examined, had initial investigations and was felt to have a potential diagnosis of pulmonary embolism. He was transferred to the Acute Medical Assessment Unit (AMU), where there was agreement with the differential diagnosis on the ward round the following morning, and a Ventilation Perfusion (V/Q) Scan was booked.

The request was collected by the porters later that day but by the time it was received by Radiology it was too late in the day to carry out. With no weekend service, the next available slot was Monday. He received his investigation on the Monday afternoon. However, the results were not available until after 5 pm, by which time the medical staff had gone home. The discharge decision was therefore delayed until the following day.

As ANPs within acute medicine, it was quickly obvious to us that this was a frequent scenario, frustrating to both patients and clinicians. As a team, we examined the issues around this group of patients – their flow through the system and the effect of such delays both on them and on the organisation as a whole. It seemed clear that the availability of diagnostics seven days a week would have a huge impact on all patient flow, and also on staff, and costs within the acute sector.

The areas we focused on were:

- Length of time between consultant review and request of V/Q scan
- How the V/Q scans were delivered
- Communication with Nuclear Medicine
- Reporting of V/Q scans

The ANP targeted patients who presented to AMAU with symptoms requiring exclusion of pulmonary embolus. On admission, once these patients had been reviewed by a senior, the request of a V/Q scan was confirmed at the same time. We negotiated with Nuclear Medicine to acknowledge a faxed copy of the request form, which reduced the time taken to deliver the request. Booking of the V/Q diagnostic test was then made by Nuclear Medicine on the Radiology system, thus allowing clinicians to see the date and time of the test. We were then able to expedite the results, ensure rapid review or criteria-led discharge, and complete the discharge letter and prescription. This enabled the patient to be discharged in the evening, without the need for medical review, rather than having to wait till the following morning.

Case study 2

A 25-year-old man was admitted with sudden-onset severe headache; he had no previous history of headaches and was otherwise well. He was seen by both junior and senior medical staff and it was felt that a diagnosis of subarachnoid haemorrhage needed to be excluded, and a CT scan was ordered in the late afternoon.

The scan was done the following day. The scan was normal, and a lumbar puncture (LP) needed to be carried out to examine for Xanthochromia. The medical staff dealing with this patient were busy and unable to carry out the LP before the cut-off time of 4 pm for analysing for Xanthochromia. The procedure was done the following day, and the result was reviewed by medical staff. The result was normal and he was discharged home. This patient's length of stay was three days.

The opportunity for ANPs to manage this common presentation was explored. It was felt that early recognition after admission, rapid requesting of tests, and moving patients to the Medical Short Stay Unit to complete their episode of care, would improve the quality of care and reduce their length of stay. We were trained in carrying out lumbar punctures, which enabled us to reduce unnecessary delays in the patient pathway and progress through criteria-led discharge.

In this case, the ANP role could offer the following benefits:

- The patient would be satisfied that he had been fully investigated quickly and safely
- The medical team would be satisfied
- There would be effective management of patient pathway from admission
- It would ensure a delay-free, planned discharge process
- It would reduce the patient length of stay
- It would impact upon bed occupancy
- By reducing length of stay, it would reduce the financial impact on the AMU

This type of case would require ANPs to have the following skills:

- Venepuncture
- Cannulation
- ECG interpretation
- Investigation requesting
- History taking
- Physical examination

- Assessment of the critically ill
- Prescribing
- Referral to specialties
- Discharge planning
- Providing discharge documentation
- Liaison with primary care
- Lumbar puncture

Conclusion

Making these small changes locally has made a huge difference to length of stay for this group of patients. As ANPs, it is imperative that we think about discharge on the patient's arrival and then work to consider everything affecting the patient's journey, to examine how we can have a positive impact on the patient's length of stay and provision of service during their stay in hospital. We can also see opportunities for ANPS to extend their scope by managing these patients further on an outpatient basis.

Future additions to the ANP role could include:

- Targeting more condition-specific roles such as DVT, low-risk chest pain, pyelonephritis
- Providing education for these patients at the time of presentation and diagnosis
- Managing the patients from the time of admission to time of discharge
- Taking on a key role in training other healthcare professionals, including doctors, within the team
- Addressing the needs of patients with frequent recurring admissions who require a more holistic, multidisciplinary approach

Making the most of the skills of ANPs can ensure that they have a key role in providing and promoting timely discharge. By involving ANPs in training, enabling them to support both medical and nursing staff on a day-to-day basis, and allowing them to play a role in service development and making strategic decisions, they can contribute significantly to effective and quality discharge planning.

Developing these roles has been extremely rewarding, not just for the patients but also for the individual staff members involved. The scope for extending practice further is extremely exciting and already a group of Medical Support Nurses have been introduced, in the hope that we can continue to grow our ANP workforce for the future.

References

Nursing and Midwifery Council (2005). 'Definition of the Advanced Nurse Practitioner'. London: NMC.

Royal College of Physicians (2007). 'Acute medical care: The right person, in the right setting – first time'. London: RCPL.

Scottish Government Health Directorates (2008). 'The Advanced Practice Toolkit'. SGHD. http://www.advancedpractice.scot.nhs.uk

Part C

Cases from primary care or involving multi-agency partners

Chapter 29

Emergency patient placement from Acute Medical Unit (AMU)

Liz Lees

This is a case study that represents a smooth transfer of patient care from an Acute Medical Unit (AMU) to emergency residential care placement. The aim is to demonstrate the process used and the considerations likely to be involved for staff working in similar clinical areas, notably clinical decision units, emergency departments and surgical emergency admission areas. Bracketed numbers appear throughout the text and these relate to the numbered key learning points explained at the end of the case. This case is quite unusual. Not many patients can be discharged on the day of presentation to an emergency residential placement – unless the relevant knowledge and support systems/processes are available.

Situation

It was a busy Monday afternoon in the AMU. Jim, an 85-year-old with a short history of worsening confusion, had been transferred from the emergency department (ED) to the AMU for a medical review, pending a decision regarding admission or transfer of care. The AMU has an area where patients are assessed and decisions are made regarding whether to admit or discharge from hospital.

Prior to transfer, Jim had been brought into the emergency department by ambulance. Passers-by had alerted the police, having found him wandering a main shopping street in a state of undress. The police were told where Jim was thought to live, and they had managed to make contact with his daughter via a helpful neighbour.

Relevant past medical history

From Jim's medical records and the ED handover documents, the acute medical team understood that he had experienced a short history of worsening confusion and had a long-standing history of vascular dementia. He had been fit and well with no previous recent admissions to hospital apart from two episodes of surgery when he was a young man. His daughter had earlier stated that she felt her father was becoming intermittently quite aggressive and that his carers had complained the outbursts were making him increasingly unpredictable and difficult to manage at home. He was prone to outbursts[1] of frustration that were felt to be related to the times when carers were leaving.

Social history

Nursing staff on the AMU obtained a social history from his daughter over the telephone, which revealed that he had been receiving a care package[2] at home, via social services, for two years. The package comprised three calls to his house per day, except for the weekends – when both his daughters were the main carers[3]. A comprehensive geriatric assessment is appropriate at this stage and has been recommended as 'standard practice' in an emergency admissions department (Stuck & Illife 2011). This process provides a 'rounded' assessment of function, environment, psychosocial and medical problems.

The two daughters both had young families and worked full time. One daughter had accompanied Jim to the emergency department but needed to leave prior to his transfer to acute medicine, to collect her child from school. Consequently, staff relied upon information documented in the medical records and from the telephone conversation with his daughter. Such telephone contact with service providers, GP, nursing home and neighbours and friends (particularly in the absence of relatives) is essential to piece together social information and can often be overlooked in a busy department. The records included mobile telephone numbers for both daughters. The emergency department staff also documented that the daughters felt they could no longer cope with caring for their father at weekends, and that even during the week, notwithstanding the care package, they could not cope with Jim's increasing demands.

Presentation

Jim was mobile safely (not prone to falls) and verbally distressed. He wandered around the unit from the moment of arrival and was not able or content to sit in a chair, seeming quite agitated. An abbreviated mental test[4] was performed by nursing staff and this revealed a score of 1 out of 4 (Swain & O'Brien 2000). Jim knew and responded to his name but was disorientated, and did not respond to questions about his birthday or what year it was. He was able to ask for the toilet and was assisted (directed) to the toilet with a member of AMU nursing staff. At mealtimes Jim refused to eat, throwing his meals on the floor. He also removed all his bedding from his bed, and warned any nurse away by brandishing his walking stick. Jim's daughter was contacted by telephone for a second time, to inform her of the situation and seek support/advice. His daughter decided to come to the hospital. He responded well when his daughter arrived, and she was able to persuade him to settle and to eat.

Progression to discharge

The medical team (junior doctors and consultant) examined him for chest infection, urinary infection and dehydration. Jim was well nourished, had not fallen and had no injuries, and the team assessed him as medically fit to go home.

At this point, nurses referred Jim to the intermediate care service based at the hospital. The team visited the AMU shortly after referral and deemed him inappropriate for rehabilitation at home or in the intermediate care unit itself. It was suggested that the nursing team should contact social services for reassessment. It was also suggested that Jim should be referred to a psycho-geriatrician for a psychiatric assessment[5] to explore his current behavioural issues, especially as this was the main concern of both the family and his carers.

Jim was known to the locality-based social services team and his case was 'open' to them[6]. The locality-based team were not able to visit the hospital until the next working day. When this was explained to his daughter, she agreed to continue to support him at home in preference to his remaining in hospital, provided that the social services reassessment could be done speedily. A referral/request was made through the single point of access, known as 'SPA', based in the primary care trust (PCT) for additional support in his home environment, while further assessments[7] were made, with the involvement of the family and carers. It was acknowledged that the family were under stress.

At the same time, an assessment of his immediate needs for handover and transfer[8] was made by nursing staff on the AMU with the full support of his daughter. This included his activities of daily living, with particular attention to his mobility, elimination, washing and dressing, and dealing with medication. His carers were also contacted to ascertain his usual levels of ability to function at home and carry out his activities of daily living, with help. It was soon established that he needed significant prompting to wash and dress. He was able to go to the toilet alone and enjoyed his food, eating unaided. It was decided that ongoing assessment[9] would take place after he left the hospital.

Despite initially being informed that an assessment would not be available until the next day the social worker visited the AMU at 4.30 pm after liaising/briefing with the locality-based team. After talking to Jim and his daughters, it was agreed that a transfer to emergency respite care was most appropriate. Many telephone calls were made to find available beds appropriate for his care needs in the locality. A bed was eventually located. His daughter left the unit to go home and have dinner, with the intention of visiting him later with clothes and a wash bag at the residential home.

Concurrently, an alternative route to support (emergency respite care) was also pursued, via the emergency duty team. This is a department of social services that is available outside normal working hours via a duty line. The usual details, including address, GP, and (importantly) that the case was 'open' with social services, were passed on to emergency duty team staff.

When hospital staff attempted to discharge Jim from the AMU, he became very distressed and uncooperative, as he was unable to understand where he was going. His daughter was telephoned again to ask if she was able to accompany him in the ambulance. On the arrival of his daughter, he was calm and left the unit without question. A discharge checklist[10] was completed, together with a nursing letter documenting the nursing/functional assessment undertaken by staff (DH 2010a).

Conclusion to this case

Jim was followed up[11] at the residential home a week after his transfer. He had not settled at all, and his daughters had decided to arrange transfer of his care to live with them at one of their homes, where they preferred to try to accommodate his needs with adequate ongoing support/care package. They found that they could not cope with the distress of seeing their father in his vastly altered state in the home. It is understood that they were planning to give up work and they would be in receipt of enhanced allowances to provide personal care.

Key learning points

1 The outbursts of anger may be triggered by being in an unfamiliar (and therefore frightening) environment or they may be caused by anxiety due to his situation, which he was unable to express verbally. His ability to have a conversation was diminished and he only used key words to express his needs. Up-to-date screening tools and protocols for patients presenting to emergency care with dementia-related issues are available and should be engaged at this stage of care – in this example the social worker was trained to use appropriate assessment tools to determine an appropriate referral to services (DH 2010b, NICE 2010).

2 It is critical to find out whether the care package is meeting the needs of the individual. The total time spent on each visit may be no more than 30 minutes and can be as little as 15. In this case, it may mean that the person is alone for up to 21 hours a day. The problems could be occurring at night, or only when carers are with the person, or in between the carers' visits. Getting a history of what has been happening will indicate where further help may be required. In some areas of the country tele-monitoring is also used to observe the person at key points of the day in their own home.

3 Involving the family carers from the outset is essential, even if the patient is not accompanied to hospital. This will enable you to gather important information about the home situation, which can make the difference between a successful and unsuccessful discharge. This information also highlights the central role that carers play in supporting people like Jim. If there are no main carers, phoning the person's GP will reveal sources of information that will be valuable to the process (DH 2010a). Understanding and being empathetic to the feelings and needs of the carers is critical to the discharge pathway. Family members with a caring role may be exhausted, anxious about the future of their relative and in need of reassurance about 'what comes next'.

4 Wherever possible, the family and carers should be placed at the centre of the discussions and ultimately any decisions that are being made. In a busy department or ward, this may be overlooked, in favour of expediting a process that involves professionals in the planning – and family as an afterthought. In some areas of the country, 'tele-care' can be provided, to supplement care by support staff or family carers. This could include a pendant alarm to summon help in an emergency, pressure pads (under carpets) to switch lights on if the individual gets up in the night to go to the toilet, or alerts if they open the front door and go outside at inappropriate times (DH 2009).

5 Assessment by a psychiatrist in this case was to differentiate between depression and other psychiatric illnesses or disorders. Older people are particularly prone to depression and delirium, and it can be difficult to differentiate these conditions from dementia. In some cases, this may also be carried out by a liaison service (nurses). An assessment is therefore a very useful way of identifying co-morbidities and ensuring that the patient's pathway is appropriate. Aggressive outbursts may have been a sign of an underlying psychosis and would have changed the care pathway and placement that was judged to be right for Jim.

6 People whose needs have been assessed by adult social care and who require ongoing monitoring and review are referred to as 'open cases'. This means they should have a named social worker allocated to them. A closed case, in contrast, will need a referral for a new assessment. But you should be able to request background information on file about the individual.

7 An assessment of the person in their home environment is always preferable to hospital in order to gain an insight into the person's 'normal' behaviour. In hospital, there are multiple distractions, noises, emergency situations and a large multi-professional team

who are assessing patients behind curtains. All this makes close observation impossible, if a situation should arise where an individual were to wander and try to leave the unit. This raises huge safety issues and highlights the person's vulnerability.

8 An assessment of activities of daily living is essential for handover; at this stage it is important to establish whether the transfer is to a residential or nursing home, as they each provide entirely different levels of support. The critical difference is that nursing (health needs) are met at nursing homes and personal care (social care needs) are accommodated at residential homes. As with any assessment, regular reassessment is vital and reimbursement systems require that a comprehensive geriatric assessment is undertaken (Stuck & Illiffe 2011). Assessments do not stand the test of time, especially when there are multiple transfers. Lack of up-to-date assessment information may negatively impact upon the person being moved, especially in terms of adapting to another new environment (Ward & Reuben 2011).

9 A further change of environment is likely to cause some distress and disorientation to a patient suffering from vascular dementia. Their needs may change and will need to be reassessed. When assessing the activities of living, an ongoing assessment of other factors (apart from essential functions) will be undertaken by social workers with experience in this area. For example, a financial assessment will be necessary for future care needs. This is a step beyond the initial assessment in the AMU.

10 The transfer of patients is another stage in the discharge process. A discharge checklist will enable staff to trace what time a patient left an area, what transport they used, whether they were accompanied, and so on. The aim is to provide a safe patient transfer, in which essential aspects of discharge practice are not overlooked. In this case, a familiar face (Jim's daughter) was critical to the process of transfer. Involvement of relatives and carers, whenever possible, should always be central to care in such cases. Communication of the medications that are to be transferred is essential in all cases; especially so, in the case of transfer to a residential home where the care staff (usually unregistered) may be responsible for overseeing or helping the patient to take medication themselves.

11 Follow-up at the residential home demonstrated that staff had employed strategies to try to get to know Jim, and to understand the potential causes of his behavioural outbursts. They were keeping behaviour charts to observe, communicate and try to manage his challenging behaviour. In addition, they had used a document originated from the Alzheimer's Society called 'This is me', to obtain a history of the person and their preferences prior to the dementia (www.alzheimers.org.uk). Once completed, this document can be transferred with the patient between settings to provide continuity of information, and prevent the family and patient enduring repetitive questions during admission or transfer of care. Moving a person into a residential home can be a daunting experience – hence the decision by this family to take him home. For the individual involved, the impact will inevitably exacerbate behavioural issues displayed prior to transfer – and these behavioural issues may never be resolved in this unfamiliar environment.

References

Department of Health (2009). 'Telecare'. London: HMSO.

Department of Health (2010a). 'Ready to go? Planning the discharge and the transfer of patients from hospital and intermediate care'. London: HMSO.

Department of Health (2010b). 'Revised Dementia Plan'. London: HMSO.

National Institute for Health and Clinical Excellence (2010): 'Quality Standards for Dementia and Liaison Services'. www.nice.org.uk

Stuck, E. & Illiffe, S. (2011) Comprehensive geriatric assessment for older adults. *British Medical Journal.* **343**, 1029–1030.

Swain D.G. & O'Brien, A.G. (2000). Cognitive assessment in elderly patients admitted to hospital: the relationship between shortened version of the AMT and the Abbreviated Mental test and Mini Mental State Examination. *Clinical Rehabilitation.* **14**, 608–610.

Ward, K.T., & Reuben, D.B. (2011). 'Comprehensive Geriatric Assessment'. www.uptodate.com

Chapter 30

District nurses working with hospitals to expedite patient discharge
Anne Strafford

This chapter describes the role of the district nurse and looks at a case study of a patient who was discharged from a local hospital, in the context of a busy team providing a community nursing service in an urban setting. Lessons learned are listed, to illustrate aspects that could be improved in the discharge of patients from hospital settings.

Context

The district nursing team described in this chapter is based in the eastern district of Birmingham in the West Midlands. The team comprises 19 staff (some full-time and some part-time). Some are registered nurses and some non-registered (known as healthcare assistants). The size of teams throughout Birmingham varies according to the size of the local population. Services are aligned to GPs' surgeries, which provide nursing care mainly for housebound patients living in the community in their own homes. The definition of being 'housebound' is important in order to allocate resources to those in most need. Patients who are not housebound, and able, are encouraged to attend for treatments, such as dressings, in a clinic setting. Patients who live in residential homes also fall within the remit of the district nursing team. Residential homes generally do not employ registered nurses, whereas nursing homes do. This care could involve end-of-life care, dressings or insulin administration.

The district nursing (DN) service operates over 24 hours, seven days a week, including bank holidays. Out-of-hours needs, from 10 pm to 8.30 am, are covered through a service known as Badger (Birmingham and District GP Emergency Rooms). This is a consortium of local (West Midlands-based) doctors. In addition to the overnight service, they also provide a district nursing messaging service.

Referral mechanisms

The team handles an average of 50 referrals per week; these may be new patients, or patients already being cared for by the team who develop increased or new needs. Referrals are received via a central message service from patients ('self-referrals'), carers and relatives, as well as from hospitals discharging patients with DN needs, GPs and via other healthcare professionals. Interdisciplinary referrals to practice nurses also occur when patients' needs can be met in a clinic setting during normal working hours.

Organisation of workload

District nurses triage patient referrals as they are received, in order to prioritise and manage their caseload effectively. Workload can change frequently throughout the day, with ongoing referrals requiring triage. This has to be balanced alongside the need to provide timely care and consideration of patients' safety (for those at home alone, waiting for daily visits). For example, a new referral for a complex assessment can take up to two hours to complete. Likewise, an urgent referral, such as 'a blocked urinary catheter', will also need to be dealt with quickly, usually within four hours. The daily workload is therefore ever-changing; and allocation of patients (following triage) has to take into account the experience, skills and competence of the staff members on duty, not to mention the logistics of getting to and from the locations, working alone or in pairs as required.

There are similarities between the dynamic nature of the district nurse's caseload and that of a hospital ward nurse. However, the crucial difference lies in the autonomy and the level of responsibility required of the district nurse, as well as the district nurse's obvious need to travel between patients.

What does district nursing involve?

This is often where confusion arises, particularly with healthcare professionals not working in the community setting. An appreciation of the district nurse's work will assist understanding of the breadth of the role. The following list summarises healthcare needs for which referral to a district nurse is entirely appropriate:

- Complex and non-complex assessments of nursing needs
- Wound assessment and ongoing treatment
- Pressure ulcer assessment and care
- Palliative care and support and end-of-life care
- Carers' support and bereavement support
- Sign-posting and referral to voluntary, statutory and private agencies

- Continence care (including catheters and associated care), continence assessment and bladder retraining programmes
- Injections and administration of medicine via oral, naso-gastric and PEG tube feeds
- Monitoring of patients with long-term conditions in conjunction with community matrons
- Health promotion

In addition to the clinical aspects of the work, a big part of the district nurse's role is to look after students – both pre-registration community placements and post-registration district nursing students. This involves assessing, mentoring and teaching. In some cases this can be for up to 12 months' preceptorship, or for the duration of a course, such as the prescribing qualification.

A typical day

A district nurse's day consists of stipulated morning visits, such as diabetic care (administration of insulin and/or teaching of diabetic care or self-administration). Wound care (non-complex and complex compression bandaging, including doppler assessments where workload allows) are also usually carried out in the mornings. Then it's on to new assessments for the latter part of the morning, and possibly afternoon, depending on the needs of the patient and the nurse's workload. The last visits of the day are usually those that have to be done at a specific time, such as administration of early evening insulin or eye drops.

It is important to meet up as a team to promote good communication and shared learning opportunities. This meeting generally occurs either before or after lunch, when the team get together, check for messages, act upon them and divide the workload as appropriate. At this stage, the next day's work will be allocated. Liaison is also a large part of the district nursing role, involving communication with GPs, patients, social services, and other community services and managers.

As in a hospital ward, the district nursing team will allocate one staff member as a coordinator each day. In addition to holding a caseload (list of patients), this staff member will carry the team mobile, which allows contact via the message service for urgent new referrals. It is that person's responsibility either to merge any new referrals into their caseload or allocate them appropriately to another member of the team.

What district nurses *don't* do

Healthcare reforms, some dating back as far as 1991, have meant that district nursing has focused its service on 'nursing needs' while working closely in support of other services such as chronic disease management, intermediate care and palliative care.

In doing so, the district nurse's expertise is utilised appropriately – as a finite resource.

This list is offered as a guide for those less familiar with district nursing, to provide clarity about the role.

District nurses do *not* deal with:

- Medical emergencies
- Mobile patients who can get to a GP's surgery or local clinic (unless they have complex wounds, e.g. venous leg ulcers requiring compression therapy)
- Patients under 16 years of age
- Patients 28 days post-partum (who are cared for by midwives)
- Routine washing and dressing (role of social care assistants)
- Housework and shopping (social carers)
- Post-surgery 'check visits'

Case study: A referral to district nurses

This is a case study of a patient discharged from hospital to the care of the district nursing team.

A referral was made to the district nursing service on a Friday afternoon, arranging a visit to an 86-year-old woman. The referral requested a continence assessment and dressings for a pressure ulcer on the right shin. The visit was requested for the following day.

The ward was contacted the next day to obtain further information and clarify details regarding the shin. The district nurse's concern was that a wound on a shin would not usually have been caused by pressure damage. In addition, the district nurse wanted to know about the reason for hospital admission and any other relevant information, such as past medical history and the patient's ability to carry out activities of daily living.

The staff nurse was unable to share much information, as the patient's medical notes had already left the ward for filing and no one on duty knew much about Mrs P. Consequently, the reason for Mrs P's admission remained unclear, but it was confirmed that Mrs P had no further wounds and was self-caring and mobile. She also advised that Mrs P's husband was the main carer, and provided any assistance required, and that their son also lived with them.

On assessment the following day, a brief discharge letter from the ward stated that Mrs P had been admitted for emergency surgery on a strangulated hernia. She had developed a wound infection, post surgery, resulting in an abdominal cavity wound, approximately 5 cm deep and 100 % sloughy. A holistic assessment was carried out and several nursing needs identified, which contradicted the telephone information and referral via the message service.

She had a wound to her inner maleolus, which Mrs P's daughter-in-law stated had occurred when a cannula had been left in situ, and become infected. Mrs P was found to be in a confused state, doubly incontinent, with no continence supplies. In addition, she was immobile and at risk of pressure area damage, with no pressure-reducing equipment in place.

Mrs P's husband was elderly and also quite confused.

Their daughter-in-law had travelled an hour to settle Mrs P back into her home. Their son, who also lived an hour's drive away with his wife (not with his parents) was actually away, working in another country!

Mrs P's medication had not been sent home with her, as it was not ready at the time of discharge. The family were asked to return to the hospital on Friday night to collect the prescribed medication.

This case study illustrates fragmented working practices and a lack of appreciation of the post-discharge needs of the patient, Mrs P. The district nursing team were not given any opportunity to allocate nursing or equipment resources in advance of the discharge from hospital. The notion of planning discharge from the point of admission was by no means evident; nor were any of the core principles of discharge planning, such as wound assessments, district nursing letter, discharge checklist or involvement of the family and carers. The issues identified pointed to a risky discharge home.

Immediate actions of the district nursing team

A referral to intermediate care was completed, requesting an assessment to provide a rehabilitation programme for Mrs P.

A urine sample was taken as part of the initial continence assessment, and Mrs P was later diagnosed with a urinary tract infection, which probably accounted for her confusion.

Mrs P, despite the best efforts of the district nursing team, was readmitted to hospital a week later with pneumonia.

This case is not intended to reflect negatively upon any professionals involved but to identify areas that can be improved in order to ensure smooth discharge from acute services and successful transition into primary care.

Lessons learned

In this case, there are four key changes that would significantly improve the process of discharging patients with district nursing needs:

1. An improvement in the quality of information communicated via the initial telephone referral from the hospital ward; a follow-up telephone conversation to clarify issues might also be helpful.

2. A comprehensive discharge letter could have improved the transition from hospital to community, ensuring timely, appropriate communication of care needs. Standardisation of the information in this letter would also be useful, to prompt consideration of key issues.

3. The use of a discharge checklist is fundamental to successful discharge planning. This would also ensure that a named nurse was accountable for a safe discharge. Moreover, it would enable contact from the community with a named nurse following discharge from hospital.

4. Inviting district nurses to a multidisciplinary team meeting before the hospital discharge would be beneficial for all health professionals. It would improve communication and enhance timely collaborative working between the hospital and community services.

Conclusion

In the future there will be opportunities to improve communication by developing a single shared electronic system to access medical and nursing records – integrated in a contemporaneous manner as the patient progresses through the care pathway towards home. It is perfectly feasible that, through such a system, services could be aligned to individuals' needs in advance of discharge, giving care providers time to install any services or equipment required for a safe discharge home. Furthermore, professionals engaged in discharging patients from hospital settings need to be made more accountable for their decisions and actions.

If these changes were made, the system would be more cohesive, with the patient's needs at the centre of service planning. Currently, there is little, if any, consideration of a district nurse's caseload, to ensure that there is adequate 'service supply' prior to discharge. This also needs to change.

Chapter 31

Multi-professional working with complex patients and long-term conditions
Maggie Shepley and Sheila Kalanovic

Since 2005, there has been a drive to address the care needs of patients with long-term conditions and to do so in a proactive way. The current health and social care strategy is to use a self-management model with individuals who have lived with their conditions for many years. To do this effectively, there is a need to build a more functional way of working across primary and secondary care, and also to have a much more integrated approach with our colleagues in social services.

This chapter looks at a case study in Calderdale, West Yorkshire, where a 'virtual' team works operationally across different organisations. It discusses the role of a multi-professional complex discharge team, and considers in-reach into the Acute Hospital Trust to achieve more timely discharges. This case study illustrates the difficulties and complexities that staff sometimes faced in discharge planning, as well as solutions and changes made to the process.

Context

Calderdale has a population of over 200,000 inhabitants and primary healthcare is provided by NHS Calderdale Provider Services. Calderdale Royal Hospital is the one site of secondary care, which is part of an Acute Foundation Trust with Huddersfield Royal Infirmary. Community matrons (CMs) were introduced into Calderdale early in 2005 and they originally worked with a caseload attached to a GP's practice. The community matron's remit is to work with patients with long-term conditions and complex needs, who are high-intensity users of healthcare services. Community matrons were given an opportunity to work within the hospital to engage with patient flow issues; and it was recognised that there was a greater need for more integrated working with secondary care.

Case study

This case involved a patient with an inpatient length of stay exceeding 160 days.

The patient's wife continually refused to engage with hospital staff to consider her husband's discharge plan. Eventually it became clear that the existing transfer of care arrangements were no more than a suggested process. In fact, there was no policy to support any plan for discharge to another place of care or to the patient's home.

This situation was escalated up to director level within the Acute Trust, where the question was asked: 'What are the discharge processes and what action has been taken to resolve the difficulties regarding discharge planning?' The role of 'Matron for Patient Flow' was piloted in order to look at systems and processes that could develop communication channels between all the organisations potentially involved with the individual. These systems and processes could then be applied to future instances of a similar nature.

Statistics covering length of stay (LOS) and bed days within the hospital were explored, to look for delays, and then used as a measure for audit purposes. From this data, it was possible to make a weekly list of patients with an LOS of 14 days or more, for further review. (Initially, a seven-day LOS was suggested. However, this was unworkable, as most patients were discharged or moved onto another area within this period.)

The process that developed was that a matron from the hospital and a social worker reviewed each of these longer-term cases and allocated a key worker who would act as coordinator with each individual patient and their family. This was so successful that, within a short space of time, we changed the focus to patients with an LOS of 10 days or more in order to further drive down the length of stay by exploring problems that came up earlier in the hospital stay.

In addition, the commissioners requested a focus on the most complex of these patients – particularly the 40 patients who, at that time, had an LOS of over 100 days. More often than not, these were patients on the rehabilitation wards, where allied health professionals would request further time to help their patients reach higher levels of ability. There appeared to be no sense of urgency about discharging these patients to continue their rehabilitation within their own home environment.

Complex discharge team

The concept of a complex discharge team (CDT) emerged from a whole systems approach. This type of approach commonly involves several different organisations, and several disciplines from these organisations working together across a care pathway. The aim was to provide safe and timely discharge of patients from an acute episode of care, ensuring that patients receive the Right care, at the Right time and in the Right place (DH 2008). It was anticipated that the vast majority of inpatients (80%) would be managed and discharged or transferred by the ward teams, with the remaining 20% of complex patients being supported and managed by the CDT.

In response to this more innovative way of working, an Urgent Care/Emergency Services Collaborative Board was formed. This included members from Calderdale & Huddersfield NHS Foundation Trust, NHS Calderdale, Calderdale Council, Kirklees Council, NHS Kirklees and South and West Yorkshire Mental Health Trust, which gave wide-ranging endorsement of the proposed principles and practice. This was further embedded by commissioning a strategic report, called the Tribal Report, to review a more integrated approach to discharge planning.

In late 2006, Tribal Consulting undertook a review of discharge planning – the 'back end' of the care pathway. The report was presented to the Calderdale & Huddersfield Foundation Trust in January 2007 and provided a review of progress, to ascertain the extent to which the recommendations had been implemented. The following issues were considered in the report:

- Multidisciplinary working and communication – who 'owns' the patient journey?
- Interaction with social services
- Rehabilitation – where does/should this occur?
- Patient choice – where should patients decide on or wait for home care or residential/nursing home placement?

The report's key recommendations were:

- The major bottleneck, and the one that is easiest to address, is the lack of coordinated MDT working and processes.
- We recommend that the Trust and its partner organisations establish a project team to standardise MDT processes.
- This project could be initiated immediately and would rapidly drive improvement and standardisation of associated documentation.
- As medium-term projects, we recommend that the Trust and its partner organisations undertake an option appraisal around rehabilitation service provision and developing a policy with regard to patient choice in the discharge process.

- We recommend the development of a single discharge facilitation service to develop the interface with ward-based staff, primary care and community services.
- We recommend a clear decision-making process, which will be linked to a central policy agreed at Board level to support front-line staff (DH 2003)

A review of hospital discharge policy, and the roles and responsibilities of each organisation, led to the development of Transfer of Care Policy 2008. Transfer of care and discharge policies are commonplace and are mandated by the Clinical Negligence Scheme for Trusts (CNST). CNST requires that all Trusts are regulated according to national criteria, which must be met (albeit at different levels) to ensure safe practice, and against which they are assessed. Principles from the 2008 policy are quoted below.

1. PURPOSE

1.1 This policy is intended to eliminate all delays in the transfer of care of acute patients, aiming to ensure the right patient is in the right place at the right time:
- It ensures that people are cared for in the most appropriate environment.
- It sets out the principles of reimbursement.
- It recognises that a whole system agreement is necessary to eliminate delayed transfers of care.

1.2 The protocol supports the ED indicators and quality of care frameworks and ensures best use of overall bed capacity, which in turn supports a well-organised admission and discharge process.
[Whilst the major focus is upon integrated working, the freeing up of acute beds was an additional bonus of the CDT process. The same principle is transferable to other areas of care, where delays are experienced.]

1.3 This policy recognises that systems and processes may be slightly different for out of Calderdale and Huddersfield hospitals; however, the principles remain the same.

2. PRINCIPLES

The policy is based on the following principles:
- That joint working and the sharing of responsibility for the transfer of care of patients across agencies is key to eliminating delayed transfers of care
- The joint working of all agencies delivers decisions within the framework of Safeguarding Adults and is in compliance with the Mental Capacity Act and standards set out in the Deprivation of Liberty Safeguards
- All health and social care organisations are committed to a whole systems approach, whereby responsibility for effective patient care and the discharge process is shared across organisational boundaries

- Planning of patients' transfer/discharge should commence on or before the day of admission to hospital, although acute unplanned admissions do not have the luxury of pre-planning. The expectation is that, once a patient is medically predictable, an estimated date of discharge should be set, following a multidisciplinary meeting and decision-making process.
- The transfer of care process will focus on the person's needs, and both they and their carers should be involved and kept informed of what is happening at all times.
- The management (including assessment) of a person's health and social care needs should be a single process. Duplication of effort is time-consuming for professionals and frustrating for patients.
- A commitment to the development of community resources to avoid inappropriate hospital admissions and to prevent the ED being used as the main gateway to health and social care services.
- Optimum use of bed capacity resources for appropriate patients.
- Acute hospital beds are for people with acute medical care needs. People who do not have acute medical care needs should not be admitted to acute beds; and those who have acute medical care needs on admission should be transferred as soon as they are medically fit and safe for discharge.
- On transfer from acute care, the first consideration should be for the patient to return home, safely and with the appropriate support. If necessary, a transitional/interim placement will be offered, whilst appropriate support, adaptations or alternative accommodation is put in place.
- Only in exceptional circumstances should patients transfer directly to long-term residential or nursing home care. In the majority of cases, the community care assessment should be completed in a non-acute environment.

Processes developed so far

The hospital matrons are currently leading weekly meetings to discuss delays on each site, and responsibility to action complex discharges is identified. The discussion of each case involves both social services and hospital matrons.

Social workers on both sites have been encouraged by the complex discharge team to produce identical documentation. This will alert ward staff to their involvement with a patient. It will also provide instant access for the ward team, to identify what discharge plans are in place.

Building on our increased integration with the hospital matrons and ward staff, we have held teaching sessions for ward staff, centred around the launch of a patient information leaflet called 'Moving on', which explains the discharge process (locally developed leaflet within the Trust) In addition, a rolling programme of teaching sessions is now mandatory. These sessions are aimed at Band 5, 6 and 7 nurses but also include AHP staff and occasionally ward clerks who have expressed an interest in learning more about the process. They include information on Continuing Care Assessment, particularly the Nursing Report. They also offer information on the roles of physiotherapist, occupational therapist, social worker, district nurse, community matron and mental health liaison staff; as well as the process around expected date of discharge; and criteria-led discharge, and the discharge lounge and pharmacy.

This training assists staff in achieving accurate completion of the continuing care documentation, which is used at the weekly multidisciplinary team (MDT) meetings to determine funding. We have also encouraged senior ward staff to attend on a rotational basis so that they can share learning and cascade this to their team members.

In addition, for a short period of time during the winter of 2009–2010, a pilot scheme to provide five 'step down' beds was based in a local nursing home. These beds provided care in the community in a nursing setting, which were used to facilitate earlier discharge plans for patients who were to be measured against continuing care criteria. Patients had instant access to nursing care, and their medical needs were addressed by the GP who provided their services at the home. This came about as a result of winter pressures on bed availability and because the Specialist Services Department found that patients were opting for placement into 24-hour care from an acute setting.

Each patient had to have an allocated social worker and CM, and the placement was for a period of up to six weeks, with a plan for reassessment after ten weeks. They were then presented to the MDT for a funding decision. A further meeting was arranged with the patient and family to discuss the funding outcome and the long-term care plan. This enabled the patient to make this important decision outside the hospital setting. Due to its success, this scheme is to be re-introduced in 2011, as it also takes into account the need to put the patient at the centre of the discharge process.

We then formulated several work streams, in which experts from the six organisations contributed their knowledge and expertise. This gave us access to decision-making at a much higher level. The work streams were:

- Criteria (nurse)-led discharge; to improve discharge arrangements of all adult patients
- Complex care; improve patient flow and reduce LOS of complex care patients
- Rehabilitation; improve LOS and appropriateness of admission to rehab wards
- Expected date of discharge (EDD); to enable appropriate and timely discharge planning
- Multidisciplinary team working; to ensure safe, effective and timely discharges

through MDT working

- Discharge medication; aid effective and timely discharge and reduce delays with prescribed discharge medications

For example, for Work stream 2 – Medical/Elderly Discharges Group, the purpose was:

- To deliver sustainable improvements in patient flow by improving transfer of care processes from the point of discharge from medical care
- To ensure the implementation of the recommendations from the Tribal Report in the following three areas:
  - Coordinated and timely multidisciplinary team decision-making
  - Patient choice in the discharge process
  - Access to and navigation of rehabilitation and community services

The complex discharge team was responsible for:

- Improving the transfer of care process for medical/elderly admissions between partner organisations
- Improving patient flow within wards and associated areas both within and outside the two acute hospital sites
- Ensuring that patients receive timely and multidisciplinary assessments to avoid unnecessary delay in moving on to a more appropriate setting

This was all achieved mostly by ensuring that senior clinical staff were available in a timely manner to make discharge decisions. The process provided an opportunity to explore further clinical pathways to alternative care settings, as necessary. It also covered such areas as estimated date of discharge (EDD) plans, and improved inter-agency working with organisations such as Social Services and the local ambulance provider.

In-reaching

As complex discharge matrons, we based ourselves within the hospital and attended MDT meetings on the wards. The rest of the CMs in the team were also proactive in attending wards if their patients were admitted and also in attending case conferences about their patients and discharge planning.

Education days

With regard to the Tribal Report, we worked in conjunction with one of the modern matrons and established multidisciplinary educational study days. These involved nine different disciplines explaining and exploring the concept of successful and timely discharge planning.

In order to identify patients with long-term conditions who may need the services of a community matron, we liaised with our IT department. This has enabled each community matron to have an identified caseload of patients on the system. As a patient is put on the system, this generates an anonymous and automatic email to the CM, with the NHS number as the unique identifier. This also shows on the patient's front sheet to inform ward staff that this patient is known to a CM. The CM is responsible for contacting the ward in order to update staff about any change in the patient's condition.

System One

Calderdale PCT Provider Services, along with the rest of Yorkshire and Humber SHA, is currently rolling out an electronic IT system called 'System One' (S1) to its clinical staff, as an operational tool. S1 is an activity-reporting tool, a repository for management information and for sharing information with other local services providers. In a parallel project, it is also being rolled out to local GPs.

At the point of contact, the advantages of S1 are that:

- Total patient history can be viewed
- It allows for access to pathology results
- It provides greater knowledge of drug interactions
- Fuller assessment can be made as a result of the large number of templates available
- Complete assessment can be recorded

The system allows us to reduce risk around information-sharing by providing real-time information. We have seen improvement in contemporaneous record-keeping, which has a potential impact on the need for hospitalisation of patients.

With close reference to the original recommendations of 'Tribal' of a 'single portal', all referrals to CMs and intermediate care are now received into our 'Direct Referral Point' (DRP). We plan to develop this further to become the DRP for all intravenous therapy and falls referrals, and it will eventually become the intermediate tier between primary and secondary care.

With the introduction of 'Transfer of Community Services' (DH 2010a, 2010b), the commissioning arm of NHS Calderdale introduced a further review of the service. This review, in turn, focused on our role in co-operating with the intermediate care team to develop new ways of working.

Even with all this in place, the transfer of patients into a 'step down' facility within intermediate care remained problematic. The team had been set up with a rehabilitation focus and they were perceived as 'gatekeepers' to the placement of patients in a community setting. This contradicted their actual purpose – to accommodate different types of clients with many different needs (DH 2003).

Where are we now?

There are now two key roles as a result of the work described in this chapter: matron (with a clinical role) and coordinator (with a coordination role) between primary and secondary care around admission avoidance and early discharge, working more closely with staff in the Emergency Department, Medical Assessment Unit, short-stay wards and the intermediate care services. The roles are supported by a nurse facilitator within the team.

All other medical wards now have the responsibility of performing their own assessments for patients who may require some form of intermediate care. They are helped in this process by the nurse facilitator, who provides guidance on the type of information required to ensure a smooth discharge into community care. In addition to this, the district nurses and community matrons are conducting holistic assessments on patients in their caseloads who may require intermediate care provision. This ensures that the most appropriate person is carrying out the assessment and avoids the need to duplicate assessment. Duplication is time-consuming and does nothing to reassure the patient that everyone is aware of their problems and is communicating with each other to help resolve the issues.

Conclusion

We believe that our greatest achievements in encouraging more cohesive primary and secondary care working have come about because of our determination to use a very friendly style and approach when liaising with all our colleagues, at any level. Our model has been one of sharing successes and learning from our mistakes, and never adopting a punitive approach to any situation.

References

Department of Health (2003). HSC 2003/009. 'Delayed Discharge Act, Chapter 5: guidance for implementation'. www.dh.gov.uk or www.legislation.gov.uk

Department of Health (2008). 'High quality care for all: NHS next stage review'. Final report, by Lord Darzi, Department of Health: London. HMSO

Department of Health (2009). 'Transferring Community Services: Ambition, Action, Achievement – transferring services for acute care closer to home'. London: HMSO.

Department of Health (2010a). 'Transfer of Community Services'. London: HMSO.

Department of Health (2010b). 'Liberating the NHS: Legislative Framework and Next Steps'. London: HMSO.

Department of Health (2010c). 'Care Services Efficiency Delivery homecare re-ablement toolkit – Intermediate care and homecare re-ablement: what's in a name?' London: HMSO.

Chapter 32

Facilitation of hospital discharge within a community intravenous therapy service
Diana Milligan and Janet Knight

Historically, many patients receiving intravenous therapy (IVT) would have had an inpatient stay on an inpatient ward to receive the full course of antibiotic therapy – even if they were fully ambulant and independent. This practice resulted in unnecessarily lengthy stays (for some not all patients), contributing to the pressure placed upon bed capacity within acute hospitals. In the wake of reforms in emergency and primary care, there has been an impetus to expand patient services, and this has given rise to innovation in services to meet patient choice and need, as well as new roles for practitioners within the community (DH 2004, Royal College of Physicians, 2007).

This chapter demonstrates, through case examples, how facilitation of discharge for patients into new services requiring IVT can either be simple and relatively speedy to engage, or complex and inefficient. It does not analyse the current political impetus to commission services, which is the job of commissioning teams and GP clusters – and is at an embryonic stage of development. In the long term, the service principles will stand the test of time, long after the current restructures have passed – and no doubt undergone further metamorphosis! It begins by describing how the IVT service was established and key elements of this service. It also looks at key areas in which improvement can be achieved and offers tips to deliver an effective, efficient IVT service, which is both flexible and proactive.

Overview of relevant literature

Nurse-led home IVT has been developing in practice for healthcare providers, both in the United Kingdom and the United States, for many years (Grayson *et al.* 2002, Seaton *et al.* 2005). Research has shown that the benefits of IVT include: admission prevention, reduced length of hospital stay, and patient satisfaction. It is also been accepted as safe and effective practice in a community setting (Duke & Street 2003, Seaton *et al.* 2005, Lees *et al.* 2006, Lees & Sonkor 2006). The ethos of the IVT service is to prevent hospital admissions where appropriate, promote care closer to home and improve the patient experience of the NHS. Consequently, facilitating a good timely discharge is important and all parties involved must ensure they follow a proven effective pathway, with good communication. Timely discharge means discharging the patient home or transferring them to an appropriate level of care as soon as they are medically/clinically stable and fit for discharge (DH 2004). To ensure minimal delay in discharge, the IVT service accepts referrals seven days a week, including bank holidays.

Background

The IVT service was developed five years ago within an NHS primary care trust, with the aim of reducing hospital admissions and facilitating discharge from the acute sector. The service started, like many other services, treating cellulitis only. However, due to much perseverance and forward thinking, the conditions being treated have rapidly expanded and patients with conditions such as urinary tract infections, respiratory infections, post-operative infections including vascular, orthopaedic patients and exacerbations of chronic conditions such as septic arthritis have all been successfully treated.

This service is primarily nurse-led, with medical input as required from a consultant geriatrician who has a special interest in IVT. A consultant microbiologist, along with the primary care trust's medicines management team, also plays a pivotal role in the review of appropriate IVT. This enables assurance for all parties involved in the patient's care pathway that IVT is required, and oral antibiotics are not suitable, and that the type of antibiotic is appropriate.

Delivery

Key to the successful delivery is the integration of the IVT service with two other interfacing community services, namely, intermediate care and the district nursing team. There are two arms to the service – rapid intervention (at the point of referral) and a longer-term approach to the delivery of home IVT. The intermediate care service act as first responders, who will commence treatment for the first 24–72 hours. Then the district nurses continue treatment until the course is completed.

Many patients requiring IVT are discharged from acute medicine units, short-stay wards or even emergency departments (EDs), as well as medical and surgical wards. With the current ethos being 'care closer to home', direct GP referral has always been a part of the development of the service. This has since been reinforced by GP commissioning of services (DH 2011). The amount of time spent in hospital does not determine whether or not a patient has a straightforward, simple discharge. A patient could be seen in the ED within four hours and be discharged; or they could be on an acute ward for many weeks and, once they are medically/clinically stable, be discharged for further IV treatment within the community. The key is swift action, once the decision to discharge has been made, to promote bed capacity in acute hospitals. Acute staff do need to truly facilitate and aid timely discharge. To achieve this, a good understanding of the community IVT service and effective communication of arrangements are of the utmost importance.

The role of the IVT nurse

The role of the IVT nurse is to promote the ethos of the service and safely deliver IV therapy. All nurses in the IVT service are competent practitioners, working autonomously, and taking responsibility for ensuring that a holistic approach is taken to the needs of all patients. This reduces duplication of the services utilised within the patient's home environment, which can create confusion and intrude upon patient's normal routine.

Communication is at the forefront of the IVT nurse's role, as they are the gatekeepers of the patient's care. They act as patient advocates, ensuring seamless delivery of care.

Informing and reassuring patients

Many patients have commented that, although they were glad to be going home, they were anxious and unsure about how receiving IV antibiotics at home worked. They also expressed concerns regarding the cannula and how to care for it at home, especially having to wait overnight before being seen at home by the community IVT nurses.

This is where nurses in the acute sector can play an important part in helping to reassure patients. When planning discharge, the acute sector nurse should first liaise with the doctors and consultants involved, to ensure that the patient has been clinically risk-assessed according to the community IVT suitability criteria. This consultation should take place before discussing discharge and making the decision with the patient, to ensure that the patient is not given false information. The suitability criteria are easily accessible on the intranet, to aid the process of assessment and referral. The assessment process and the way the home IVT service works should both be fully explained to patients. This will reassure them and will also provide an opportunity to gain their consent to treatment away from the hospital setting. Taken together, these measures will make patients feel like active participants in their own care, with a contribution to make.

All nurses should possess the experience, knowledge and skills (NMC 2008), as well as the ability, to appreciate how bewildering it can be for a patient to receive IVT at home. In addition, nurses need to alleviate the concerns of family members, to reassure them that a clinical skill, which has historically been performed in hospital, can be achieved safely in their home environment. Both acute and community IVT nurses play an important role in educating the patient about the treatment they will be receiving, ensuring that future medication and follow-up requirements are arranged, and liaising with the responsible physician.

To assist this communication process, patient education leaflets regarding the service, frequently asked questions and information about cannulae care are all freely available on the intranet for staff to give to patients. It is pertinent to give family members this information as well, as many of them also feel anxious and bewildered when patients return home with a medical device in situ.

Arranging medication

When planning discharge, nurses should ensure that any medication and diluents are also available to be sent home with the patient. This requires forward planning by all parties involved in the patient's care. Chasing tablets to take out (TTOs) that have not been dispensed on time or written on a valid medication chart can be time-consuming and may delay discharge.

Although there are independent/supplementary prescribers within the community IVT service, certain antibiotics can only be prescribed under consultant instruction. Incomplete medication charts also increase manpower requirements, as the prescribing nurse is not allowed to prescribe and administer at the same time (DH 2005, NHS Executive 2000). In such a situation, two members of staff have to visit the patient instead of one (NMC 2010). This clearly has an effect on capacity, reducing the service's ability to facilitate discharges.

Fortunately for emergency departments, the community IVT service supplies a particular type of antibiotic that can be administered by a nurse in the community, by following a patient group direction (PGD) used for a group of patients with the same clinical situation and service circumstances. Therefore there is no need for that medication to be dispensed if it is the drug of choice, which aids a timely discharge. However, if any other, more specific type of medication is required, a TTO would be needed for the hospital pharmacy to dispense it.

Key discharge facilitation points for both acute and community services

- Communication, communication, communication!!
- All acute staff must have clear roles, responsibilities and understanding of the community IVT service when referring patients

- Documentation for the community IVT needs to be completed in full, including the medication chart
- Drugs and consumables must be provided correctly to avoid wastage and improve cost-effectiveness
- Medical responsibility should be confirmed prior to discharge, to avoid confusion with liaison and to aid patient care follow-up
- Referral to be made on any day, including weekends and bank holidays
- There should be good marketing of the community IVT service, clarifying exactly what the service offers, via presentations and meetings
- There should be a single point of referral, to avoid confusion
- Robust pathway/clear intervention criteria are needed
- Integrated service use (IC/DN) allows for rapid intervention and long-term treatment
- Equipment and drug stock levels must be adequate for service demands (lack of equipment delays treatment)
- Competent staff ensure effective care

Case studies

The majority of people, given a choice, prefer the comforts and familiar surroundings of their own home when they are ill. There are a growing number of patients with family dependants, who want to continue their familiar routine as far as possible; or they just do not wish to be admitted to hospital, especially if they can be catered for at home. In such cases, healthcare professionals should be understanding and flexible in meeting the requests of the patients.

The following case studies demonstrate how preventing hospital admission can be beneficial to all parties.

Case study 1: Admission prevention

Patient care route	Key factors that helped prevent admission
Patient diagnosed by GP with cellulitis; seven-day course of oral antibiotics given, with a review after course completed	Correct to use oral antibiotics as first line intervention Review date given
Patient re-attends GP's surgery after three days, following a deterioration of their condition	Patient re-attended GP's surgery, rather than going to hospital

GP refers patient to ED for medical review with a covering letter	The GP's letter aided communication and continuity of care, informing doctors of previous treatment, medical history, etc.
Patient is seen in ED by medical consultant, who liaises with microbiologist	Clear communication links aided diagnosis without hospital admission
Referral made to community IVT and patient is discharged on the same day without need for acute admission	Documentation, including prescription form, completed thoroughly and sent home with patient
IVT team pick referral up on same day and therapy continues next day without delay in treatment; drugs provided by primary care trust in line with cellulitis pathway	Hospital admission was prevented

Although this case study demonstrates how admission was prevented, the process could possibly have been more streamlined. The GP (following an assessment of the patient in surgery) could have liaised directly with the microbiologist to make the decision to administer IV antibiotics, thus removing the need for an ED visit. The GP could also have generated an FP10 if required and made the referral directly to the community IVT, following the existing care pathway.

Case study 2: Facilitating discharge

Patient care route	Key factors that assisted timely discharge
Patient diagnosed in acute sector with an infected vascular graft; medically fit for discharge home	Correct diagnosis and discharge pathway ascertained
Communication between vascular ID and microbiology consultant to ascertain correct drug for treatment	Communication took place with appropriate health professionals (acute)
Communication with IV lead nurse and medicines management primary care Drug was risk assessed within 24 hours and was suitable for use in the community but required weekly monitoring	Communication took place with appropriate health professionals (primary care) Risk assessment completed promptly (aiding timely discharge)

IV lead nurse liaised with primary care consultant with special interest in IV therapy, to negotiate with consultants in the acute sector regarding monitoring	Decisions were made and negotiated in direct conversations, as well as the IV team assisting in planning discharge
Weekly monitoring arranged with the ID consultant for patient to be reviewed on outpatient basis	Outpatient appointments were pre-arranged, providing clear direction for patient and health professionals; this aids planning of care delivery and monitoring of condition
Patient discharged home within 48 hours of planned discharge from the acute sector, with appropriate paperwork, medication and consumables	Safe, timely discharge and care delivery were ensured

Again, the process could have been made even more streamlined. If the medicines management team acted proactively in risk-assessing potential medicines for community use this would prompt a speedier discharge.

Case study 3: Ineffective discharge

The usual pathway for referrals to the IV community teams is to complete a referral form, found on the Trust intranet in three of the nearby acute hospitals to aid the communication process. Alternatively, acute sector staff may contact the single point of referral telephone line and request a copy of the document to be faxed over or emailed. If a pre-discharge enquiry is required, there is a direction to the nurse leads for IV therapy or to contact the consultant with special interest to assist in smooth transfer to primary care.

An enquiry referral was received from a ward in the acute hospital regarding a pending discharge. The patient had just had surgery to remove a foreign body in the stomach, which indicated a fungal growth in the culture analysis. On discussion with the consultant taking medical responsibility, as per the community IVT pathway, it was recognised that the drug of preference had not been pre-risk-assessed as being safe for use in primary care. Therefore a risk assessment was required by the community medicine management team, and on this occasion was performed within 24 hours.

However, the means by which the foreign body had entered the patient's stomach raised concern for community IVT nurses, as it was a self-inflicted condition and the patient had previously required surgery for the same condition. Therefore, even though the consultant had advised that she felt there was no cause for concern with the patient's discharge home, the community nursing staff still had to complete a risk assessment against suitability criteria to accept the patient for treatment at home. Once discharged, the patient would be at home with a peripheral line/cvc in situ, and drugs in the home, without supervision. As clinical practitioners performing and delegating tasks, IVT nurses have to be confident that the patient is suitable for safe treatment in an alternative setting and are therefore required to complete a risk assessment to ensure that they are medically stable and prepared for the discharge.

As the IVT community team have a presence in the acute hospital in order to help speed up the discharge process, they attended the ward to complete a pre-discharge risk assessment to ensure the patient's suitability for care in the community. Just because someone is apparently suitable and complying with treatment in hospital, it does not necessarily mean that they will be the same at home. At the same time, patient empowerment and understanding remain uppermost in the discharge process. As the nurse was about to complete the assessment, the infectious disease registrar visited to review the patient. Having made his assessment, he decided to commence the patient on an oral antibiotic.

Although this was a satisfactory outcome for the patient, as she could take medication orally and thus would not require IV therapy at home, it clearly wasted resources and added a layer of complication to the discharge process. It was non-productive in terms of the use of acute and community IVT time.

Key issues and learning points

- Did the patient need IV drugs?
- Length of stay was increased whilst patient was being considered for community IVT. If the review had been more timely, the patient would have been prescribed oral antibiotic therapy and discharged home sooner.
- If the infection disease consultant had been involved at the outset, referral to IVT would not have been necessary.
- Medicine management needs to be more proactive with risk-assessing drugs that are suitable for community IV administration in order to speed up the discharge process.

- Suitability criteria will not fit all patients and must not be used on their own. Clinical judgement and risk assessment should also play a part in the discharge process.
- Acute and community IVT staff all need to be aware of patient suitability criteria.

Conclusion

In conclusion, good communication between the acute service and the community IVT team can definitely facilitate and aid a timely discharge. It can also reduce the need for hospital admissions, and promote and enhance care in the alternative setting. The emphasis should be on involving the correct people early on, communicating effectively, and having flexible services and innovative practice, with awareness of what each service can and should provide.

References

Department of Health (2004). 'Achieving timely "simple" discharge from hospital: A toolkit for the multidisciplinary team'. London: HMSO.

Department of Health (2005). 'Improving patients' access to medicines: a guide to implementing nurse and pharmacist independent prescribing within the NHS in England'. [online]. http://www.dh.gov.uk/assetRoot/04/13/37/47/04133747

Department of Health (2011). 'The functions of GP commissioning consortia: a working document'. London: HMSO.

Duke, M. & Street, A. (2003). Hospital in the home: constructions of the nursing role – a literature review. *Journal of Clinical Nursing*. **12** (6), 852–859.

Grayson, M.L., McDonald, M., Gibson, K., Athan, E., Munckhof, W.J., Paull, P. & Chambers, F. (2002). Once-daily intravenous cefazolin plus oral probenecid is equivalent to once-daily intravenous ceftriaxone plus oral placebo for the treatment of moderate-to-severe cellulitis in adults. *Clinical Infectious Diseases*, **34** (11), 1440–1448.

Lees, L., Dyer, P. & Knight, J. (2006). Delivering an Intravenous Therapy Outpatient Service (Part 2). *Emergency Nurse*. **14** (5), 28–34.

Lees, L. & Sonkor, M. (J2006). Delivering an Intravenous Therapy Outpatient Service (Part 1). *Emergency Nurse*. **14** (3), 30–35.

NHS Executive. 'Patient Group Directions (England only)'. Department of Health, 9 August 2000 [HCS 2000/0261].

Nursing and Midwifery Council (2008). 'Nursing and Midwifery Council – The code: Standards of conduct, performance and ethics for nurses and midwives'. London: NMC.

Nursing and Midwifery Council (2010). 'Standards for medication administration'. London: NMC.

Royal College of Physicians of London (2007). 'Acute medical care: the right person in the right setting first time – report of the acute medicine task force'. London: RCPL.

Seaton, R.A., Bell, E., Gourlay, Y. & Semple L. (2005). Nurse-led management of uncomplicated cellulitis in the community: evaluation of a protocol incorporating intravenous ceftriaxone. *Journal of Antimicrobial Chemotherapy*. **55** (5), 764–767.

Index

Index